Atherosclerotic Plaques

Advances in Imaging for Sequential Quantitative Evaluation

NATO ASI Series

Advanced Science Institutes Series

A series presenting the results of activities sponsored by the NATO Science Committee, which aims at the dissemination of advanced scientific and technological knowledge, with a view to strengthening links between scientific communities.

The series is published by an international board of publishers in conjunction with the NATO Scientific Affairs Division

A	**Life Sciences**	Plenum Publishing Corporation
B	**Physics**	New York and London
C	**Mathematical and Physical Sciences**	Kluwer Academic Publishers
D	**Behavioral and Social Sciences**	Dordrecht, Boston, and London
E	**Applied Sciences**	
F	**Computer and Systems Sciences**	Springer-Verlag
G	**Ecological Sciences**	Berlin, Heidelberg, New York, London,
H	**Cell Biology**	Paris, Tokyo, Hong Kong, and Barcelona
I	**Global Environmental Change**	

Recent Volumes in this Series

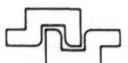

Series A: Life Sciences

Atherosclerotic Plaques

Advances in Imaging for Sequential Quantitative Evaluation

Edited by

Robert W. Wissler

University of Chicago Medical Center
Chicago, Illinois

Associate Editors:
M. Gene Bond and Michele Mercuri

Bowman-Gray School of Medicine
Winston-Salem, North Carolina

Piero Tanganelli and Giorgio Weber

University of Siena
Siena, Italy

Technical Editor:
Gertrud Friedman

University of Chicago Medical Center
Chicago, Illinois

Plenum Press
New York and London
Published in cooperation with NATO Scientific Affairs Division

Proceedings of a NATO Advanced Research Workshop on
Progress, Problems, and Promises for an Effective Quantitative
Evaluation of Atherosclerosis in Living and Autopsied
Experimental Animals and Man,
held June 3-7, 1990,
In Siena, Italy

Library of Congress Cataloging-in-Publication Data

NATO Advanced Research Workshop on Progress, Problems, and Promises
for an Effective Quantitative Evaluation of Atherosclerosis in
Living and Autopsied Experimental Animals and Man. (1990 : Siena,
Italy)
    Atherosclerotic plaques : advances in imaging for sequential
quantitative evaluation / edited by Robert W. Wissler ; technical
editor, Gertrud Friedman ; asssociate editors, M. Gene Bond ... [et
al.].
        p.   cm. -- (NATO ASI series. Series A, Life science ; v. 219)
    "Proceedings of NATO Advanced Research Workshop on Progress,
Problems, and Promises for Effective Quantitative Evaluation of
Atherosclerosis in Living and Autopsied Experimental Animals and
Man, held June 1-3, 1990 in Siena, Italy."--T.p. verso.
    "Published in cooperation with NATO Scientific Affairs Division."
    Includes bibliographical references and index.
    ISBN 978-1-4757-0440-2   ISBN 978-1-4757-0438-9 (eBook)
    DOI 10.1007/978-1-4757-0438-9
    1. Atherosclerotic plaque--Imaging--Congresses.
2. Atherosclerosis--Etiology--Congresses.   I. Wissler, Robert W.
(Robert William), 1917-   . II. North Atlantic Treaty Organization.
Scientific Affairs Division.   III. Title.   IV. Series.
    [DNLM: 1. Atherosclerosis--pathology--congresses. 2. Diagnostic
Imaging--trends--congresses.   WG 550 N27965a 1990]
    RC692.N33 1990
    616.1'36--dc20
DNLM/DLC
for Library of Congress   91-39615
                                                                          CIP

ISBN 978-1-4757-0440-2

PREFACE

The philosophy of this NATO Advanced Research Workshop and the monograph it has yielded is that if you put a small number of very talented and creative scientists of different backgrounds and documented accomplishments together in a cloistered place for a few days to consider a very important and timely topic, many new ideas will be generated. The keynote of this conference was the <u>Future</u>. By this we mean the expected future developments of highly reliable sequential quantitative measurements of atherosclerotic plaque size and components in living human subjects.

Some of the best minds and the most experienced and talented individuals at the leading edges of imaging of arteries were involved; some of the best scientists and students of the atherosclerotic plaque and its components participated; and some of the leading investigators of the cell biology or, as we call it in the USA, the pathobiology of atherosclerosis, contributed important new information. All of these individuals were actively involved in the conference and each obviously had carefully prepared and was able to communicate effectively.

Quantitative measurements of the effect of the atherosclerotic process on the artery wall at any given time in a person's life is indeed a very important area of advancing science. Atherosclerosis is one of the most important and most dangerous forms of chronic disease and mortality, leading as it does to the death of about half of all individuals in the industrialized nations of the world. It is also one of the most difficult disease processes to evaluate at the lesion level in the living individual, since it often leads to sudden death or life threatening ischemic heart attack or brain stroke or other peripheral vascular effects with little or no warning.

Today it looks more and more promising to prevent, retard, or to cause cessation of progression of this process or to reverse it substantially by relatively low risk methods. It is also a frequently performed procedure to correct the worst areas by angioplasty, endarterectomy, or bypass, and to try to prevent progression in the rest of the vascular tree, so we really need the best possible way to follow the course of the disease. That is what the NATO advanced research workshop in the beautiful Tuscany hills and this resulting monograph are all about.

As one of us (Professor Weber) recounted at the beginning of the meeting, the history of the Certosa di Pontignano and the University's role in this lovely spot where we were gathered was worth noting.

This was a charter house of a Carthusian monastary with beautiful cloisters. It was founded in 1343, and it was later suppressed in the time of Napoleon in 1810. Nevertheless, some of its devotion to worship still remains.

v

Following the Second World War, this building, which was almost in ruins, was given to the University of Siena and, little by little, much of it has been renovated.

First the University used it as a college for highly talented students of forensic sciences who came here from every part of Italy. So in those days it was a hall of residence for 30 or thereabouts. In 1968, the University changed its plans and so, also, here something changed, a much more effective restoration to renovate the old buildings. Since that time the Certosa has functioned mostly as a conference center for the University to host small group meetings like this one or for summer courses or, also, for hospitality for foreign scientists who want to stay a period of weeks or months at the University of Siena, which is a rapidly growing university in spite of its age, for it is one of the oldest in Europe. From the windows of this Certosa you can look at the new, modern, and very large polyclinic in the hills nearby.

We are very thankful to all the speakers and participants who came. We hope that this monograph will be a source of pride to His Magnificence the Rector Professor Berlinguer who made this meeting possible here in this beautiful city, and who arranged the support of the University of Siena. We are grateful for his support and the support of Professor Tosi, the dean of the faculty, a great morphometrist himself.

The host (Professor Weber) and the organizing chairman (Professor Wissler) wish to acknowledge the help of many others who have been working behind the scenes to make this monograph possible.

We are particularly indebted to Gertrud Friedman who has served as managing editor throughout the long and difficult task of the trans-Atlantic assembly of the many photo-ready manuscripts. We also acknowlege the skillful assistance of Alexander Arguelles, who prepared much of the final copy.

Drs Gene Bond and Piero Tanganelli have had a major part in organizing the program, raising the additional funds, and choosing the participants, as well as editing the monograph. Dr Loretta Resi, a pillar in the Pathology Institute, and Dr Giorgio Bianciardi, an outstanding cell biologist, have had a lot to do with the development of this meeting locally, and finally Dr Michelle Mercuri has helped in a major way with the demanding tasks of editing.

There are some great experts on atherosclerosis and on the pathobiology of atherosclerosis who have helped greatly in developing the meeting and also the funds for the meeting. These are Professor Crepaldi, Professor Paoletti, and Professor Ricci. In addition to the support of the University of Siena, the Monte dei Paschi di Siena, and the Italian National Research Council, a group of companies (the Bristol-Myers Squibb Company, Merck Sharpe and Dohme, Dupont Medical Products Department, E.R. Squibb & Sons, Hoffman LaRoche, Janssen Research Foundation, Johnson and Johnson, USA, and, along with them, McNeil Pharmaceuticals, Inc., Parke Davis, Pfizer Laboratories, Wild Leitz, and Cassa di Risparmio di Firenze of Italy) all contributed generously. So we are indebted to many sources for helping finance this meeting and this monograph in additon to the major contribution which NATO has made.

In this volume the editors have tried to maintain the spirit of creativity with an emphasis on what the future holds by including the condensed highlights of the discussion periods which followed six of the sessions. This emphasis on what we can look forward to is intensified by the contents of the summarizing session which, in a way, forms a synthesis of the most promising developments in each session.

We trust that this monograph will serve as an important indicator of the progress being made and that which can be expected soon in this important field of research. The results of these studies will, in all probablity, be the single most important factor in being able to measure the successful conquest of the atherosclerotic process by means of prevention and regression.

The Editors

CONTENTS

ATHEROSCLEROSIS: A MOVING TARGET

KEY NOTE PRESENTATION

Henry C. McGill, Jr.

Department of Pathology
University of Texas Health Science Center and the
Southwest Foundation for Biomedical Research
San Antonio, Texas

It is gratifying the see the effort and attention given here to the issue of evaluating atherosclerotic lesions, especially atherosclerosis in living persons. Pathologists who have examined the arteries of autopsied persons for many years have longed for the opportunity to observe the movement of the process. In attempts to describe that movement, we have had to reconstruct the process by measuring various qualities of the lesions in large numbers of autopsied persons, and arranging the values in age sequence.

Using that method, the work of many investigators over the last 50 years has led to the schematic diagram of the natural history of atherosclerosis shown in Figure 1 (McGill et al, 1963; McGill, 1988). The earliest lesions that we can relate to atherosclerosis with confidence are simple deposits of lipid in the aortic intima, the fatty streaks of infancy, or juvenile fatty streaks. These appear in the aortas of almost all children by three years of age, increase slowly in extent if at all until about age 10, and then often increase rapidly during adolescence. Fatty streaks appear in the coronary arteries at about age 15, and increase steadily thereafter.

At about age 20, both the abdominal aorta and the coronary artery may show many larger and thicker raised fatty plaques with discrete borders. These are smooth and pale yellow with abundant microscopically evident intracellular lipid mostly in macrophages and smooth muscle cells, but little evident increase in collagen or elastin. At about the same time, a few raised lesions with thicker pearly gray glistening fibromuscular caps overlying cores of extracellular lipid and necrotic debris appear. These lesions are called fibrous plaques because they not only contain more smooth muscle cells, but also more collagen and elastic tissue. During the third decade, fibrous plaques are, on the average, more extensive in persons from high risk populations (that is, populations with high rates of clinically manifest atherosclerotic disease) than in those from low risk populations.

In subsequent years, fibrous plaques undergo a number of changes which include vascularization, hemorrhage, and ulceration. These changes stiffen the arterial wall, reduce the size of the lumen, and predispose to thrombosis. Finally, 30 years or more after the process began, a thrombus on the intimal surface may abruptly further reduce the size of the lumen or occlude it completely, interrupt the blood

Atherosclerotic Plaques, Edited by R.W. Wissler *et al.*
Plenum Press, New York, 1991

supply, and cause ischemic necrosis (infarction) of the heart, brain, or extremities. Calcification also may occur in the base of the plaque, but this process appears to be a stabilizing component of the lesions and does not influence the likelihood of thrombosis.

Thus, atherosclerosis, with this long and complex natural history, presents a moving target. Components of atherosclerotic lesions that are useful as markers for evaluation purposes may vary among the different stages of the process. There has been a great deal of progress in the technology for hitting this target at the upper end

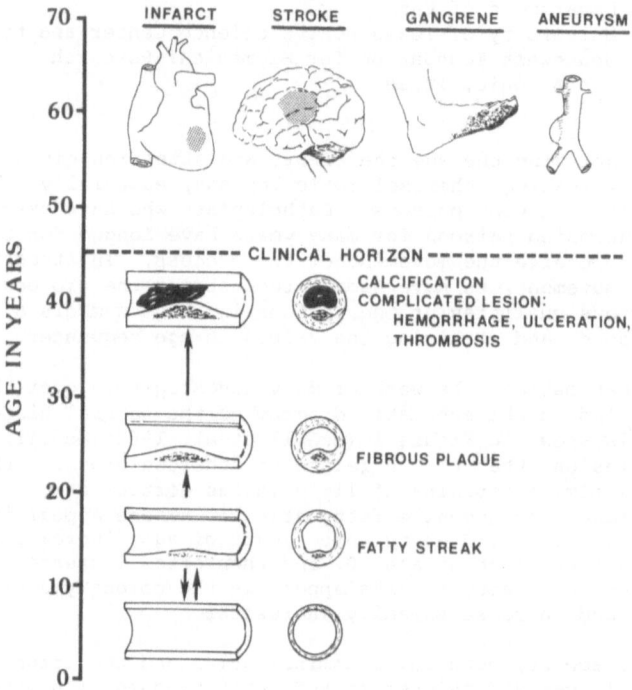

Figure 1.--Natural history of atherosclerosis (redrawn from McGill,et al., 1963)

-- that is, in the occlusive stages, because these lesion displace radioopaque contrast media, affect blood flow, or have sufficient mass to be visualized by physical methods. The need and the challenge, however, is to detect and measure lesions at the lower end -- that is, the fatty streak, the fatty plaque, and the early fibrous plaque. For example, it would be most valuable to be able to detect and define the several forms of the intermediate lesion in transition between the fatty streak and the fibrous plaque, because this intermediate lesion in some of its forms probably represents the critical stage in acceleration of atherosclerosis in young adults from high risk populations. This ability would enable us to study the environmental and genetic factors associated with atherosclerosis when the rewards of prevention and the potential for regression are maximal.

A number of studies have attempted to identify the components or characteristics of lesions that mark the transition from fatty streaks to fibrous plaques. Among the most recent is that of Stary (1989), who examined intensively a site in the coronary arteries of over 500 children and young adults from birth to 30 years of age. This site, the left anterior descending coronary artery just distal to its origin from the left main coronary artery, is well known for its predilection to develop advanced and occlusive atherosclerotic lesions in adults. It also is one of the sites where fatty streaks are most frequently seen in young persons, and consequently one would expect transitional or intermediate lesions to occur at this site if they occur at all.

Standardized microscopic sections of pressure perfused arteries showed isolated macrophage foam cells in the coronary intima at this site in young children, even in the first year of life. In children at the age of puberty, 12 to 14 years, the numbers of lipid filled macrophage foam cells were increased and many smooth muscle cells contained lipid droplets, and there were a few fine extracellular lipid particles. In older children and in some young adults the amount of extracellular lipid increased greatly and became a prominent feature of the lesions. In some young adults the masses of extracellular lipid became the cores of typical fibrous plaques with fibromuscular caps, but the predominant lesion was a fatty plaque with 90-95% of the lipid in smooth muscle cells and only a few monocyte/macrophage foam cells apparent. By age 20 years, about 20% of the subjects had lesions with substantial accumulations of extracellular lipid, making this the most prominent new feature of atherosclerosis at that age. These observations, together with other evidence, indicate that extracellular lipid accumulation is the marker for progression of the fatty streak and the several forms of fatty plaques to the fibrous plaque.

Many other components have been identified in atherosclerotic lesions at one or another stage, but few of these are unique to atherosclerosis or are associated with one of the distinctive stages of progression. Table 1 summarizes how the location of abnormal lipid, as described above, and a number of other components described in numerous recent reports on the pathogenesis of atherosclerosis, are related to the three major stages of pre-clinical atherosclerosis: early lesions, uncomplicated juvenile fatty streaks; transitional lesions, i.e., those occurring in high-risk sites in the early part of the third decade; and advanced lesions, well developed fibrous plaques (but not end stage complicated or occlusive lesions).

Abnormal lipid is a prominent feature of all three stages, but its distribution and composition change. It shifts from an intracellular (macrophages and smooth muscle cells) to an extracellular location, and it changes from predominantly cholesteryl oleate to cholesteryl linoleate as the lesion progresses (Katz, 1981).

Various apolipoproteins, particularly apo B, have been identified in lesions by immunohistochemistry, but present evidence does not indicate whether the type, amount, or location is a useful marker for progression.

Low density lipoproteins(LDL), and particularly modified forms of LDL, have also been identified in lesions. We do not know enough about the association of LDL with lesions to use the amount or location as a reliable marker, but plasma LDL exchanges with lesion LDL. Labeled LDL would be expected to accumulate in lesions, and this exchange provides a means of labeling lesions.

Mononuclear cells and macrophage foam cells dominate the cell population of lesions in the very early stages, but they become less prominent as lipid-containing smooth muscle cells and extracellular lipid increase -- not necessarily because they are decreased in number, but because they are diluted by other tissue components. Lesions also often contain lymphocytes and some of these are T-lymphocytes, but information is just now emerging regarding how they participate in lesion development and what their significance is.

Table 1. Components of Atherosclerotic Lesions by Stage

Component	Lesion stage		
	Early	Transitional	Advanced
Lipid	+++	+++	+++
Intracellular	+++	++	+
Extracellular	-	+	+++
Cholesteryl oleate	++	+++	+
Cholesteryl linoleate	+	++	+++
Lipoproteins	+	++	+++
Apolipoproteins	+	++	+++
Mononuclear cells	+++	+	+
Macrophage foam cells	+++	++	+
Smooth muscle cells	+	+++	+++
Proteoglycans	+	+	+
Collagen	+	+	+++
Elastic tissue	+	++	+++
Calcium	-	-	+
Fibrinogen/fibrin	-	++	+++
Platelets	-	-	+
Endothelial defects	-	+	++
Vascularization	-	-	++
Hemorrhage	-	-	++
Viral markers	?	?	+
Oncogenes	?	?	?
Tumor suppressor genes	?	?	?
Immunoglobulins	?	?	?
Cytokines	?	?	?
Growth factors	?	?	?

? = area of active investigation

Smooth muscle cells and connective tissue elements are present in atherosclerotic lesions at all stages, and they become more prominent in the transitional or intermediate fatty plaque where they are by far the predominant cell and they remain prominent in advanced lesions as their major synthetic product, collagen, forms the fibromuscular cap of the fibrous plaque. Smooth muscle cells are present in early lesions as part of the normal arterial structure, and those in the vicinity of clusters of macrophage foam cells accumulate lipid droplets, but proliferation of smooth muscle cells is not a prominent feature until raised fatty plaques and fibromuscular caps form. The smooth muscle cells become less active in the fibrous cap as it matures and these cells become trapped in their own synthetic products, but foci of smooth muscle cell proliferation are still often active at the shoulders of the lesions.

Proteoglycans and elastic tissue also are present in all stages but there is no evidence that either the type, the amount, or the distribution is a reliable indicator of the type of lesion or its likelihood to progress.

Calcium is a latecomer to advanced lesions and may represent healing and stabilization of advanced lesions rather than progression.

The role of the hemostatic system in the pathogenesis of atherosclerosis has long been a controversial issue. Vascularization is a hallmark of advanced lesions and may be a precursor to hemorrhage into the plaque. In turn, hemorrhage is a frequent precursor of mural or occlusive thrombi, which represent end stage disease, but many observers find evidence that most of the blood which appears in the plaque comes from fractures or tears in the fibrous caps. Platelets and fibrin may contribute to the progression of some early lesions, and attempts to identify them and to relate them to progression are under way, but they are not prominent components of most early or transitional lesions.

Endothelial defects have been proposed as the initiating event of atherogenesis, but they have never been demonstrated to precede early lesions in humans or experimental animals. Localized functional defects, not detectable by conventional techniques, may account for the initiation of lesions, but these have not been demonstrated convincingly in either experimental or human lesions.

Table 1 concludes with a selective list of tissue or cellular components that have been identified in or are suspected to be present at various stages of atherosclerotic lesions. Most of these are under active investigation. Some of them, such as markers for viral infections (Melnick et al. 1990), have been demonstrated in lesions but their roles in the natural history and pathogenesis have not been established. They may represent important mechanisms in pathogenesis, but in many instances they may be insignificant passenger viruses and so far there is insufficient evidence to make them useful as markers of progression or regression. This list is being rapidly expanded; for example, a recent report describes the presence of PDGF-B protein (Ross et al., 1990) in atherosclerotic lesions, and the evidence for involvement of immune processes (as well as the importance of cytokines and leukotrienes) in many cases of atherosclerosis is just emerging (Libby et al., 1988, 1989; Pober & Cotran, 1990).

Table 2 summarizes the dominant and distinctive features that characterize the major stages of atherosclerotic lesions. It should be apparent that the significance of each characteristic in evaluating lesions depends on the age range and the type of lesion (as classified by conventional gross and microscopic techniques).

Table 2. Markers for Atherosclerotic Lesions

Stage	Age, years	Type	Major feature(s)
Early	10-20	Fatty streak	Intracellular lipid
Intermediate	15-25	Transitional or intermediate lesions	Mostly intracellular lipid with marked proliferation of lipid filled smooth muscle cells
Advanced	20-35	Fibrous plaque	Extracellular lipid, necrotic core, and fibromuscular cap
Occlusive	35+	Complicated lesion	Thrombosis, endothelial defect, hemorrhage, neovascularization

Table 3. Selecting Evaluation Target by Objective

Objective	Measurement
Natural history	Gross lesion size and type
Pathogenesis	Component of interest related to natural history

Etiology
    Environmental agents
    Intervening variables
    Genetic variants
	Marker of progression or of advanced lesion

Regression	Gross lesion size and marker of progression
Prognosis/Treatment	Predictors of stenosis, thrombosis, or vasoconstriction

Table 3 summarizes the influence of the study objective on the choice of markers and measures of atherosclerotic lesions.

Although there are many theoretical possibilities for evaluating atherosclerosis in living persons or animals by measuring one or another lesion component, the practical choices are quite limited because of accessibility. Autopsy specimens present even more theoretical possibilities because the tissue is available for analysis, but practical choices are also limited because the significance of many of these components is not known. Size, shape, texture, and the lipid, cellular, and collagen contents as judged grossly and microscopically remain useful and valuable means of evaluating lesions in order to detect genetic or environmental effects on progression. Considerable progress can be made by using these simple measurements when they are combined with measurements of suspected etiologic agents or intervening variables.

REFERENCES

Katz, S.S., 1981, The lipids of grossly normal human aortic intima from birth to old age. J. Biol. Chem. 23:12275-12280.

Libby, P., Warner, S.J.C., and Friedman, G.B., 1988, Interleukin-1: a mitogen for human vascular smooth muscle cells that induces the release of growth inhibitory prostanoids, J. Clin. Invest. 88:487-498.

Libby, P., Salomon, R.N., Payne, D.D., Schoen, F.J., and Pober, J.S., 1989, Functions of vascular wall cells related to the development of transplantation-associated coronary arteriosclerosis, Transplantation Proc. 21:3677-3684.

McGill, H.C., Jr., 1988, The pathogenesis of atherosclerosis. Clin. Chem. 33:B33-B39.

McGill, H.C., Jr., Geer, J.C., and Strong, J.P., 1963, Natural history of human atherosclerotic lesions, in "Atherosclerosis and Its Origin," M. Sandler and G.H. Bourne, eds., Academic Press, New York.

Melnick, J.L., Adam, E., and DeBakey, M.E., 1990, Possible role of cytomegalovirus in atherogenesis. JAMA 263:2204-2207.

Pober, J.S. and Cotran, R.S., 1990. Cytokines and endothelial cell biology. Physiol. Rev. 70:427-451.

Ross, R., Masuda, J., Raines, E.W., Gown, A.M., Katsuda, S., Sasahara, M., Malden, L.T., Masuko, H., and Sato, H., 1990, Localization of PDGF-B protein in macrophages in all phases of atherogenesis. Science 248:1009-1012.

Stary, H.C., 1989, Evolution and progression of atherosclerotic lesions in coronary arteries of children and young adults. Arteriosclerosis (Supp. I) 9:I-19-I-32.

A CARDIOLOGIST LOOKS AT THE IMPORTANCE OF BEING ABLE TO QUANTIFY THE

PATIENT'S PLAQUE SIZE

J. Bonnet, Th. Couffinal, V. Tourtoulou, D. Benchimol

Department of Cardiology
University of Bordeaux
Bordeaux, France

Angina pectoris, myocardial infarction, sudden death, and heart failure following ischemic cardiomyopathy are the main clinically important areas of cardiovascular disease. It is clear that heart attacks are in fact the consequence of coronary atherosclerosis.

If we look at pathogenetic sequences in atherosclerotic coronary artery disease, the progression from the normal individual with no detectable coronary atherosclerosis and the diagnosis of coronary artery disease by the cardiologist is complicated and actually not clearly defined.

It is clear that the rate of conversion from one step to another may vary greatly from person to person and that some of the forms of atherosclerosis may possibly be independent of one another. The conversion between each step is influenced by one or more different risk factors. Coronary artery disease exhibits several clinical manifestations including ischemic chest pain, classical myocardial infarction, and sudden death. The latter two have irreversible consequences and in half of the cases are not associated with a prior diagnosis of coronary artery disease. This means that the clinical understanding of how the modification of risk factors as etiologic components may influence the formation of fibrous plaques and asymptomatic coronary stenosis is still incomplete. Therefore the primary prevention of coronary artery disease by avoiding the major pathologic changes is only partially attained.

If we analyze the practical clinical approach to coronary artery disease in our patients at present, we find that we are trying to find solutions by means of large epidemiological studies or clinical trials which indicate that modification of risk factors will influence the clinical manifestations.

This approach can be implemented in two ways. It can be used to promote primary prevention by following asymptomatic individuals who are considered to be free from coronary atherosclerosis. Or it can be used to produce secondary prevention by following patients who have a prior history of myocardial infarction. This approach has given many positive results by demonstrating the effectiveness of altering clinical risk factors of

Atherosclerotic Plaques, Edited by R.W. Wissler *et al.*
Plenum Press, New York, 1991

coronary artery disease. Some promising solutions have resulted in establishing the effectiveness of drugs lowering the cholesterol level, the value of beta-blockers, thrombolytic therapy, and the possibilities of antiplatelet drugs after myocardial infarction.

Although this approach is very interesting, we should not forget that asymptomatic patients are rarely free from atherosclerotic plaques. Many necropsy studies have clearly demonstrated that 50% or greater stenosis of one or more coronary arteries is found in more than half of those patients who died of other causes (1, 2). Moreover, the epidemiologic studies use endpoints such as mortality or new cardiac events which may be due to factors other than progression of atheroma. These can include arrhythmias, clotting tendencies, plaque hemorrhage, or coronary arterial spasm unrelated to anatomic progression.

This makes it difficult to relate the results of epidemiological studies which have clinical endpoints to effects on the main problem, which is the atherosclerotic plaque. To study the atherosclerotic process directly, we must be able to quantify the effects of the patient's atherosclerotic plaque on the coronary artery lumen. In cardiology practice, it may seem simple because we analyze several times per day the degree of coronary atherosclerotic stenosis from coronary angiograms. So, the most widely used approach to assessing coronary artery disease is to perform a study of angiographic images in patients with coronary artery disase. No matter which procedures are used for quantification, we can try in this keynote presentation to analyze the importance of this approach in cardiology practice.

In the first place we must analyze the clinical indications for doing a coronary angiogram. Since the coronary catheterization is essentially performed to determine the presence and extent of coronary artery stenoses, there should be definite indications for coronary arteriography. The first of these is to obtain, for a preoperative or preangioplasty assessment, patients with a prior diagnosis of coronary disease. The second good reason that coronary angiography is performed is to gain a better understanding of patients who are asymptomatic but who have laboratory evidence of coronary artery disease, including a positive stress ECG, silent ischemia, or Holter registration. The third indication for coronary angiography is to develop a diagnosis of coronary artery disease in patients with atypical chest pain. These indications are essential in evaluating the results and the complications of coronary artery bypass surgery, percutaneous transluminal angioplasty, or post-thrombolytic therapy of acute myocardial infarction.

In these patients, what objectives can be attained by coronary arteriography and quantification of atherosclerotic plaque stenosis?

The first goal is to study coronary atherosclerosis independently from its clincal events. Five different objectives can be defined by using this approach.

First, we can use cross-sectional data to study the association of cardiovascular risk factors with arteriographically defined coronary arteriosclerosis. Specific risk factors associated with clinical events of coronary artery disease would not necessarily be associated with extent or severity of atherosclerosis. In fact, nearly all risk factors defined in clincial epidemiological studies have been found related to the presence of coronary atherosclerosis on angiographic models (3). However, a number of studies indicated no association between hypertension and the severity of coronary artery disease as defined from angiographic evidence (4-8).

Table 1. Clinical and angiographic factors associated with
progression of coronary artery disease.

Clinical and angiographic factors	References
Time	Moise (8)
	Kramer (9)
	Bruschka (10)
	Vanhaecke (11)
Severity of coronary atherosclerosis	Bruschke (10)
	Kramer (9)
	Palac (12)
	Moise (13)
Unstable angina	Kimbiris (14)
	Moise (15)
Age	Moise (15)
	Kramer (16)
HDL cholesterol	Arntzenius (17)
Glycemia	Vanhaecke (11)
	Bemis (18)
Cholesterol level	Bemis (18)
	Moise (19)
Smoking habits	Moise (19)
	Raichlen (20)
Hypertension	Raichlen (20)
Type of vessel: RC	Kramer (9)
Type of vessle: LAD	Bruschke (10)
Length of left main artery	Gazetopoulos (21)
Coronary artery bypass	Palac (12)
PTCA	Hwang (22)
	Benchimol (23)

Second, segmental catheterizations permit the direct study of risk
factors associated with the progression of coronary atherosclerosis or the
appearance of new plaques. Many clinical and angiographic factors
associated with progression of coronary atherosclerosis have been found
(Table 1). The time separating the two angiographic assessments is a major
factor in measuring atherosclerosis progression (7-10), but severity and
extent of coronary atherosclerosis (8, 9, 12, 13), unstable angina (14,
15), age (15, 16), cholesterol level (18, 19), and HDL cholesterol (17),
hyperglycemia (11, 18), smoking habits (19, 20), type of vessel (9, 10),
length of left main artery (21), coronary artery bypass (12), and
percutaneous coronary angioplasty (PTCA) (22, 23) all appear directly
associated with angiographically defined coronary atherosclerosis
progression.

Third, accurate and reproducible methods of determining the rate of disease progression by quantitative angiographic measurements allow clinical trials to evelute the effects of drugs and other interventions on the rate of progression and even their effects on regression of coronary atherosclerosis. For example, two studies show that nifedipine seems to suppress substantially the appearance of new lesions detectable by quantitative coronary arteriography (24, 25).

Fourth, quantitative assessment of atherosclerotic plaque lumen narrowing makes it possible to identify patients whose disease may be progressing rapidly, and who can be followed with pathophysiological evidence of changing functional status.

Finally, in the future, growth factors, their expression, and their receptors or manifestations of local inflammatory processes, will certainly be studied by means of the many biotechnological approaches being developed.

The second main goal of atherosclerotic plaque quantification is the independent study of coronary artery disease and its clinical manifestations.

Four different objectives can be recognized in the definition of the natural history of coronary artery disease and five in treatment assessment.

First, the follow-up of patients with angiographically defined atherosclerosis allows identification of subgroups of patients who are at particularly high risk of morbid or mortal events (26).

Second, risk factor analysis for clinical manifestations independent of the atherosclerotic process can be performed. So, Hartz et al. have demonstrated by stratifying the extent of coronary atherosclerosis angiographically that cigarette smoking, after the development of coronary atherosclerosis, may induce acute myocardial infarction in addition to its effect on the atherosclerotic process (27). Using a similar approach, two catheterizations separated by substantial intervals allowed Moise et al (28) to define clinical and angiographic factors associated with the appearance of a new coronary occlusion, as well as the major plaque complications associated with the acute myocardial infarction. New occlusions can be predicted by a combination of two angiographic factors associated with the severity and extent of coronary atherosclerosis and two clincial characteristics, namely smoking status and male gender (28).

Third, by stratification of coronary atherosclerosis extent, a pathophysiological approach to the study of clincial events can be developed. For example, in our group we have associated the preoperative myocardial infarction during coronary artery bypass to a clotting tendency (29).

A fourth utilization of quantitative angiography is that it facilitates the study of the relationship of anatomic stenosis to functional effects. The quantitative assessment of coronary artery lumen dimensions can predict the physiologic significance of a coronary stenosis. Zulstra et al. report a study of the regional flow reserve as measured by digital substraction cineangiography before and after intracoronary administration of papaverine. They assessed the coronary artery dimensions quantitatively and demonstrated that coronary flow reserve is curvilinearly related to minimal luminal cross-sectional area (30).

The patient's plaque quantification in coronary artery disease is useful in other ways. It permits therapeutic assessment of vasoactive drugs and new procedures of revascularization. The cross-sectional area determination of normal lumen or atherosclerotic stenosis has made it possible to clearly demonstrate vasodilatation of atherosclerotic stenosis. By means of this approach, the coronary vasomotion of normal, prestenotic, stenotic, and post-stenotic segments following vasoactive drugs can be determined (31, 32). Moreover, the quantification of the atherosclerotic plaque can be performed before and after a new procedure of revascularization, such as thrombolytic therapy, percutaneous coronary angioplasty (33), or laser or rotative angioplasty, have been carried out in the clinic. It appears that this approach may help to explain some difficult problems like the role of medial injury in these revascularization procedures or the definition of some of the pathophysiological approaches to explain the thrombotic tendency in the restenosis process.

It appears that plaque quantification is becoming very important in cardiologic practice. It appears that the definition of the effects of risk factors on coronary atherosclerosis and on its progression, as well as the study of long-term drug intervention, are greatly facilitated by this development. But independently of the atherosclerotic process, the effects of risk factors, the pathophysiological approach to the study of clinical events like thrombotic occlusion can be studied with the aid of angiographic methods. The physiologic significance of coronary stenosis and the assessment of medical or instrumental treatment of coronary artery disease can be greatly facilitated.

However, the angiographic data have their limits. The main limit is surely the bias in selection of study participants. Many biases are in fact possible. Among them are prevalence and incidence of disease, the clinic admission population and rate, cigarette comsumption status, and non-respondent diagnostic suspicion biases (34). The ethical limits make the acceptance of some of these biases necessary.

Moreover, the angiographic approach to the study of the atherosclerotic process constitutes only an indirect measurement of lesions. It never permits the analysis of the lesion components in the artery wall. The major reason for angiographic underestimation of coronary narrowing is the widespread presence of the atherosclerotic process throughout the coronary arteries. This makes it difficult to develop a real definition of a normal control artery for any study. Angiographic quantification also requires costly and sophisticated equipment. Angiographic approaches to the study of the atherosclerotic process, while not without risk, greatly decrease the necessity for surgical procedures, which carry a much greater risk and a 0.1% to 0.2% risk of death.

The main ongoing problem with the angiographic approach to atherosclerotic plaque quantification is to obtain an optimal detection of coronary artery disease. Visually assessed change in percent coronary stenosis is associated with a fairly large inter- and intra-observer variablity (8% to 18%). Only objective measurements from angiograms with advanced imaging technology assisted by computers permit a substantial reduction in these variability measures.

Moreover, to avoid biases in the recruitment of patients for cross-sectional studies it appears necessary to define controls with arteriographically normal coronary arteries and neighbourhood controls, without symptoms of coronary disease. But the main problems of recruitment in the angiographic approach of atherosclerosis quantification and study are in fact the usual problems connected with studying a chronic disease in free-living persons. New diagnostic approaches to atherosclerosis quantification are developing at a swift pace for peripheral arteries, and it remains to be seen whether some of these can, with the innovative technologies which are so pervasive, be adapted to coronary artery imaging and quantification to yield less invasive and more informative results.

REFERENCES

1. V. T. Rinassen. Coronary atherosclerosis in cases of coronary death as compared with that occuring in the population. Clin. Res. 7:412 (1975).
2. J. K. Mason. Asymptomatic diseases of coronary arteries in young men. Brit. Med. J. 2:1234 (1963).
3. T. A. Pearson. Coronary arteriography in the study of the epidemiology of coronary artery disease. Epid. Rev. 6:140 (1984).
4. Y. Hasin, S. Eisenberg, J. Friedlander, B. Lewis, M. Gotsman. Relationship between extent of coronary artery disease and correlative risk factors. Am. Heart J. 98:555 (1979).
5. A. J. Anderson, J. J. Barboriak, A. A. Rimm. Risk factors and angiographically determined coronary occlusion. Am. J. Epidemiol. 107:8 (1979).
6. M. H. Frick, G. Dahlen, K. Berg. Serum lipids in angiographically assessed coronary atherosclerosis. Chest 73:62 (1978).
7. K. A. Franck, S. S. Heller, D. S. Kornfeld. Type A behavior pattern and coronary angiographic findings. JAMA 240:761 (1978).
8. A. Moise, P. Théroux, Y. Taeymans, D. D. Waters, J. Lesperace, P. Fines, B. Descoings, P. Robert. Clinical and angiographic factors associated with progression of coronary artery disease. JACC 3:659 (1984).
9. J. R. Kramer, H. Kitazume, W. L. Proudfit. Progression and regression of coronary atherosclerosis: relation to risk factors. Am. Heart J. 105:134 (1983).
10. A. V. Bruschke, T. S. Wijers, W. Kolters, J. Landmann. The anatomic evolution of coronary disease demonstrated by coronary arteriography in 256 non-operated patients. Circulation 63:527 (1981).
11. J. Vanhaecke, J. Piessens, F. Van de Werf. Angiographic evolution of coronary atherosclerosis in non-operated patients. Eur. Heart J. 4:547 (1983).
12. R. T. Palac, M. H. Hwang, W. R. Meadows. Progression of coronary artery disease in medically and surgically treated patients 5 years after randomization. Circulation 64:suppl II, 17 (1981).
13. A. Moise, B. Clement, J. Saltiel. Clinical and angiographic correlates and prognostic significance of the coronary extent score. Am. J. Cardiol. 61:1255 (1988).
14. D. Kimbiris, A. Iskandrian, H. Saras, G. Inder, G. E. Bemis, B. L. Segal. Rapid progression of coronary stenosis in patients with unstable angina pectoris selected for coronary angioplasty. Cathet. Cardiovasc. Diagn. 10:101 (1984).
15. A. Moise, P. Théroux, Y. Taeymans, J. Lespérance, D. D. Waters, G. B. Pelletier, M. G. Bourassa. Unstable angina and progression of coronary atherosclerosis. New Engl. J. Med. 309:685 (1983).
16. J. R. Kramer, Y. Matsuda, J. C. Mulligan. Progression of coronary atherosclerosis. Circulation 63:519 (1981).

17. A. C. Arntzenius, D. Kromhout, J. D. Barth, J. H. C. Reiber, A. V. G. Bruschke, B. Buis, C. M. Van Gent, N. Kempen-Voogd, S. D. Strikwerda, E. A. Van der Velde. Diet, lipoproteins, and the progression of coronary atherosclerosis. The Leiden Intervention Trial. New Engl. J. Med. 312:805 (1985).

18. C. E. Bemis, R. Gorlin, H. G. Kemp. Progression of coronary artery disease. A clinical arteriographic study. Circulation 47:36 (1973).

19. A. Moise, P. Théroux, Y. Taeymans, D. D. Waters. Factors associated with progression of coronary artery disease in patients with normal or minimally narrowed coronary arteries. Am. J. Cardiol. 56:30 (1985).

20. J. S. Raichlen, B. Healy, S. C. Achuff, T. A. Pearson. Importance of risk factors in the angiographic progression of coronary artery disease. Am. J. Cardiol. 57:66 (1986).

21. N. Gazetopoulos, P. J. Ionnidis, A. Marselos. Length of main left coronary in relation to atherosclerosis of its branches: a coronary arteriographic study. Brit. Heart J. 38:180 (1976).

22. M. J. Hwang, P. Sidhu, I. Pacold, S. Johnson, P. J. Scalon, H. S. Loeb. Progression of coronary artery disease after percutaneous transluminal coronary angioplasty. Am. Heart. J. 115:297 (1988).

23. D. Benchimol, H. Benchimol, J. Bonnet, J. F. Dartigues, T. Couffinhal, H. Bricaud. Risk factors for progression of atherosclerosis six months after balloon angioplasty of coronary stenosis. Am. J. Cardiol. 65:980 (1990).

24. A. Loaldi, A. Polese, P. Montorsi, N. De Cesare, F. Fabbiocchi, P. Ravagnani, M. Guazzi. Comparison of nifedipine, propranolol and isosorbide dinitrate on angiographic progression and regression of coronary arterial narrowing in angina pectoris. Am. J. Cardiol. 64:433 (1989).

25. P. R. Lichtlen, P. Hugenholtz, W. Rafflenbehl, H. Hecker, S. Jost, J. W. Deckers, Retardation of angiographic progression of coronary artery disease by nifedipine. Lancet 335:1109 (1990).

26. J. O. Humphries, L. Kuller, R. Ross. Natural history of ischemic heart disease in relation to arteriographic findings: a tewlve-year study of 224 patients. Circulation 49:489 (1974).

27. A. J. Hartz, P. N. Barboriak, A. J. Anderson, R. G. Hoffman, J. J. Barboriak. Smoking, coronary artery occlusion, and non-fatal myocardial infarction. JAMA 146:851 (1981).

28. A. Moise, J. Lesperance, P. Théroux, Y. Taeymans, C. Goubet, M. G. Bourassa. Clinical and angiographic predictors of new total coronary occlusion in coronary artery disease. Analysis of 313 non-operated patients. Am. J. Cardiol. 54:1176 (1984).

29. N. Oysel, J. Bonnet, C. Vergnes, D. Benchimol, M. R. Boisseau, C. Moreau, P. Bernadet, E. Baudet, J. Larrue, H. Bricaud. Risk factors for myocardial infarction during coronary artery bypass graft surgery. Eur. Heart J. 10:806 (1989).

30. F. Zulstra, J. Van Ommeren, J. H. Reiber, P. W. Serruys. Does the quantitative assessment of coronary artery dimensions predict the physiologic significance of a coronary stenosis? Circulation 75:1154 (1987).

31. K. F. Hossak, G. Brown, D. K. Stewart, H. T. Dodge. Diltiazem-induced blockade of sympathetically mediated constriction of normal and diseased coronary arteries: lack of epicardial coronary dilatory effect in humans. Circulation 70:465 (1984).

32. P. W. Serruys, T. E. Hooghoudt, J. H. C. Reiber, C. Slager, R. W. Brower, P. G. Hugenholtz. Influence of intracoronary nifedipine on left ventricular function, coronary vasomotility, and myocardial oxygen consumption. Brit. Heart J. 49:427 (1983).

33. P. W. Serruys, J. H. C. Reiber, W. Wijns, M. Brand, C. J. Kooijman, H. J. ten Katen, P. G. Hugenholtz. Assessment of percutaneous transluminal coronary angioplasty by quantitative coronary angioplasty: diameter versus densitometric area measurement. Am. J. Cardiol. 54:482 (1984).

34. D. L. Sackett. Bias in analytic research. J. Chronic Dis. 32:51 (1979).

ULTRASOUND IMAGING OF ATHEROSCLEROTIC LESIONS IN ARTERIES OF ANIMALS:

VALIDITY AND REPRODUCIBILITY

M. Gene Bond,[1] Alan S. Berson,[2] and Fred A. Bryan[3]

[1] Bowman Gray School of Medicine, Winston-Salem, NC
[2] National Heart and Blood Institute (NIH), Bethesda, MD
[3] Research Triangle Institute. Research Triangle Park, NC

INTRODUCTION

The study of atherogenesis and the time course of atherosclerosis progression in animal models is a research area which has led to significant advances in knowledge about the human atherosclerotic process. Ultrasound B-scan imaging is one of the few noninvasive procedures which may be used to quantitatively assess the presence and severity of arterial lesions. Its advantages, which include ease of application, low cost, and repeated use without adverse consequences, make ultrasound imaging a preferred modality.

Ultrasound methods have been used with increasing frequency to noninvasively detect carotid artery atherosclerosis in human subjects since first described by Olinger (1969) and Blue et al. (1972). Previously, these studies and others by Giddens et al. (1982) and Spencer and Reid (1979) have focused on hemodynamically significant lesions and/or lumen diameter measurements (Chin et al. (1985)). Early attempts at validating and determining the reliability of artery wall thicknesses highlighted the need to develop and test criteria for what tunics could be visualized and measured using B-mode ultrasonography (Ricotta et al., 1987). Subsequently, Pignoli et al. (1986) validated B-mode ultrasound measurements of intima-media thickness in far walls.

A disadvantage of the method has been the lack of data on validity and reliability to document the resolution with which total arterial wall thicknesses, i.e., intima, media, and adventitia, may be identified. The study, some results of which are reported here, had as its objective the determination of the accuracy, precision, and repeat variability of B-mode ultrasonography in imaging total wall thicknesses from both near and far walls at the site of atherosclerotic lesions in arteries of monkeys. In vivo arteriographic studies and measurements from excised vessels were used to validate the ultrasound findings.

Atherosclerotic Plaques, Edited by R.W. Wissler *et al.*
Plenum Press, New York, 1991

METHODS

Experimental Design

Experiments were designed that would produce a wide range of arterial wall lesions, from modestly involved carotid arteries and abdominal aortas to those severely affected with atherosclerosis. The animal, the adult male Macaca fascicularis (cynomolgus) monkey, was selected because of its known propensity to develop atherosclerotic lesions within a reasonable time interval when fed a high cholesterol containing diet. The methods used to exacerbate the disease included hypertension created by coarctation of the descending thoracic aorta. Three groups of experimental animals were established. Group 1 (n = 11) had thoracic aorta coarctation to induce hypertension, and these animals were fed a high cholesterol containing diet. Group 2 monkeys (n = 12) were fed the high cholesterol containing diet, and Group 3 (n = 5) consisted of animals with modest hypercholesterolemia induced by feeding a butter control diet without added cholesterol.

All animals had blood drawn for determination of total serum cholesterol concentration every three months during the 26 month experiment. Prior to necropsy each animal had two B-mode ultrasound examinations of the carotid arteries and aorta, and on the day of necropsy, arteriographic examination of the same vessels was acomplished.

In Vitro Experiments

Initial studies were aimed at developing criteria for instrument gain settings, and for establishing those arterial interfaces that could be identified for subsequent measurements. The approach was to establish what was to be measured and how best to measure it and was based on a series of in vitro experiments using excised and opened human abdominal aortas removed at the time of autopsy. Twenty sites in these vessels were selected with the conscious bias that a wide range of lesions would be present. The periadventitial tissue was removed, and each segment was mounted in a heated water bath (38°C). The thickness of each lesion site was measured with ultrasound using 9 different gain settings ranging from 1 (low) to 9 (high). Measurements of total wall thicknesses that included combined intima, media, and adventitia were made at each gain setting. The measurement made at the target site was the linear distance from the first interface (nearest the transducer) observed to the distal edge of the outer echogenic region (farthest from the transducer). At the end of each experiment, a metallic pin was positioned adjacent to the site interrogated with ultrasound and the specimen cross-sectioned at this level. Without knowledge of the B-mode ultrasound results a second investigator sectioned the specimens at the point of ultrasound measurement, and using a 7X magnification micrometer reticle graduated in 0.1 mm increments, measured the total arterial wall thickness directly from the cut surface of the specimen. The instrument gain settings and criteria for making arterial measurements for use in the subsequent in vivo animal studies were based on the information and data derived from this set of experiments.

Animal Ultrasound

For all in vitro and in vivo studies, the HRL SCANNEX (Horizon Research Laboratory, Inc., Fort Lauderdale, Florida) ultrasound unit with a 10 MHz mosaic transducer was used. Animals were anesthetized with Ketamine (IM) and were placed in the supine position on a heated water blanket. The skin regions of the neck and abdomen were shaved to reduce image artifacts. The areas of interrogation were restricted to the region of the abdominal aorta between the renal arteries and the common iliac bifurcation and to the common carotid arteries. The flow divider of the common iliac artery at peak systole was used as a reference, and all measurements of aortic lumen diameter and wall thickness were made 5.0 and 10.0 mm superior to this site. The lowest possible gain setting which demonstrated arterial interfaces was chosen in order to reduce the artifacts that occur with higher settings. With the image in focus during real-time scanning, the sonographer depressed the "freeze frame" button and captured an image as close to peak systole as possible. The captured image was critically evaluated by the interpreter, and if the above described criteria were not met, the scan was repeated. Several attempts were usually necessary before an image of acceptable quality was obtained. When this image was obtained, the interpreter recorded several cardiac cycles on 3/4" video tape. Similarly, the segment of the single frame chosen for measurement was also recorded. Information and measurements, made directly from the monitor using the internally calibrated electronic cursor, included lumen diameter, wall thickness, instrument gainsetting, and depth of near artery wall from skin surface.

Four angles of view were attempted for the abdominal aorta: anterior-posterior (AP), right anterior oblique (RAO), left anterior oblique (LAO), and either right or left lateral views (RL or LL, respectively). All animals were prepared and anesthetized in the manner described for the abdominal aorta prior to beginning the common carotid artery scan. In each case the carotid arteries were examined during the same scanning session; however, in randomly selected cases the carotid arteries were studied prior to the aortic evaluation. The extracranial carotid arteries presented unique and challenging problems because of their small size, i.e., lumen diamters 2 mm or less, and because of their location. The relatively short distance between the mandible and clavicle, combined with high bifurcations and small lumen diameters, precluded evaluation of the internal carotid arteries, or establishing definitive intra-arterial reference sites.

We examined several animal colonies twice. In order to establish the reliablity of B-mode ultrasound, measurements using the techniques and methods described were made. The second examination was performed within three weeks of the initial scan, and the last exam occurred within twenty-four hours of animal sacrifice. Since the goal of these experiments was to determine the reliability and validity of B-mode ultrasound, the decision was made to focus measurement techniques on specific arterial sites with the rationale that lesions would be present at these highly predisposed sites. Our criteria were developed because it was important to be able to return to the same site for replicate measurements, and to a site that could be defined from both arteriographic images and pathology specimens for comparison. Therefore the interpreter, at the beginning of the second examination, was presented a list of "localizing" data that consisted of the following: (1) arterial segment to be examined (aorta, right or left carotid artery); (2) angle; (3) intra-arterial reference; (4) distance from reference point to the target site; (5) depth of near wall adventitia-periadventitia interface from skin surface; and (6) instrument gain setting used during the first examination. The second examination for each arterial site was done using this information.

Arteriographic Methods

Prior to necropsy and after the final B-mode ultrasound examination, animals that were included in the validation protocols were examined arteriographically. Under Ketamine anesthesia, surgical anesthesia was induced with intravenously administered pentobarbital. A femoral arteriotomy was performed, and the artery was cannulated with a 0.045 inch diameter, barium impregnated, 40 cm long polyethylene catheter with a single curve one centimeter from the distal tip. Four-to-six mls of meglumine iothalamate (injection USP 60%) was injected by hand into the aortic arch with a single exposure in a Schonander changer with a 0.6 mm focal spot x-ray tube. After evaluation of the subsequent AP aortic x-ray (resolution - 7 line pairs), the catheter was moved using fluoroscopy to the origin of the right brachiocephalic artery and a small amount of contrast media injected at this point to confirm the position of the catheter. An AP arteriograph was then taken which demonstrated the extracranial portion of the carotid arteries, bilaterally. The animal was turned on its side and a lateral arteriograph of the carotid arteries was performed. The carotid arteriographs were recorded on 2:1 magnification film, and were obtained by hand injection of 2-3 ml of meglumine iothalamate. Magnification was measured geometrically and checked by comparison with a dimensional marker of known size which was placed on the skin surface within the field of view.

Arteriographic images were evaluated by a technician who was unaware of the B-mode ultrasound findings. The position of the common iliac flow divider was determined from the AP aortogram, and sites to be measured 5.0 and 10.0 mm proximal to this reference were marked on the x-ray. Arteriographic measurements of the lumen diameter were made at both target sites using a 7X micrometer reticle graduated in 0.1 mm increments. Arteriographic measurements of wall thickness were not made because of the inability of this method to visualize the outside boundary of the artery, i.e., adventitia-periadventitia interface.

The AP x-rays of the carotid arteries were evaluated by first defining the position of the flow divider(s) which identified the origins of the right and left common carotid arteries. In order to find the midpoint of the common carotid artery, the flow dividers separating the internal from external carotid arteries within the bulb region were identified in each vessel, and a mark was placed on both right and left common carotid arteries at the midpoint between the origin and the carotid bifurcation. Measurements were made of lumen diameters at this midpoint. The lateral films proved more difficult to evaluate because the left and right carotid arteries occasionally overlapped near the origin of the vessels. In order to solve this problem, the lateral and AP views x-rays were overlaid and the midpoint of the artery was determined by positioning the lateral view on the AP view using extra-arterial landmarks such as the clavicle or vertebral column. Once this was established a mark was made on the lateral x-ray using the mark that had already been determined for the midpoint of the artery from the AP film. After all arteriographic measurements were made, each was converted to absolute in vivo measurements by using a calibration factor determined from the dimensional marker which had been placed on the skin surface, and which was present in the x-rays.

Pathology Evaluation

Necropsies were performed immediately after the last ultrasound examination, or in the case of those animals that had an arteriograph, immediately after that procedure. The peritoneal cavity was entered through an incision along the linea alba and the inferior vena cava identifed and mobilized. The diaphragm and pericardium were incised, and an 18 gauge needle, attached via tubing to a pressure perfusion chamber, was inserted into the apex of the left ventricle. Perfusate, either normal saline or phosphate buffer (pH 7.0), was then infused into the cardiovascular system at 100 mm/Hg pressure. The inferior vena cava was immediately incised and the perfusate allowed to circulate through the cardiovascular system for approximately 10 minutes. When formalin fumes were noted emanating from the incised cava, this vessel was clamped, and the pressure within the cardiovascular system maintained at 100 mm/Hg for 60-90 minutes, i.e., the time necessary to insure fixation of arterial structures. The aorta and extracranial carotid arteries were then marked in situ. A line was drawn along the anterior (ventral) midline of the abdominal aorta from the renal bifurcation to the iliac bifurcation and two additional marks were made horizontally, the first 5.0 mm and the second 10.0 mm superior to the flow dividers separating the common iliac arteries, i.e., the reference point used for in vivo studies. Each common carotid artery was also marked along its anterior midline for orientation purposes, and a single mark was made midway between the origin of each vessel and the origin of the carotid bulb. The arteries were then removed and the periadventitial connective tissue was cleaned from the outer surface of the vessel.

An experienced pathology technician who was not involved in the B-mode ultrasound scanning or the arteriographic procedures then made measurements directly from the specimens. The abdominal aorta was cross-sectioned 5.0 and 10.0 mm superior to the common iliac bifurcation, and measurements of near artery wall thicknesses and lumen diameters were made from each of the AP, RAO, LAO, and RL or LL angles. RL and LL measurements were made perpendicular to the AP orientation. In the carotid arteries a mark was made along the anterior wall in situ for angle orientation. The entire length of the artery was measured, and a second mark was made on the vessel midway between its origin and the bulb. All pathology measurements were made directly from gross specimens using a hand held 7X magnification micrometer reticle.

RESULTS

The baseline observations for body weight, total serum cholesterol and HDL cholesterol concentrations of the three groups of M. fascicularis are presented in Table 1. Mean values for each parameter were comparable among the groups. The observations during the 26 months experimental period are shown in Tables 2A and 2B. Body weights and direct blood pressure measurements are single values that were determined prior to necropsy. The lipid values, total serum cholesterol, and HDL cholesterol concentrations represent mean values averaged over the 26 month experimental period. Body weights at the end of the experiment were similar among the three groups, and were also similar to baseline values, indicating that signficant growth did not occur during the experiment. Total serum cholesterol concentrations in Groups 1 and 2 increased markedly over baseline values. This same parameter was elevated in Group 3 when compared to baseline, and on a group basis was approximately 50% of the value observed in Groups 1 and 2. HDL cholesterol concentrations decreased in Groups 1 and 2, but did not change significantly in Group 3 when this value was compared with the baseline observations. Direct, mean blood pressure was highest in Group 1 animals, followed by Groups 3 and 2, in that order. Most of this difference results from larger systolic pressures since mean group diastolic pressures were comparable. The lipid and pressure values indicate that considerable variability was present within each of the three experimental groups, thereby allowing us to evaluate the effect of a wide range of risk factor dosage on lumen diameters and artery wall thicknesses in these models.

Table 1. Baseline Observations

	Body Weight (kg) Mean ± SD	Total Serum Cholesterol (mg/dl) Mean ± SD	HDL Cholesterol (mg/dl) Mean ± SD
Group 1	4.4 ± 0.9	107 ± 37	47 ± 10
Group 2	4.1 ± 0.8	121 ± 20	51 ± 12
Group 3	4.2 ± 0.4	115 ± 8	49 ± 9

Table 2A. Experimental Observations

	Body Weight (kg) Mean ± SD	Total Serum Cholesterol (mg/dl) Mean ± SD
Group 1	4.5 ± 0.4	731 ± 106
Group 2	4.3 ± 0.5	753 ± 119
Group 3	4.3 ± 0.5	376 ± 182

Table 2B. Experimental Observations

	HDL Cholesterol Concentration (mg/dl) Mean ± SD	Blood Pressure (Direct) Systolic	Blood Pressure (Direct) Diastolic Mean ± SD	Blood Pressure (Direct) Mean
Group 1	28 ± 8	148 ± 30	87 ± 13	121 ± 21
Group 2	27 ± 6	130 ± 26	82 ± 13	96 ± 29
Group 3	49 ± 18	136 ± 41	83 ± 22	110 ± 31

Effects of Gain Setting on Ultrasound Wall Thickness Determined From B-Mode Ultrasound

Instrument gain setting had an appreciable effect on total arterial wall thicknesses in vitro. Increasing instrument gain setting in increments of 1, resulted in an almost linear increase in measured apparent wall thicknesses made from B-mode images. At a gain setting of 0, arterial structures were not well visualized. At a gain setting of 1 (low) artery walls measured 2.6 mm in average thickness when determined from B-mode ultrasound, and continued to apparently increase in size to 4.0 mm at high gain settings. At the highest gain setting possible, the total image was "whited" out, and it was impossible to reliably identify any arterial interfaces. Since the same specimens were used for all serial gain studies, the group measurement variability was similar at all settings. The mean total wall thicknesses of the pathology specimens when measured directly at the end of the studies was 2.7 mm, which corresponded most closely with the lower B-mode gain settings, i.e., between 1 and 3. Because of this correspondence, the in vivo measurements of total artery wall thickness in vivo was performed at low gain settings, usually between 1 and 2. In all replicate studies however, the initial gain setting used to measure wall thickness was used for subsequent scans.

The in vivo studies on gain settings demonstrated two additional important findings. First, increase in gain did not substantially affect the position of the adventitia-water boundary resulting in increased ultrasound estimates of wall thickness. Higher gain settings used to evaluate wall structure and to define interfaces masked the adventitial-water interface required to measure arterial thickness. The in vitro arteries in this study were measured with the intimal surface closest to the probe, and were comparably oriented to the far arterial wall when studied in vivo. If the in vitro arteries were turned over in the water bath, and evaluated with the adventitial side closest to the transducer, i.e., comparable spatially to the in vivo view of the near artery wall, the principal artifactual effect would occur on the deeper lying intimal interface. In these tests the in vitro experiments aided us in defining the quantitative ramifications of high gain settings on lumen diameter measurements. The higher the gain the smaller the apparent lumen diameter would be; this was due to the artifactual thickening of the near wall intimal surface when studied in vivo. Also the acoustical characteristics of normal artery walls and atherosclerotic lesions changed considerably with increasing gain settings. Specifically, we observed qualitative changes with higher gain settings that obscured intralesion tissue layers and inreased gray scale heterogeneity within and among layers of these vessels.

Validation Studies and Animal Models

The data comparing B-mode ultrasound with pathology specimen measurements of carotid arteries and abdominal aortas are presented in Table 3. Two hundred arterial sites were evaluated for total wall thickness and lumen diameter using the methods described previously. Almost all wall thicknesses measured by B-mode ultrasound were larger than those from pathology specimens with a resulting mean absolute difference of 0.3 mm. The maximum mean wall thickness found by examining pathology specimens in a single animal was 1.1 mm, which compared to 1.8 mm of this vessel when measured from B-mode ultrasound images. In general, the lumen diameters measured from B-mode ultrasound images were also larger than those measured from pathology specimens with an absolute difference of 0.56 mm. In Table 4, the last series of B-mode measurements (n = 76 sites) were evaluated to demonstrate the effect of learning in making these measurements. The absolute difference between lumen diameters measured between B-mode ultrasound and pathology was 0.36 mm, which was comparable to the absolute difference observed between the methods for total wall thickness. In part, we believe some of this difference can be explained by learning which took place during this study. The reason for the remaining relatively small absolute differences between the two methods is unclear, but could be the result of several factors, including the 0.15 mm axial resolution of the ultrasound instrument used, changes in arterial size that occurred when the animal was sacrificed and during the time the cardiovascular system was being pressure fixed, the difficulty in trimming vessels and making gross measurements as precisely as 0.1 mm, or to small errors in identifying spatially specific ultrasound arterial interfaces in small arteries. The complete data base suggests that it is feasible to noninvasively measure wall thicknesses and lumen diameters with mean group absolute differences between 0.3 - 0.4 mm when compared to pathology specimens. Measurements from B-mode and arteriography are compared in Table 5. In almost every comparison, the arteriographic lumen diameters were larger than those measured from B-mode ultrasound images with an absolute difference of 1.0 mm. Arteriographic lumen diameters were also larger than those made from pathology specimens as can be seen by comparing Tables 4 and 5. The principal reason which might explain most of this difference may have been the hand generated pressures used to inject the contrast media in these small elastic arteries. Although not measured,

Table 3. Ultrasound - Pathology Validation

	Lumen Diameter (n = 200 sites)	
	B-mode (mm)	Gross Pathology (mm)
X ± SD	2.71 ± 0.66	2.39 ± 0.78
Absolute Difference	0.56	
r	0.41	

	Wall Thickness (n = 200 sites)	
	B-mode (mm)	Gross Pathology (mm)
X ± SD	0.80 ± 0.23	0.51 ± 0.20
Absolute Difference	0.30	
r	0.42	

Table 4. Lumen Diameter: Ultrasound-Pathology Validation

	B-mode (mm)	Gross Pathology (mm)
X ± SD	2.60 ± 0.49	2.73 ± 0.50
Absolute Difference	0.36	
r	0.57	
n	76	

Table 5. Lumen Diameter: Ultrasound-Arteriography Validation

	B-mode (mm)	Arteriography
X ± SD	2.61 ± 0.50	3.61 ± 0.75
Absolute Difference	1.0	
r	0.69	
n	68	

these pressures are usually considerably higher than blood pressure and probably resulted in transient arterial dilatation which was subsequently captured on the arteriogram.

Reproducibility Studies in Animal Arteries

The reproduciblity of B-mode ultrasound measurements of wall thickness and lumen diameter is presented in Table 6, which uses data from the replicate and "blinded" examinations of the abdominal aorta in Macaca fascicularis. The absolute difference in lumen measurements comparing first and second scans from these animals was 0.23 mm. Similar comparison of wall thicknesses resulted in an absolute difference of 0.17 mm. These small absolute differences may have resulted from slight changes in the cardiovascular status of the animals which occurred between evaluations, or from the difficulties encountered in capturing single B-mode ultrasound frames at exact peak systole. Since these differences are absolute, i.e., the positive and negative signs have not been used to determine the mean differences, and since the mean absolute differences in measuring both parameters approaches the axial resolution of the instrument used, we believe these studies demonstrate the error of the method when evaluating small vessels in animal models.

Table 6. Reproducibility: B-Mode Ultrasound
Macaca fascicularis Abdominal Aorta

	Lumen Diameter (mm)		
	1st Observation		2nd Observation
X ± SD	2.52 ± 0.41		2.52 ± 0.51
Absolute Difference		0.23	
r		0.81	
n		60	

	Wall Thickness (mm)		
	1st Observation		2nd Observation
X ± SD	0.98 ± 0.25		1.03 ± 0.21
Absolute Difference		0.17	
r		0.47	
n		60	

CONCLUSIONS

The validity results demonstrate that arterial lumens and walls of small animals (4kg) can be detected with B-mode ultrasound, and can be measured with a precision of 0.3 - 0.4 mm, i.e., appoximately twice the axial resolution of the instrument used. This appears to be a conservative estimate of the methodological error because the arteriography and pathology methods, which were the standards against which the ultrasound was validated, also changed arterial dimensions to some degree.

Excellent reproduciblity was demonstrated and approached the resolution of the instrument when used to measure wall thickness and lumen diameters in animals.

The procedures used for these B-mode ultrasound studies are similar to those used for imaging human carotid and peripheral arteries, except that greater care was exercised in precise positioning and repositioning of the transducer, and in fine tuning instrument controls. It is reasonable to expect equivalent levels of accuracy and precision for human studies with this level of care.

ACKNOWLEDGEMENTS

We wish to thank Mrs Diana Swain and Mrs Janet Kaduck-Sawyer for technical assistance, Marshall Ball, MD, for the arteriographic examinations and Ms. April Comer for manuscript preparation.

This work has been supported by grant NHLBI N01-HV-12916 from the National Institutes of Health.

REFERENCES

Blue, S. K., McKinney, W. M., Barnes, R., Toole, J. F., 1972, Ultrasonic b-mode scanning for study of extracranial vascular disease, Neurology, 22:1079-1085.

Chin, H. P., Curry, P., Low, G., Nessim, S., Blankenhorn, G. H., 1985, Autopsy callibration of carotid artery b-mode ultrasound imaging: Effects of pressure on residual lumen size, <u>J. Lab. Clin. Med.</u>, 105:120-123.

Giddens, D. P., Khaliffa, A. M., 1982, Turbulence measurements with pulsed doppler ultrasound employing a frequency tracking method, <u>Ultrasound Med. Biol.</u>, 8:427-437.

Olinger, C. P., 1969, Ultrasonic carotid echoarteriography, <u>AJR</u>, 106: 282-295.

Pignoli, P., Tremoli, E., Poli, A., Oreste, P., Paoletti, R., 1986, Intimal plus medial thickness of the arterial wall. A direct measurement with ultrasound imaging, <u>Circulation</u>, 74:1399-1406.

Ricotta, J. J., McKinney, W. M., Bryan, F. A., Bond, M. G., Kurtz, A., O'Leary, D. H., Raines, J. K., Berson, A. S., Clouse, M. E., Calderon-Ortiz, M., Toole, J. F., DeWeese, J., Smullens, S. N., and Gustafson, N. F., 1987, Multicenter validation study of real-time (b-mode) ultrasound: Arteriography and pathology, <u>J. Vasc. Surg.</u>, 6:512-520.

Spencer, M. P., Reid, J. M., 1979, Quantitation of carotid stenosis with continuous-wave (C-W) doppler ultrasound, <u>Stroke</u>, 10:326-330.

HETEROGENEOUS MORPHOLOGICAL PATTERNS OF THE FIBROATHEROMATOUS PLAQUE

AND RISK FACTORS

Luigi Giusto Spagnoli, Alessandro Mauriello,
Giampiero Palmieri, Augusto Orlandi, Giuseppe Santeusanio

Cattedra di Anatomia ed Istologia Patologica
II Universita' di Roma "Tor Vergata"
Via Carnevale - 00173 Roma (Italy)

INTRODUCTION

Vascular changes in human atherosclerosis are heterogeneous in both architecture and histocytological composition of the lesions (1-3). The histological characterization of the fibroatheromatous plaques and their histogenesis are, however, still to be defined. Factors responsible for the evolution of intimal lesions and the mechanisms and stages of fibro-atheromatous plaque formation are still largely obscure.

There are a number of drawbacks involved in the study of the histogenesis of the disease and possible causative factors at the morphological level. The disease process is characterized by a long course so that factors acting in the clinical stage may not be the same as those operating as initiating factors (4). However, the clinical stage of atherosclerosis has been reported to correspond to the appearance of complicated plaques in the arterial tree (5).

Focusing as it does on symptomatic plaques, the aim of this study is to answer the questions whether plaque heterogeneity is the result of a haphazard clustering of various components or an organized pattern in response to risk factors. To this end, histocytologic components of the plaque were quantified and correlated by statistical analysis.

MATERIAL AND METHODS

Plaques

A hundred and eighty carotid plaques from patients affected by transient ischemic attack (TIA) or by stroke, with angiographic stenosis equal to or greater than 50%, were studied after endoarterectomy.

Atherosclerotic Plaques, Edited by R.W. Wissler *et al.*
Plenum Press, New York, 1991

Sampling and Light Microscopy

The segment of maximal stenosis, angiographically or ultrasono-graphically documented, was sampled from each carotid. This constitutes the target on which any risk factors present have produced maximum response and is the area causing the maximum clinical consequences. The stenotic tract was identified in the surgical specimen by comparison with the angiographic or ultrasonographic findings, taking the carotid bifurcation as the reference point. Once the plaque had been identified, a number of transverse serial sections were made.

Arterial slices, fixed in formalin and methanol-Carnoy and embedded in paraffin, were sectioned and stained with hematoxylin-eosin, Weigert-Van Gieson, Alcian blue-PAS and Movat pentachrome (6).

The semiquantitative light microscopy observations were collected according to a morphological protocol, previously described (7), in which the histological and cytological components of the fibroatheromatous plaque were analytically reported. The plaque components were graded at a magnification of 40x. The staining intensity of the interstitial component was arbitrarily graded as absent, +, ++ and +++. The plaque and interstitial components were quantified by two independent pathologists without knowledge of the clinical data of the patients. The inter-observer reproducibility was 96%.

Validation Methods

In order to validate the light microscopic findings we used electron microscopy and immunohistochemistry on selected samples with the following primary antibodies: HHF35 (subunits alpha and gamma of smooth muscle actin) (8), HAM56 (human macrophages and histiocytes) (9), L26 (lymphocyte B) (10), OK M1 (monocytes/macrophages) (11), collagen type IV (basal membranes). The data obtained on a smaller number of cases will be published elsewhere.

Clinical Data Protocol

The patients were grouped according to age, sex and presence or absence of the risk factors listed in Table 1.

Statistical Analysis

Data, digitized and stored in an Olivetti M28 PC, were analyzed by SPSS (Statistical Package for the Social Sciences). Two different kinds of statistical analysis were applied.

The chi-square test was applied to all possible pairs of variables of the fibroatheromatous plaque in order to evaluate the relationship between two histocytological components. The values of chi-square distribution were both uncorrected and corrected using Sidak's multiplicative inequality (13). Sidak's tables were applied so as to avoid the random associations occurring in multiple comparisons.

TABLE 1

Risk factors

===

HYPERTENSION (12)
a) BORDERLINE: diastolic pressure between 95 and 105 mmHg
b) SEVERE: diastolic pressure ⟩ 105 and/or systolic pressure ⟩ 160 mmHg
DIABETES
a) INSULIN-DEPENDENT
b) TREATED WITH DIET AND/OR ORAL AGENTS
HYPERLIPEMIA
a) MILD: plasma triglycerides or cholesterol between 200 and 239 mg/dl
b) SEVERE: plasma triglicerides or cholesterol ⟩ 240 mg/dl
SMOKING HABIT
a) MODERATE: between 10 and 20 cigarettes/die
b) HEAVY: more than 20 cigarettes/die

===

Student's T-test for unpaired samples was applied in order to
evaluate the effect of the single risk factor on the various histocytological components of the plaque. Thus, each group with a risk
factor was compared with a control group defined as all other patients
without that particular risk factor.

Values with P⟨0.05 were considered statistically significant.

RESULTS

Patients

The mean age of the 180 patients studied was 62.57 ± 7.44 years.
Sixteen were under 50 and 29 over 70. Of the 36 (20%) female patients
only 2 were under 50.

A hundred and five patients were hypertensive (25 with borderline
hypertension and 80 with severe hypertension), 56 diabetic (38 undergoing
treatment with oral and dietetic agents and 18 insulin-dependent), 74
hyperlipemic (37 with mild hyperlipemia and 37 with severe hyperlipemia)
and 115 were smokers (31 moderate and 84 heavy smokers).

All of the four risk factors considered were absent in only 7
patients. One factor was present in 57, and two or more in the
remainder. In 9 patients all four risk factors were present
simultaneously.

Histologic Examination

In 163 patients (90.56%) we found multiple and often confluent
fibroatheromatous plaques. In the reamaning 17 (9.44%) there was a
single plaque. The dimension of the atheroma, the thickness of the cap
and the cellular composition varied from one plaque to the next. The cell

component consisted of varying numbers of smooth muscle cells (SMC), foam cells (FC), mononuclear cells (MC) and, more rarely, multinuclear giant cells (MGC). SMC were present in all plaques, FC in 89.44%,, MC in 67.12% and MGC only in 18.89%. The SMC of the plaque differed partially from those of the tunica media but maintained some typical ultra-structural characteristics such as the presence of the basement membrane, micropinocytic vescicles and intracytoplasmatic anchoring maculae (14,15).

Immunohistochemically the SMC were positive to the antibody anti-actin HHF35 (8), and the anti-collagen type IV antibody showed a thick shell of basement membrane which encased each SMC. There were two types of FC. The first was elongated with a fusiform nucleus and showed the ultrastructural and immunohistochemical characteristics of SMC (HHF35-positive). The cytoplasm was, however, largely or totally occupied by lipid droplets. The second type was larger and roundish or oval, with a round, often eccentric, nucleus and cytoplasm entirely filled with lipid droplets associated with a varying number of dense lisosomal bodies. These cells showed the ultrastructural features of the macrophagic cells and were positive to the anti-macrophage antibody HAM56 (9). The MC were positive to the anti-lymphocyte B antibodies (L26) (10) and monocytes/macrophages (OK M1) (11).

Complications were present in 80% of the plaques, with the following incidence: calcification 67.4% of cases, hemorrhage of the vessel wall 44.44% and thrombosis 22.78%. In agreement with lmparato et al. (16) and Lusby et al. (17), intramural hemorrhage in the plaques studied by us seems to play a greater role than thrombosis in the occurrence of vascular stenosis and symptoms.

Relationship Between the Histocytologic Components of the Plaque

As previously reported (18) the various histocytologic components of the fibroatheromatous plaques displayed statistically significant non-random associations, as demonstrated by the chi--square test based on Sidak's multiplicative inequality (Table 2).

A positive correlation was demonstrated between the presence of thrombosis and the size of the atheroma. Whereas only 14% of plaques (6 out of 43 cases) with an atheroma occupying less than 30% of the plaque were associated with thrombosis, 49% (21 out of 43 cases) of those with an atheroma larger than 60% of the plaque were associated with thrombosis.

The inverse relationship between cap thickness and size of the atheroma is closely linked with the relationship between thrombosis and the size of the atheroma (p⟨0.01). Progression towards the surface of the atheroma, together with mechanical stress, is the premise for a discontinuity in the fibrous cap covering the atheroma (19). The ulcerated plaque is particularly exposed to vascular thrombosis, even though hemodynamic disturbances favoring the accumulation of activated coagulation factors and platelet aggregating factors are necessary for

TABLE 2
Correlation between histocytologic components of the fibroatheromatous plaque, using chi-square based on Sidak's
multiplicative inequality.

		correlation	p
Thrombosis	Thickness of cap	negative	< 0.01
Thrombosis	Atheroma	positive	< 0.01
Thickness of cap	Atheroma	negative	< 0.01
Thickness of cap	Connective tissue	positive	< 0.01
Connective tissue	Atheroma	negative	< 0.01
Pas-positivity	Alcianophilia	negative	< 0.05
Foam cells	Mononuclear cells	positive	< 0.01
Giant cells	Mononuclear cells	positive	< 0.01

its formation (19). In our study the thickness of the cap was inversely
related to thrombosis (p<0.01). In 94% of the ulcerated plaques (in which
the cap was very thin or not clearly visible) thrombosis was present. In
those having a cap equal to 30-60% or more of the plaque, thrombosis was
observed in 12% or 13% of cases, respectively.

The amount of connective tissue present in the plaque was inversely
related to the size of the atheroma (p<0.01), in keeping with the
observations of Tracy et al. (20), who suggested that only the cap and
not the base participate in the decrease of connective tissue with
increasing atheronecrotic mass. This is in agreement with our observation
that cap thickness is directly proportional to the amount of connective
tissue in the plaque (p<0.01).

It is worth noting that there is a positive correlation between MC
and FC. Of the 19 plaques without FC, in 14 MC were absent and in 4
there were very few. On the contrary, when there were numerous FC,
numerous MC were also present. This result is consistent with the
knowledge derived from studies on human and experimental atherosclerosis
(21-23). Moreover, we observed a direct relationship between MC and MGC.
When MC were absent MGC were also absent.

Relationship Between Single Plaque Components and Various Risk Factors

The effect of the single risk factor on the morphologic parameters
of the fibroatheromatous plaque, separately considered, are listed in
Tables 3 to 8.

Aging (Table 3) was associated with a significant increase in
vascularization (p<0.03). After the age of 70 the connective tissue also
increased (p<0.01). The plaques of young patients were also characterized
by a greater number of SMC, MGC and MC than the plaques of patients over
50. The difference was not, however, statistically significant in that
the two extreme groups (young and over 70) contained very few patients.

TABLE 3

Correlation between single histocytologic components of the plaque and aging. (Statistically significant values only. Mean ± SEM).

(No.patients)	AGE		
	<= 50 years (16)	50 - 70 years (135)	>70 years (29)
GIANT CELLS *	1.37 + 0.15	1.19 + 0.03	1.14 + 0.08
	I-----p<0.05----I		
	I-----------------p<0.05-------------I		
CONNECTIVE *	2.31 + 0.18	2.53 + 0.07	2.86 + 0.15
	I----------------p<0.01------------I		
VASCULARIZATION **	1.62 + 0.12	1.82 + 0.03	1.76 + 0.08
	I-----p<0.03----I		

(score = *: 1 absent, 2 +, 3 ++, 4 +++; **: 1 absent, 2 present)

TABLE 4

Correlation between single histocytologic components of the plaque and sex. (Statistically significant values only. Mean ± SEM).

(No.patients)	SEX	
	MALE (144)	FEMALE (36)
MONONUCLEAR CELLS *	2.23 + 0.09	2.75 + 0.18
	I-----p<0.004----I	
FOAM CELLS *	2.64 + 0.08	3.00 + 0.16
	I----p<0.03-----I	
GIANT CELLS *	1.17 + 0.03	1.30 + 0.08
	I-----p<0.05----I	
ATHEROMA *	3.06 + 0.06	2.75 + 0.12
	I-----p<0.007---I	
HEMORRHAGE **	1.50 + 0.04	1.33 + 0.08
	I----p<0.04-----I	

(score = *: 1 absent, 2 +, 3 ++, 4 +++; **: 1 absent, 2 present)

Differences in cellular composition and size of the atheroma were present between the plaques of males and females (Table 4). The plaques females were richer in MC (P<0.004), FC (p<0.03) and MGC (p<0.05), whereas the number of SMC was unvaried. In males the atheroma were larger and was associated with an increase in the incidence of intramural hemorrhage (p<0.04).

TABLE 5

Correlation between single histocytologic components of the plaque and hypertension. (Statistically significant values only. Mean $\pm$ SEM).

===

(No.patients)	HYPERTENSION			
	ABSENT (75)	PRESENT (105)	BORDERLINE (25)	SEVERE (80)
MONONUCLEAR CELLS *	2.16 $\pm$ 0.12	2.45 $\pm$ 0.10	2.40 $\pm$ 0.19	2.47 $\pm$ 0.12
	I---p<0.03----I			
FOAM CELLS *	2.53 $\pm$ 0.11	2.84 $\pm$ 0.09	2.76 $\pm$ 0.20	2.87 $\pm$ 0.11
	I----p<0.02-----I			
GIANT CELLS *	1.12 $\pm$ 0.03	1.25 $\pm$ 0.04	1.32 $\pm$ 0.11	1.24 $\pm$ 0.05
	I----p<0.02-----I			
ELASTIC TISSUE *	2.22 $\pm$ 0.07	1.99 $\pm$ 0.07	2.20 $\pm$ 0.16	1.92 $\pm$ 0.08
	I----p<0.02-----I			

===

 (score = *: 1 absent, 2 +, 3 ++, 4 +++)

TABLE 6

Correlation between single histocytologic components of the plaque and diabetes. (Statistically significant values only. Mean $\pm$ SEM).

===

(No.patients)	DIABETES		NON INSULIN-DEPENDENT (38)	INSULIN-DEPENDENT (18)
	ABSENT (119)	PRESENT (56)		
SMOOTH MUSCLE CELLS *	2.24 $\pm$ 0.06	2.23 $\pm$ 0.07	2.32 $\pm$ 0.09	2.06 $\pm$ 0.10
			I----p<0.04---I	
CONNECTIVE *	2.46 $\pm$ 0.08	2.68 $\pm$ 0.10	2.71 $\pm$ 0.14	2.61 $\pm$ 0.14
	I----p<0.05-----I			
THROMBOSIS **	1.29 $\pm$ 0.04	1.11 $\pm$ 0.04	1.05 $\pm$ 0.04	1.22 $\pm$ 0.10
	I---p<0.003----I		I----p<0.03---I	
	I---------p<0.0009----------I			

===

 (score = *: 1 absent, 2 +, 3 ++, 4 +++; **: 1 absent, 2 present)

The plaques of patients with borderline and severe hypertension (Table 5) showed a marked increase in cells due to the statistically significant increase in the number of FC, MC and MGC associated with the statistically significant decrease in the content of elastic fibers (p<0.02). A comparison of patients with borderline and severe hypertension did not show statistically significant differences.

In diabetic patients (Table 6) there was a lesser incidence of thrombosis (p<0.003) and an increase in connective tissue (p<0.05). The comparison between insulin-dependent and non dependent patients showed a greater number of SMC in the plaques of the latter (p<0.04), along with a lesser incidence of thrombosis as compared with insulin--dependent and non diabetic patients.

In hyperlipemic patients (Table 7) there was a statistically significant increase in FC and alcianophilia (p<0.004), as compared with the controls, along with a slight decrease in connective tissue.

In the plaques of smokers (Table 8) MGC and calcifications were significantly decreased (p<0.03 and p<0.04, respectively). No differences were observed between the plaques of moderate and heavy smokers.

TABLE 7

Correlation between single histocytologic components of the plaque and hyperlipemia. (Statistically significant values only. Mean $\pm$ SEM).

| | HYPERLIPEMIA | | |
	ABSENT	MILD	SEVERE
FOAM CELL *	2.48 + 0.16	2.81 + 0.15	2.97 + 0.16
	I------------P<0.01-------------I		
ALCIANOPHILIA *	2.10 + 0.12	2.22 + 0.11	2.54 + 0.11
	I------------P<0.004-----------I		
		I----P<0.02-----I	

(score = *: 1 absent, 2 +, 3 ++, 4 +++)

TABLE 8

Correlation between single histocytologic componnets of the plaque and smoking habit. (Statistically significant values only. Mean $\pm$ SEM).

| | SMOKING HABIT | | MODERATE | HEAVY |
| | ABSENT | PRESENT | SMOKERS | SMOKERS |
(No.patients)	(39)	(115)	(31)	(84)
GIANT CELLS *	1.33 + 0.08	1.15 + 0.03	1.16 + 0.06	1.15 + 0.04
	I----p<0.03----I			
	I----------P<0.05-------------I			
	I-----------------------P<0.0001-------------------I			
CALCIFICATION **	1.82 + 0.06	1.68 + 0.04	1.64 + 0.09	1.70 + 0.04
	I---p<0.04----I			
	I----------P<0.05-------------I			
	I--------------------------P<0.05------------------I			

(score = *: 1 absent, 2 +, 3 ++, 4 +++; **: 1 absent, 2 present)

DISCUSSION

Our study has demonstrated the utility of a semiquantitative approach to human atherosclerotic lesions. Despite the limits intrinsic to light microscopy, the method used has proven to give some insight into the heterogeneous features of the human fibroatheromatous plaque. The correlations obtained strongly suggest that the clustering of various plaque constituents is not a statistically haphazard phenomenon. Moreover, some of the correlation patterns are consistent with the knowledge derived from studies on human and experimental plaques. Some of the pattern observed may reflect the effects of the food fats fed (24,25). The increased cell content of the plaques of hypertensive patients is consistent with the hyperplasia of SMC observed in the tunica media as well as in the vascular intima of different species of hypertensive animals (26,27). We cannot, however, say whether the increased number of MGC and FC we observed arose from SMC or from macrophages.

In conclusion, we have demonstrated a positive correlation between morphological patterns of human atherosclerosis and risk factors. In aging and diabetic patients plaques were rich in fibrous tissue and contained fewer cells (fibrous plaque), in females and in hypertensive patients they were rich in giant and foam cells (granulomatous plaque) and in hyperlipemic patients they showed numerous foam cells and extensive alcianophilia (xanthomatous plaque).

ACKNOWLEDGEMENTS

The authors thank Alfredo Colantoni and Renzo Bernabei for technical assistance. This work was supported by CNR grants (88.00398 and 89.01081).

REFERENCES

1. M.D. Haust, The natural history of human atherosclerotic lesions, in: "Vascular Injury and Atherosclerosis," S.Moore ed., Marcel Dekker, Inc, New York, 1, (1981)
2. L.G. Spagnoli, Storia naturale della placca fibroatheromasica umana (morfologia della progressione e regressione), Giorn Arterioscl 8:117 (1983)
3. R. Ross, The pathogenesis of atherosclerosis. An update, New Engl J Med 314: 488 (1986)
4. T.R. Dawber, The Framingham Study. The epidemiology of atherosclerotic disease, Harvard University Press, Cambridge, London, (1980)
5. H.C. McGill, J.C. Geer, J.P. Strong, in: "Atherosclerosis and Its Origin," M. Sandler, G.H. Bourne, eds, Academic Press, Inc, New York, Ch. 2 (1963)
6. H. Z. Movat, Demonstration of all connective tissue elements in a single sections, Arch Path 60: 289 (1955)

7. L.G. Spagnoli, A. Mauriello, Y. Sambuy, E. Bonanno, A. Orlandi, G. Palmieri, A computerized coding system for processing basic histopathological changes. Application to vascular pathology, Meth Inform Med 25: 139 (1986)

8. T. Tsukada, D. Tippens, D. Gordon, R. Ross, A.M. Gown, HHF35, a muscle-actin-specific monoclonal antibody. I.Immunocytochemical and biochemical characterization, Am J Pathol 126: 51 (1987)

9. A.M. Gown, T. Tsukada, R. Ross, Human atherosclerosis. II. Immunocytochemical analysis of the cellular composition of human atherosclerotic lesions, Am J Pathol 125: 191 (1986)

10. Y. Ishii, T. Tahami, H. Yasa, Six distinct antigen system of human B cells as defined by monoclonal antibodies, in: "Leucocyte typing II.", E.L. Reinherz, B.F. Hayes, L.M. Nadler, I.D. Berstein, eds, Springer Verlag, New York, 109 (1986)

11. J. Bread, E.L. Reinherz, P.C. Kung, G. Goldstein, S.F. Schlossman, A monoclonal antibody reactive with human peripheral blood monocytes, J Immunol 124: 1943 (1980)

12. G.H. Williams, P.I. Jagger, E. Braunwald, Hypertensive vascular disease, in: "Harrison's Principles of Internal Medicine", K.J. Isselbacher, R.D. Adams, E. Braunwald, R.G. Petersdorf, J.D. Wilson, eds., McGraw-Hill Kogakusha, Ltd, Tokyo, Sidney, 1167 (1980)

13. F.J. Rohlf and R.R. Sokal, Statistical Tables (2nd ed.), W.H. Freeman and Co, New York, 101 (1981)

14. J.U. Balis, M.D. Haust, R.H. More, Electron microscopic studies in human atherosclerosis. Cellular elements in aortic fatty streaks. Exp Mol Path 3: 511 (1964)

15. J.C. Geer and M.D. Haust, Smmoth muscle cells in atherosclerosis, in: "Monographs on Atherosclerosis," S. Karger, Basel: 80 (1972)

16. A.M. Imparato, T.S. Riles, F. Gorstein, The carotid bifurcation plaque: pathologic findings associated with cerebral ischemia, Stroke 10: 238 (1979)

17. R.J. Lusby, L.D. Ferrell, W.K. Ehrenfels, R.J. Stoney, E.J. Wylie, Carotid plaque hemorrhage. Its role in production of cerebral ischemia, Arch Surg 117: 1479 (1982)

18. L.G. Spagnoli, A. Mauriello, S. Villaschi, G. Santeusanio, E.Bonanno, G. Palmieri, A morphometric approach to the atherosclerotic plaque (with an assay of clinical correlations), in: "Biology of arterial wall. Interaction in the arterial wall and atherosclerosis," CIC Edizioni Internazionali, Roma, 219 (1988)

19. I. Gore, Ulceration and embolization by atheromate, in: "Evolution of the atherosclerotic plaque," R.J. Jones, ed, The University of Chicago Press, 315 (1963)

20. R.E. Tracy, J.P. Strong, V.T. Toca, C.R. Lopez, Atheronecrosis and its fibroproliferative base and cap in thoracic aorta, Lab Invest 41: 546 (1979)

21. R.G. Gerrity, The role of the monocytes in atherogenesis. II. Migration of foam cells from atherosclerotic lesion, Am J Pathol 103: 191 (1981)

22. G. Majno, I. Joris, T. Zand: Atherosclerosis: new horizons, Hum Pathol 1: 3 (1985)

23. H.C. Stary, Macrophages, macrophages foam cells, and eccentric intimal thickening in the coronary arteries of young children, Atherosclerosis 64: 91 (1987)

24. D Vesselinovitch, R.W. Wissler, T.J. Schaffner, J. Borensztajn. The effects of various diets on atherogenesis in rhesus monkeys. Atherosclerosis 35: 198-207 (1980)

25. R.W. Wissler, D. Vesselinovitch, H.R. Davis, T. Yamada. The composition of the evolving atherosclerotic plaque, in: "Vascular diseases: current research and clinical applications", D. Strandness, P. Didisheim, A. Clowes, J. Watson, eds, Grune and Stratton, Orlando, 241-256 (1987)

26. G.K. Owens, S.M. Schwartz, Alterations in vascular smooth muscle mass in the spontaneously hypertensive rat, Circ Res 51: 280 (1982)

27. A.V. Chobanian, The arterial smooth muscle cell in systemic hypertension, Am J Cardiol 60: 94I (1987)

ULTRASONOGRAPHIC AND HISTOMORPHOMETRIC EVALUATION OF ENDARTERECTOMY
SAMPLES FROM CAROTID LESIONS: NEW PERSPECTIVES IN QUALITATIVE
EVALUATION OF B-MODE ULTRASOUND IMAGES

*P. Tanganelli, G. Bianciardi, M. Salvi, V. Attino,
C. Simões, G. Weber, **U. Senin, A. Susta, D. Tazza,
M. Mercuri, S. Ventura, ***P.G. Cao, L. Moggi

*Ist. Anat. Patol., Ctr. ATS., Univ. Siena, Via delle Scotte 6
**Clin. Med. II, Ger., Ctr. Ecotom. Carotid
***Clin. Chir., U.O.Chir.Vascol., Univ. Perugia, Italy

INTRODUCTION

Since the beginning of the 1980's, various biomedical scientists
have faced the problem of measuring and validating atherosclerotic lesion severity, extent and composition by ultrasound in large and medium
arteries: aortas and carotid arteries were both studied "in vitro" and
"in vivo" by B-mode ultrasonographic devices and histopathology, often
making use of endarteretomy samples from the carotid arteries.

Experimental studies have given significant correlations in detecting the severity of lesions as determined by ultrasonographic images and histology (5-11). Schenk et al. (12) were able to replicate
measures with an error equal to 0.2 mm., and moreover they demonstrated
the technological competence of B-mode imaging in detecting a mean maximum intima media thickness variation of about 0.4 mm.

Few investigators have contributed evaluations of human atherosclerotic lesion composition on living patients, usuing a routine ultrasonographic apparatus (13-16). These studies have supplied and will continue
to supply observations following some basic rules for good data reproducibility: 1) eliminating patients with particular anatomic neck alterations, cases with insufficient scanning, cases in which the anatomic
material for the comparison was fragmented, and finally and perhaps most
importantly, 2) to provide controls in order to obtain constant and equal
calibration of the ultrasonographic apparatus.

Our experience in validation studies of B-mode "in vivo" analysis
with human carotids collected at surgery, (endarterectomy) has been aimed
at determining atherosclerotic lesion severity (quantitative study) and
lesion composition (qualitative study), evaluated by computer-assisted
devices (16).

This kind of approach has required the measurement of the degree

Part of this work was supported by CNR Research Grant 89.02852.04 and
part by NATO Grant 446/86.

of shrinkage that the histopathologic samples presented with respect to the "in vivo" ones, and in reconstructing a bidimensional transversal image from the linear longitudinal ones, obtained by B-mode imaging. New non subjective criteria for peforming qualitative analysis by image processing are also proposed.

MATERIAL AND METHODS

Seventy two carotid endarterectomies including flow divider have been performed on male and female subjects. Each of these patients was preliminarily studied, before surgery, with a B-mode ultrasonographic instrument (Biosound-Biodynamic, Indianapolis, U.S.A.) which generates a broad-pulsed medium frequency ultrasonic band (8 Mhz). For each subject, longitudinal sections (anterior, 0° to the surgical plane; lateral 90°; and posterior-lateral, 150°-170°) as well as transverse sections, exploring the whole length of the vessel (2 cm. from the common carotid below the flow divider to the internal carotid for 1-2 cm above the flow divider), were registered on video-tape (3-4" Video Cassette Recorder). For the validation study, 50 endarterectomy samples were immersion fixed in 10% buffered formalin and decalcified with Ethylene-diammino-tetra-acetic acid (EDTA). The vessels were then divided into 3mm-thick transverse slices, numbered and paraffin embedded. Histological sections were obtained from the slices where maximum luminal stenosis was present. Sections, 5μm thick, were obtained at intervals of 400 μm and stained with hematoxylin-eosin.

1) Morphometrical Measures and Mathematical Models

For shrinkage effect evaluation, 22 vessels, divided in 3 mm-thick slices, were photographed before and after fixation, and the histological samples were drawn at light microscopy by means of a camera lucida.

The transverse length of the vessel lumen and the atherosclerotic lesion areas were corrected for shrinkage that occurs during fixation, calcification and embedding. This was obtained applying correction factors by multiple linear regression in which the independant variables were atheroma and calcium percentages of the lesion.

Measurement of the fresh and fixed samples (on photographs) and histologic transevrse sections (on drawings by camera lucida) were obtained by a computerized device (Videoplan Kontron-Zeiss, FRG). On the fresh and fixed sample photographs, the internal and the external borderlines were measured. On the drawings of the histologic sections, calcium and atheroma percentages of the atherosclerotic lesions, lumen circumference length (LCL) and internal elastic lamina (IEL) were measured. The following mathematical models were used:

$$Z = a + bx + cy$$

(where Z = correction factor of LCL or IEL, x = percentage of calcium, y = percentage of atheroma), setting $Z \geq 1$ (4). The degree of stenosis (%St) was calculated by the following formula:

$$\%St = (1 - \text{lumen area} / \text{area surrounded by IEL}) * 100$$

2) Ultrasonographic Measures and Mathematical Models

a) Quantitative Evaluation. The quantitative study was carried out on ultrasonographic images taken in 2-3 longitudinal planes fitting the transverse lengths of the lumen and of the intima-media interface (IMI), using Newton's method of divided differences. The successive numerical integration produced a transverse bidimensional image in which the degree of ultrasonographic stenosis was calculated by the following formula:

%St = (1 - lumen area / area surrounded by IMI) * 100

b) Qualitative Evaluation. The qualitative study was performed using subjective criteria at first. The major or minor eco-reflection of the observed lesions, classified as either "hard", "soft" or "mixed" by the ultrasonographer, was correlated with the calcium, atheroma an fibrosis percentage contents, which were evaluated at histology.

A second approach was provided by a non-subjective method, using a morphometric parameter evaluated by the grey level distribution of the B-mode ultrasonographic images, registered on videotape, and obtained by a computerized image processing system. (IBAS II Kontron-Zeiss, 256 grey levels).

Nine soft and/or mixed transverse ultrasonographic images, chosen at the maximum stenosis level, were correlated with the corresponding histologic samples, made up of atheroma and calcium (the latter being less than 10%). The grey level distribution, obtained by image processing, was followed by "noise cutting" (2.5% tail cutting at the right and at the left of the distribution curve).

Finally, in order to determine the symmetry of the grey level distrubution curve, the third moment (m3) was calculated according to the following formulas:

$$m3 = 1/N \sum_{i=1}^{n} f_i \left(\mathbf{X_i - \overline{X}} \right)^3$$

$$\text{where } N = \sum_{i=1}^{n} f_i$$

3) Statistical Analysis

The linear regression test (F test) was applied to determine the correlation between histologic and ultrasonographic quantitative measures as well as the correlation between histologic and ultrasonographic non-subjective qualitative measures. The chi-squared test was used to compare histologic and ultrasonographic subjective qualitative measures.

RESULTS

1) Morphometric Study

The vessel shrinkage study has shown that the retraction of the external circumference of the endarterectomy sample (medial layer of the vessel) is greater than the lumen circumference itself (Tab. 1, b & c). Also, in the presence of calcium, the retraction of the lesion area is less.

Table 1.   REGRESSION PLANES TO EVALUATE CORRECTION FACTORS FOR SHRINKAGE IN ENDARTERECTOMY SAMPLES. $z \geq 1$

---

a) INTIMAL THICKENING

Fixing $z = 1.61 + 0.001x - 0.016y$

Embedding $z = 1.1 - 0.01x + 0.002y$

b) EXTERNAL CIRCUMFERENCE

Fixing $z = 1.055 + 0.007x - 0.002y$

Embedding $z = 1.25 - 0.006x + 0.001y$

c) LUMEN CIRCUMFERENCE

Fixing $z = 1.004 + 0.008x - 0.0002y$

Embedding $z = 1.022 + 0.002x + 0.001y$

---

x = % CALCIFICATION   y = % NECROTIC CORE

2) Quantitative and Qualitative Studies

a) Quantitative Analysis. The quantitative study showed significant correlation between ultrasonographic stenosis (bidimensional mathematical reconstruction from the longitudinal sections) and histological stenosis corrected for shrinkage.

$$y = 0.47x + 42.4, \quad n = 50, \quad P < 0.001$$

Ultrasonographic measures differed from the histomorphometric measurement < 10% in 66% of the cases (corresponding to a linear measure < 0.5 mm.), by 20-30% in 6% of the cases. Finally, the average of the ultrasonographic stenosis percentages was overestimated (9%) compared to the histologic one.

b) Qualitative Analysis. The hard, soft and mixed subjective criteria showed correlation with calicum content (P < 0.03), relatively poor correlation with atheroma content (P < 0.06) (Tab. 2) and no correlation with fibrosis.

Table 2. QUALITATIVE SUBJECTIVE ANALYSIS OF ULTRASONOGRAPHIC IMAGES.

CALCIFICATION

ULTRASONIC CRITERIA	No. CASES	No. CASES WITHOUT	No. CASES < 10%	No. CASES > 10%
SOFT	8	6	2	0
MIXED	26	13	13	0
HARD	16	3	8	5

P < 0.03

Note the significant correlation between ultrasonic criteria and calcification % in carotid atherosclerotic lesions.

ATHEROMA

ULTRASONIC CRITERIA	No. CASES	No. CASES < 25%	No. CASES > 25%
SOFT	7	3	4
MIXED	27	20	7
HARD	16	11	5

P < 0.06

Note the relatively poor correlation between ultrasonic criteria and atheroma % in carotid atherosclerotic lesions.

The new particular method used in order to get non-subjective criteria gave rise to significant correlation between the morphometric parameter obtained by image processing (m3) (expressed as the cubic root of m3, linearizing data) and the histologic measurements (fibrosis and atheroma) (P < 0.001). The variation coefficient appeared to be equal to 15% (Fig. 1).

Fibrosis % Vs. morphometric parameter (m3) from ultrasound images

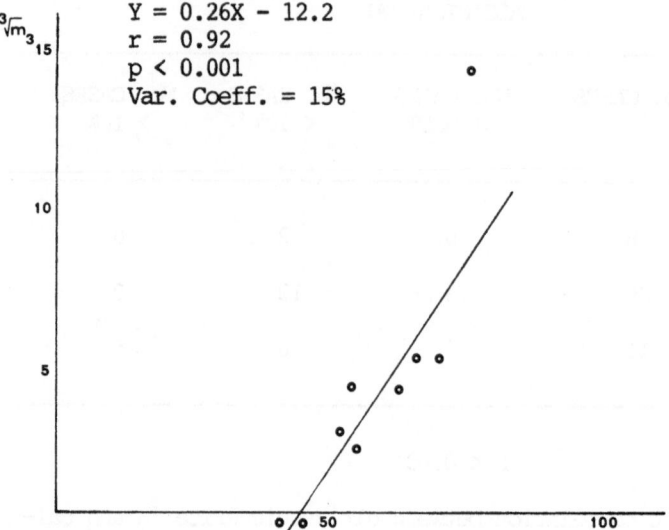

$$Y = 0.26X - 12.2$$
$$r = 0.92$$
$$p < 0.001$$
Var. Coeff. = 15%

Atheroma % Vs. morphometric parameter (m3) from ultrasound images

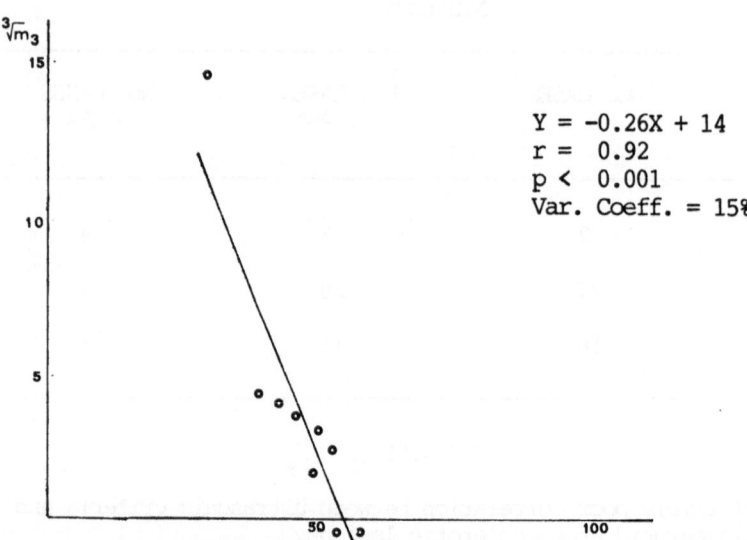

$$Y = -0.26X + 14$$
$$r = 0.92$$
$$p < 0.001$$
Var. Coeff. = 15%

Fig. 1. NON-SUBJECTIVE QUALITATIVE ANALYSIS OF ULTRASONOGRAPHIC IMAGES
BY IMAGE PROCESSING

Significant correlations between the parameter obtained by the grey
level distribution, after image processing, (m3) and histologic data
(fibrosis and atheroma).

DISCUSSION

The use of bidimensional ultrasonography, for detecting and measuring atherosclerotic lesions of selected peripheral vessels, is a valid
method, especially for evaluating lesion severity. Even in this "ex

vivo" study, linear regression and the variation coefficient are similar to those described by others in experimental and human studies (9, 12, 17). The scattering of the values may be caoused by a number of factors: problems in routine ultrasonography for recognizing the intima-media borderline, inaccurate determination of lumen vessel geometry caused by vessel movement and difficulties in determining the same cross section level in ultrasonography and histology (9, 12).

Lesion composition evaluation is of primary importance in following the evolution of arterial lesions in man. The use of subjective parameters assumes a real significance only in determining the presence of calcium in the lesions, while at present it does not permit discrimination of other components including atheroma and fibrosis.

Image processing, used by us for the first time for arterial lesion composition determination, appears to be quite promising in the near future. Other authors presented another interesting approach using the ultrasonic backscatter amplitude analysis (18). The variation coefficient degree (15%) observed in our study, has not yet allowed a more precise lesion composition evaluation. This induces us to consider further advanced results: 1) grabbing images directly from the ultrasonographic probe, 2) using image processing with more than 256 grey levels, 3) exploring arterial lesions not only constituted by atheroma and fibrosis, but also by fat, thrombus and so forth. With these technical improvements, results of this computer-assisted approach are expected to acquire more and more significance.

ACKNOWLEDGEMENTS

We would like to thank Miss Lucy Anna Bonelli for her editing assistance.

REFERENCES

1. A.J. Camerota, J.J. Cranely and S.E. Cook, Real time B-mode carotid imaging imaging in diagnosis of cerebrovascular disease, Surgery. 89: 718-729 (1981).
2. M.G. Bond, J.F. Gardin, S.K. Wilmoth, J.K. Sawyer and R.W. Barnes, Noninvasive, high resolution, B-mode ultrasound imaging of arteries, in: "Atherosclerosis Reviews" Vol. 12, R.J. Hegyeli, ed., Raven, New York, (1984).
3. A. Poli, E. Tremoli, A. Colombo, M. Sirtori, P. Pignoli and R. Paoletti, Ultrasonographic measurement of the common carotid artery wall thickness in hypercholesterolemic patients, Atherosclerosis. 70: 253-268 (1988).
4. P.Tanganelli, G. Bianciardi, L. Centi, M.Salvi, G. Weber, A. Susta, G. Ciuffetti, M.Mercuri, L. Parnetti, U. Senin, A. Tazza and L. Moggi, B-mode imaging and histomorphometric evaluation of carotid atherosclerosis, Angiology. in press (1990).
5. M.G. Bond, J.K. Sawyer, B.C. Bullock, R.W. Barnes and M.R. Ball, Animal studies of atherosclerosis progession and regression, in "Clinical Diagnosis of Atherosclerosis", M.G. Bond eds. Springer-Verlag, New York, pp. 435-449, (1983).
6. M.G. Bond, R.W. Barnes, J.K. Sawyer, M. Ball and W.A. Riley, Preliminary data on validation noninvasive techniques for arterial imaging, in "Atherosclerosis Reviews", Vol. 10, R.J. Hegyeli, ed., Raven Press, New York, pp. 175-179 (1983).

7. A.J. Camerota, Correlation of B-mode ultrasound of the carotid artery with arteriography and pathology, in: "Clinical Diagnosis of Atherosclerosis" M.G. Bond, eds., Springer-Verlag, New York, pp. 351-367, (1983).

8. M.G. Bond, W.A. Riley, R.W. Barnes, J.M. Kaduck and M.R. Ball, Validation studies of a noninvasive real time B-scan imaging system, in: "Noninvasive Techniques for Assessment of Atherosclerosis in Peripheral, Carotid and Coronary Arteries", T.F. Budinge, eds., Raven Press, New York, pp. 197-203, (1982).

9. P. Pignoli, E. Tremoli, A. Poli, O. Oreste and R; Paoletti, Intimal plus medial thickness of arterial wall: a direct measurement with ultrasound imaging, Circulation. 74: 1399-1406 (1986).

10. J.L. Dutreix, O. Genre, C. Moneger du Sorbier, P. Arbeille, F. Lapierre, A.C. Benhamou, A. Autret and L. Pourcelot, Correlations ultrasoniques, arteriographiques et anatomopathologiques dans 59 cas d'atherosclerose carotidienne, Rev. Neurol. 141: 128-136 (1985).

11. H.P. Chin, P. Carry, G. Lo, S. Nessim and D.H. Blanckenhorn, Autopsy calibration of carotid artery B-mode ultrasound imaging: effects of pressure on residual lumen sides, J. Lab. Clin. Med. 105: 120-123 (1984).

12. E.A. Schenk, M.G. Bond, T.H. Aretz, J.N. Angelo, H.Y. Choi, T. Rynalski, N.F. Gustafson, A.S. Berson, J.J. Ricotta, M.W. Goodson, F.A. Bryan, B.B. Goldberg, J.F. Tool and D.H. O'Leary, Multicenter validation study of real time ultrasonography, arteriography and pathology: pathologic evaluation and carotid endarterectomy specimens, Stroke. 19: 289-296 (1988).

13. A.C. Benhamou, J.L. Dutreix, O. Genre, P. Arbeil, C. Marchal, L. Pourcelot, F. Lapierre and C. Dusorbier, Validaiton des donnes quantitatives et qualitatives de l'echotomographie carotidienne (en temps real) par confrontation avec celles l'examen doppler standard, de l'arteriographie et de l'anatomopathologie, J. des Mal. Vasc. 9: 185-194 (1984).

14. L.G. Spagnoli, E. Zanette, V. Faraglia, A. Mauriello and C. Butinelli, Validazione istopatologica dei reperti ecotomografici di placche carotidee, Gior. Arterioscl. 2: 95-108 (1985).

15. G. Bianciardi, P.G. Cao, L. Centi, E. Mannarino, L. Moggi, M.T. Novelli, U. Senin, A. Susta, P. Toti, P. Tanganelli, D. Tazza, and G. Weber, Quantitative and qualitative evaluation of histomorphometric and ecographic data on endarterectomy samples, Paper presented at the International Congress of Angiology, Athens, June 1985.

16. G. Weber, G. Bianciardi, L. Centi, M.T. Novelli, L. Resi, M. Salvi, P. Toti and P. Tanganelli, Comparative studies of cerebral atherosclerosis: observations on endarterectomy in men, in: "Atherosclerosis VII", N.H. Fiedege, eds., Elsevier, Amsterdam, pp. 593-596 (1986).

17. M.G. Bond and D. Morley, New perspectives for the clinical evaluation of atherosclerosis, Drug Dev. Res. 6: 127-134 (1985).

18. P. Piano, L. Landini, F. Lattanzio, A. Mazzarisi, R. Sernelli, A. Distante, A. Benassi and A. L'Abbate, The use of frequency histograms of ultrasonic backscatter amplitudes for detection of atherosclerosis in vitro, Circulation, 74: 1093- 1098 (1986).

HOW DOES THE CLINICIAN EVALUATE THE ATHEROSCLEROTIC PLAQUE QUANTITATIVELY?

J. Bonnet, D. Benchimol

Department of Cardiology
University of Bordeaux
Bordeaux, France

The human atherosclerotic plaque, unlike some of the experimental models, can be associated with complications such as thrombotic or embolic processes, fissuration, intraplaque haemorrhage, and spasm. The evolution, risk factors, and complication rates vary depending on the arterial segment and affected organs. The problem of detection and quantification of the atherosclerotic disease is in fact linked to the specific atherosclerotic target. The problem for peripheral arteries is different from that for coronary arteries. Therefore the quantitative approaches, as well as the social and medical care implications of studies of the severity of atherosclerosis are different. The high prevalance of ischemic heart disease led us to study problems associated with the detection of the severity of the atherosclerotic process in coronary arteries.

The first aim was to differentiate the atherosclerotic process from its complications, thereby allowing us to study atherosclerotic stenosis and its progression. In living man coronary atherosclerosis is usually quantitated by coronary angiography and this will probably continue in many centers until new approaches can be validated in clinical practice.

Coronary angiograms constitute only an indirect assessment of lesions. However, even if it is difficult to distinguish the true atherosclerotic process from its complications, the best approach to minimize such limits is patient selection for such a study.

The first aim is to define exclusion criteria to eliminate the problem of thrombotic events associated with the atherosclerotic process. Two main clinical events are associated with a high frequency of thrombotic occlusion, acute myocardial infarction (1) and unstable angina (2, 3). Such patients are often excluded from angiographic studies which are designed to measure progression or regression of coronary atherosclerosis.

In studies of the progression or regression of coronary stenosis due to atherosclerosis it is, in our experience, wise to exclude patients who are recognized as having a high risk of life threatening cardiovascular events during the period when patient recruitment is taking place.

Lesions with lumen stenosis of 75% or greater are often excluded because the future natural history of these plaques may not reflect the primary atherosclerotic processes. Such stenoses have a reasonably high

Atherosclerotic Plaques, Edited by R.W. Wissler *et al.*
Plenum Press, New York, 1991

probability of becoming subject to interventional procedures such as bypass surgery or angioplasty or to thrombus formation thus modifying their natural history (4). Furthermore, patients whose cardiac function includes low ejection fraction or disorders limiting life expectancy or contraindications for repeated coronary angiograms must be excluded from such studies.

Another major problem is the exclusion of a spastic component of coronary stenosis. Coronary spasm can be partially excluded by using calcium antagonists before catheterization and nitrate derivatives intravenously or sublingually and even intracoronary medication during angiographic procedures. (5, 6).

Another consideration in patient selection is to define other important criteria which are associated with atherosclerosis progression. These factors must be clearly analyzed to avoid an irregular distribution, like hypercholesterolemia, diabetes, age, smoking habits, hypertension, severity of coronary atherosclerosis, localisation of coronary artery stenosis, in different comparable groups participating in a clinical trial. Moreover, atherosclerotic progression associated with aorto-coronary bypass surgery or restenosis after angioplasty have led some investigators to exclude patients who have had such treatments.

How may the atherosclerotic plaques on angiographic models be quantified? Shortcomings of visually assessed changes in the percent reduction of coronary lumen diameter are well recognized, and interobserver variablity for each determination of percent stenosis ranges from 5% to 18% (7, 8). These shortcomings have been partially overcome with quantitative assessment using a computer-assisted system. The main problem is to obtain at different times, two angiograms under comparable condition, i.e., relative to angiographic technique or radiographic imaging variables including film speed, electrocardiographic marking of cineframes, kilovolts, milliamps, contrast product volume, and beam incidence. The quantitative assessment of each angiogram involves solving the problem of computerized edge detection and making the choice between geometric diameter analysis or photodensitometric diameter analysis.

The morphology of stenosis appears, in the majority of cases, to be regular, with circular, elliptical, or D-shaped lumens. Irregular stenoses are observed in unstable clinical situations associated with unstable angina or myocardial infarction.

As a result of x-ray beam angle, elliptical or D-shaped forms of lumen may induce great variability in geometric diameter analyses. A photodensitometric, monoplanar approach to diameter analysis partially solves this problem as does the use of a biplanar visualization with a three-dimensional reconstruction analysis. On the other hand, irregular stenoses cannot be reproducibly quantified by photodensitometric monoplanar analysis, and must be evaluated using either biplanar geometric or densitometric analysis.

The computer-assisted method developed in our hospital by Nichols et al. (10) allows such quantification of atherosclerosis. An optical system using a Tagarno 33XR projector, focuses and magnifies (x2) a selected part of the frame containing the stenosis. This part of the frame is projected onto a CCD-charge couple device using a video camera which, along with a Matrox image processor (512x512 pixels, 256 grey levels), converts the analog signal to digital form. Hard copies are printed on a video printer from a control video monitor to ensure that the same segments are analyzed on consecutive angiograms. The digital images are stored and processed using an IBM PC AT computer. The operator selects points within the coronary segment containing the stenosis and the general axis and the direction of the vessel. Lumen edges are then automatically detected along the defined segment, perpendicular to its axis, the monoplanar videodensitometric profile using a first derivative algorithm.

Among the various calculated lumen parameters, minimal diameter, minimal area, length of stenosis, percentage stenosis (area), and densitometric percentage stenosis (diameter), only the last photodensitometric percentage stenosis diameter was usually used in lesion assessment. We tested the accuracy of the method in plexiglass phantom models filled with contrast medium (12 holes made in a block of plexiglass with a diameter ranging from 3.5 mm to 0.5 mm). In diameter, the accuracy was 0.08 ± 0.12 mm and in area 0.30 ± 0.49 mm^2. To evaluate percent diameter stenosis, the intra- and interobserver variability in the analysis of angiograms, respectively 80 and 72% stenoses, were assessed at random a second time, 3 months later. The linear correlations were respectively r=0.97, standard error of the estimate 4.7% and r=0.97, standard error of the estiate 5.4% (Figure 1).

The determination of severity of stenosis referenced to an adjacent normal artery may be inherently unreliable because of the diffuse nature of coronary artery disease. Absolute luminal diameter may be a better measure of stenosis using the catheter tip as reference.

With the controlled criteria of patient selection considered earlier in this paper, standardized coronary angiographic procedures, using computer-assisted methods, is a reliable indirect assessment of the coronary atherosclerotic stensosis. This approach has several potential advantages over trials using mortality as an endpoint. However, the method has limits, the main one being the fact that this approach is an indirect one. (11)

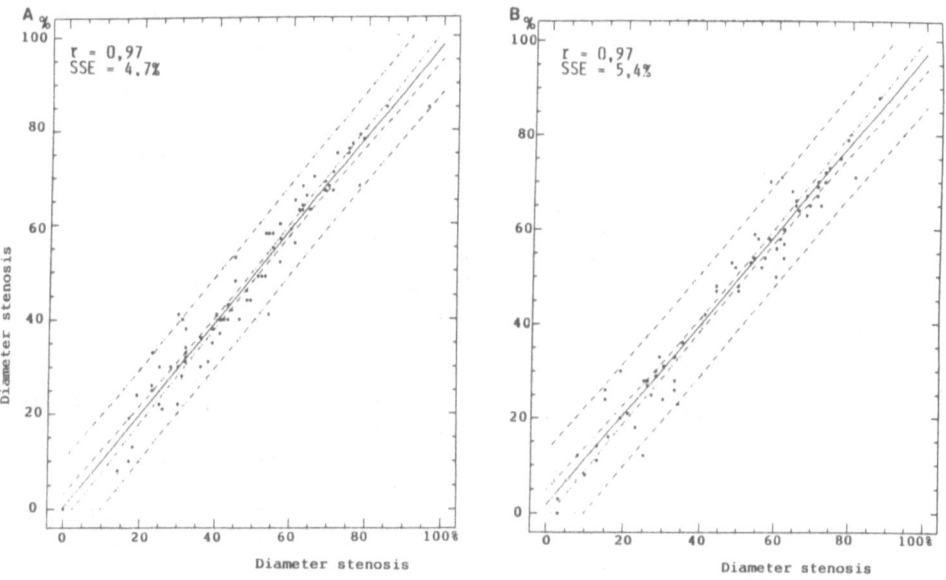

Figure 1.   Intraobserver variablity (A) and interobserver variability (B) in the analysis of angiograms determined respectively in 80 and 72 stenoses, assessed at random a second time, 3 months later. The analyses were performed in % of diamter stenosis.

Technical developments such as vascular echocardiography, endovascular echocardiography, nuclear magnetic resonance imaging, computer axial tomography, and immunoscintography, might allow a different approach to evaluating the atherosclerotic process. These approaches provide new possibilities in the atherosclerosis assessment and must be validated more completely in order to define their place in the clinic. Nonetheless, they are still indirect approaches to the quantification of the atherosclerotic process. Moreover, the coronary artery disease which is responsible for the majority of cardiovascular deaths will continue to present a difficult problem since it involves the visualization of relatively small and inaccessible arteries which are attached to a highly mobile heart.

Detection and measurement of coronary artery progression is and will continue to be one of the main challenges for the cardiologist.

REFERENCES

1. M. A. De Wood, J. Spores, R. Notske, L. T. Mouser, R. Burroughs, M. S. Golden, and H. T. Lang, Prevalence of total coronary occulusion during the early hours of transmuralmyocardial infarction, N. Engl. J. Med. 303:897 (1980).

2. K. Gotok, T. Minamion, O. Katoh, Y. Hamano, S. Fuki. The role of intracoronary thrombus in unstable angina: angiographic assessment and thrombolytic therapy during ongoing anginal attack, Circulation 77:526 (1988).

3. V. Furster, R. L. Frye, D. C. Connolly, M. A. Danielson, L. R. Elveback, and L. T. Kurland, Arteriographic patterns early in the onset of the coronary syndromes, Brit. Heart J. 37:1250 (1975).

4. A. Moise, J. Lesperance, P. Théroux, Y. Taeymans, C. Goubet, and M. Bourassa, Clinical and angiographic predictors of new total coronary occlusion in coronary artery disease: analyses of 313 nonoperated patients, Am. J. Cardiol. 54:1176 (1984).

5. V. Forstermann, A. Mugge, V. Alheid, A. Haverich, and J. C. Frolich, Selective attenuation of endothelium-mediated vasodilation in atherosclerotic human coronary arteries, Circ. Res. 62:185 (1988).

6. K. F. Hossack, B. G. Brown, D. K. Stewart, and H. T. Dodge. Diltiazem-induced blockade of sympathetically mediated constriction of normal and diseased coronary arteries: lack of epicardial coronary dilatory effect in humans, Circulation 70:465 (1984).

7. M. E. Sanmarco, S. H. Brooks, and D. H. Blankenhorn, Reproducibility of a consensus panel in the interpretation of coronary angiograms, Am. Heart J. 96:430 (1978).

8. T. A. De Rouen, J. A. Murray, and W. Owen. Variability in the analysis of coronary angiograms, Circulation 55:324 (1977).

9. A. C. Thomas, M. J. Davies, S. Dilly, N. Dilly, and F. Franc, Potential errors in the estimation of coronary arterial stenosis from clinical arteriography with reference to the shape of the coronary arterial lumen, Brit. Heart J. 55:129 (1986).

10. A. B. Nichols, C. F. O. Babrieli, J. J. Fenoglio Jr., and P. D. Esser, Quantification of relative coronary arterial stenosis by cinevideodensitometric analysis of coronary arteriograms, Circulation 69:512 (1984).

11. S. Ellis, W. Sanders, C. Goubet, R. Miller, K. Cain, J. Lesperance, M. Bourassa, and E. Alderman. Optimal detection of the progression of coronary artery disease: comparison of methods suitable for risk factors intervention trials, Circulation 74:1235 (1986).

Summary of Discussion following Session 2

Cornhill asked Bond about the percent of variance with which he felt comfortable in measuring artery wall thickness. Bond responded that in the case of animal models there was very little spread of data and that a plaque 0.4 mm thick in a monkey constituted a large lesion. Under these circumstances correlation coefficients are not very reliable. Burnstock was impressed with the data presented by Bond demonstrating the rather severe vasodilatation occurring as the cynomolgus monkey lesions develop, in view of the evidence to be presented later that T-compensatory vasodilatation takes place in early atherosclerosis. Bond indicated that some of these effects might be due to the vasa vasorum which penetrates into the underlying base of the plaque and which could release vasodilatory substances. Finally, Kramsch reported that some of the measurements made by Selzer at the University of Southern California Atherosclerosis Research Institute indicated that for certain types of arteries ultrasound is a much more quantitative method but for coronary arteries only an angiographic record appears to yield the quantitative results that are needed.

Following Berglund's presentation, Wissler asked for the names of the investigators, namely Inger Wendelhag and Jerker Persson, whose work Berglund had summarized but which, at the moment, could not be included in the printed volume.

Following Spagnoli's presentation, Wissler asked two brief questions. He inquired about the cutoff point which Spagnoli used to delineate hyperlipidemia, and how he classified individuals who had no risk factors. Spagnoli indicated that they had used 300 mg% of cholesterol as the point above which they defined hyperlipidemia. He indicated that they had not yet been able to define the individuals with advanced lesions but no classical risk factors. Kramsch also asked a number of questions about the components of the plaques which Spagnoli had studied with particular reference to diabetes and hypertension. He was impressed with the increased amounts of connective tissue in the diabetic lesions and with the finding that collagen in diabetes is often glycated and that the proteoglycans which are increasingly deposited in diabetes also trap LDL avidly. Kramsch indicated that the lesions in patients with hypertension might have had more foam cells because these individuals tended to develop prominent fibromuscular thickenings before they develop the lipid laden plaques. His studies in rabbits indicate that macrophage invasion in arterial lesions developing in hypertensive patients is a major precursor for the full development of atherosclerotic lesions. Heistad voiced his hope that imaging might aid in the prediction of thrombosis based on the thickness of the fibrous plaque. Spagnoli indicated that B mode imaging accompanied by densitometry might, in the future, aid in analyzing the morphologic material in such a way as to help define those lesions which were likely to lead to thrombosis.

Tanganelli's presentation was followed by comments indicating that the types of lesions which might be most dangerous were not necessarily the big ones. Wissler pointed out that in many instances the relatively small plaques with thin fibrous caps and large, soft, cholesterol rich centers constitute some of the most threatening plaques because their surfaces are likely to ulcerate and lead to thrombosis. Therefore, any methodology which makes it possible to learn more about the lesion components from imaging approaches might be of great value in recognizing in the artery wall those situations which are most likely to lead to clinical effects. Cornhill also indicated that automated edge detection and histograms of the different intensities of grey might help in the classification of fibrous tissues. Tanganelli responded that they were moving in the direction of being able to automate the analysis of the intensity of greyness and to make a more accurate determination of the interface between blood and plaque.

Following Bonnet's presentation, Wissler expressed surprise that the diagram of the right coronary artery which Bonnet had presented showed more severe disease distally rather than proximally. He was also surprised that Bonnet had eliminated from his studies the patients with more than 90% of their arterial lumen narrowed, based on angiography. Bonnet responded that in his experience the right coronary progression often appears to be more severe in the second segment than it is in the proximal part of the artery. He attributes this to the relatively low pressure in the underlying right ventricle. He went on to indicate that they eliminated the very severe complicated lesions from their study because these advanced plaques are not the ones which they attempt to influence with intervention by means of anticoagulant or antiplatelet drugs. Wissler pointed out that the difference in localization of plaques as compared to the right coronary arteries which Cornhill is studying in PDAY may be mainly a function of the age of the individuals, and may indeed indicate that, as the disease progresses in the right main coronary artery, there is a tendency for the lesions to progress distally.

Bini asked about the immunofluorescent studies which Bonnet presented and asked what the antibodies were directed towards and what type of rabbit model Bonnet had studied. He indicated that these were pictures which had been taken using antibodies to the smooth muscle cells of the rabbit artery wall and that the lesions were ones developing in a cholesterol-fed rabbit with no genetic abnormalities. Kramsch indicated his agreement that one can see differences between what appear to be recent plaques and old established ones in the angiograms and that one can often influence the formation of new lesions if one uses drugs that interfere with calcium metabolism. Bonnet agreed that it is very important to be able to differentiate between a chronic lesion and a recently developed plaque. Heistad asked how often Bonnet had observed catheter-induced spasm in individuals treated with nitroglycerin as compared to the currents of spontaneous spasm and how to detect differing degrees of increased tone which would affect an estimate of stenosis. Bonnet agreed that that is a big problem; every effort is made with calcium antagonists and the use of nitrates intravenously to attempt to rule out the fluctuations of vascular tone.

Liu then entered this part of the discussion by indicating how important it is to have a normal segment as a reference standard in determining stenosis and that serial progression is perhaps a more important variable to measure in these kinds of studies. He suggested that if one uses agents to test for endothelial function at the time of coronary angiography, it may bring out some of the physiological abnormalities of early atherosclerosis and that it might be advantageous to combine these studies with quantitative angiography. Bonnet replied that this is a very important problem and that measurements of the catheter within the vessel might frequently be of value as a reference to help avoid some of the fluctuations due to arterial tone. Bond noted that some of the phenomena being observed in the angiographic study of coronary atherosclerosis might be explained on the basis of the low shear rates which are observed just distal to a plaque. Barbieri indicated his interest in the stenoses which occur after balloon dilatation coronary angioplasty. He wondered whether these patients should be treated surgically or medically and whether the coronary angioplasty patients should be treated with beta blocking drugs. He further noted that in his experience perfusion with calcium channel blockers such as Verapamil was more likely to be helpful than beta blocking agents if one wants to protect the patient from a change in vessel motility, especially after dilatation. Bonnet said that he agreed with that statement and that he generally accepted that it was difficult to predict the patients who were going to develop a very rapid stenosis after angioplasty. Apparently the relation between progression of atherosclerosis and restenosis after angioplasty appears only during a relatively short period of time and disappears after the restenosis process is complete.

During the general discussion period, McGill asked whether the high resolution results with increased information about what is going on in the carotid artery wall, which had been presented by Bond and several of the other ultrasonographers, could soon be applied to the abdominal aorta. Bond indicated that there are some technical difficulties in getting good scans of the abdominal aorta and that in most individuals one has to use a lower frequency transducer. As a result one will not be able to make measurements of differences less than 0.8 or perhaps 0.7 mm. In thinner people it is possible to see the aorta clearly, particularly its near wall, because it is close to the skin surface. If one avoids flatulence and has an ideal instrument it is possible to make valid measurements of intimal medial thickness using longitudinal scans. Furthermore Bond indicated that there are ongoing studies which indicate that it is possible to visualize the superficial femoral, the profunda, and the popliteal. Volpe asked Bond about the use of angiography for regression studies following cholesterol lowering regimens. Bond said that radio-opaque arteriography is excellent for detecting the presence of a plaque when there is a relatively large lesion but that many of the smaller lesions really do not bulge into the arterial lumen. He pleaded for methodologies that will yield more information in quantitative terms about the lesion components in the arterial wall; one must always keep in mind that one of the main characteristics of the progressive atherosclerotic plaque is the dilatation of the artery as the disease progresses.

Paulin noted that intravascular ultrasonography might soon be applicable to the aorta and, although invasive, it can probably be done rather safely. The magnitude of atherosclerotic lesions is likely not only to be detectable but should be measurable, including precise measurements of intimal thickening. He referred to a presentation by a research group from San Diego, California, at the last annual meeting of the North American Society for Cardiac Radiology in Washington, DC, on clinical coronary atherosclerosis measured by means of intravascular ultrasonography . Both Bond and Hay indicated that it would be useful to extend the discussion to both intravascular and transesophageal echocardiography and possibly to a pseudoinvasive procedure such as mediastinoscopy. Bond emphasized that at the present time about 10-15% of the cases can be accurately imaged in some of the better laboratories around the world and that usable coronary angiography images can be obtained in these laboratories by means of transesophageal ultrasound examination. He also pointed out that although imaging can be done in these laboratories, no real quantitative data have been obtained thus far and the methods involving gating the pulse and the respiratory rhythms are still being perfected. The discussion also emphasized the major problem of examining the arteries with the transducer in the same position when one is conducting sequential studies via the transesophageal route with several months or years between the examinations.

Soma then entered the discussion to enumerate the problems encountered in judging the morphological components of the lesions using ultrasound. Several of the participants, including Spagnoli and Berglund, indicated that progress is being made in overcoming these problems but that so far the results are not very definitive, so that the variations between consecutive examinations were relatively high. Kramsch returned to the subject of imaging the abdominal aorta and pointed out that recent reports from Japan have indicated that using 3.5 megahertz transducers, one could find a difference in compliance which appeared to correlate rather well with coronary artery disease in the same individual. He went on to indicate that some of the statements about calcium channel blockers made by <u>Bond</u> might not reflect some of the more recent results. He stated that there is a need for a systematic ultrasound study which will establish both in animal models and in human subjects what actually happens in terms of suppression of atherogenesis by treatment with calcium antagonists. <u>Bond</u> also indicated that some of the studies performed on the young people in Bogalusa had associated decreases in compliance with changes in traditional risk factors. He indicated that the B-mode ultrasound image probably needs to be exploited more thoroughly to increase our understanding of what changes in compliance indicate.

<u>Bonnet</u> asked whether the ultrasound technique yields results which are really quantitative enough to be used to help with clinical decisions and <u>Bond</u> replied that, in his opinion, the technology is already available for the carotid artery and that endovascular ultrasound should soon be able to provide equally quantitative data for the coronary arteries. He added that mineralization constitutes no problem and that the results thus far indicate that ultrasound can detect the presence of mineral with very high reproducibility and validity. Both he and <u>Wissler</u> called for more attention to the two major components of the advanced lesions, namely the size of the necrotic center and the thickness of the fibrous cap. The early observations indicate that the ratio between the thickness of the plaque and the fibromuscular cap may be of great value. The general discussion terminated with the observation by <u>Bond</u> that the dilatation of the arteries which occurs with progressive disease is not mainly an age-related phenomenon, but that it is primarily related to medial weakening due to progressive atherosclerosis.

QUANTITATIVE MEASUREMENT OF ATHEROSCLEROSIS BY ANGIOGRAPHY: IMPLICATIONS

FOR PRIMARY PREVENTION

Dieter M. Kramsch*, Robert H. Selzer**, and David H. Blankenhorn*

*University of Southern California School of Medicine, Los Angeles, CA; **Jet Propulsion Laboratory, Pasadena, CA

There are two ways to test therapy for atherosclerosis in man: trials which measure cardiovascular death rates and trials that measure the rate of change in atherosclerotic lesions. Mortality-based trials require large study groups and relatively long periods of observation. Lesion tracking trials require fewer study subjects and shorter periods of observation, but are dependent on valid reliable assessment of lesion changes. To date, coronary angiography has been the major endpoint measure used in lesion trials. This review covers factors which influence the performance of angiography.

Inherent limitations to x-ray imaging include image mottling caused by a combination of x-ray noise and non-uniform blood contrast mixing, which is a major problem when only single frames of cine angiograms are measured,[1,2] as is the case in most trials to date. Efforts to reduce the effect of image mottling have included spatial filtering,[1] averaging of densitometric profiles from adjacent scanlines along a segment, or averaging of diameter profiles from sequential cine frames.[2-4] Measurement of multiple frames during the cardiac cycle has been proposed by Spears[2] and Selzer.[3] Figure 1 shows a plot of diameter and stenosis measurements over two cardiac cycles for a segment of an unbypassed circumflex artery and illustrates the effect of frame averaging on four computer derived measures {D(90), D(3), DAVG, and % Diameter Stenosis} in 100 sequential frames of a left circumflex coronary artery. The darker lines show diameters after 5 point averaging filter. In theory, measurement error due to random effects, such as quantum mottle and contrast mixing, should be reduced in proportion to the number of averaged frames. In practice, three sequential frames appears to be the best number to average because of vessel motion during the cardiac cycle.[5]

Other limitations to angiography are of biological origin, such as differences in vasomotor tone and vessel motion and non-uniformity of blood contrast mixing. The latter has been shown to strongly affect both visual and automatic edge tracking.[6-10] Changes in size of the vessel image during the cardiac cycle have been attributed to differential magnification from vessel translation or rotation, pressure increase due to the injection itself, and arterial pressure pulsation. Periodic variations in vessel diameter have been shown in both animals and man[6,11-13] which are of the same order of magnitude as annual progression/regression rates of atherosclerosis.[14,15] In addition, from the work of Glagov et al.[16] it is known that because of compensatory vessel wall dilatation coronary artery stenosis

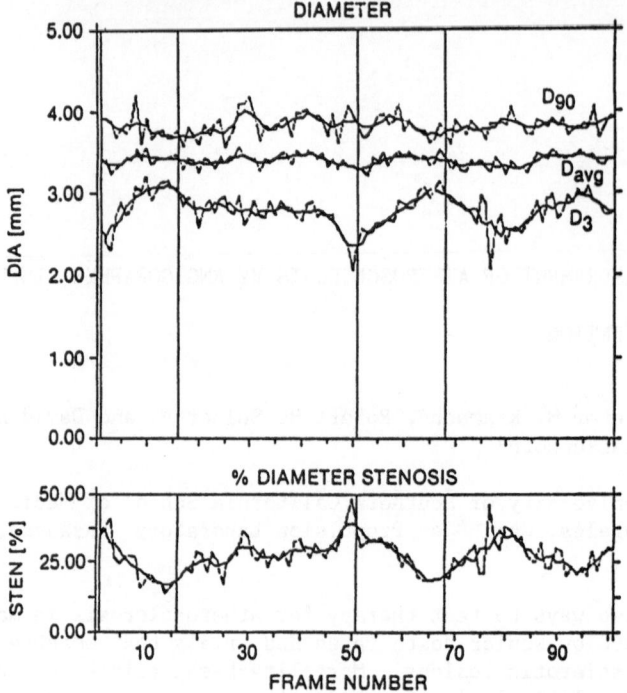

Fig. 1. Plot of diameter and stenosis measurements
over two cardiac cycles for a segment of
an unbypassed circumflex artery. From
top to bottom, plots show D(90), DAVG, D(3),
and STEN. Darker lines show diameters
after five-point averaging filter.

by plaques may be delayed until the lesion occupies 40% of the internal
elastic lamina area. Percent stenosis measured by angiography, therefore,
not necessarily reflects the actual size of the atherosclerotic lesion.

Quantitation of atherosclerosis has been by panels of human readers and
computer-assisted quantitation or computerized image processing. For
computer-assisted quantitation, coronary angiograms are projected and vessel
outlines are hand traced with a digitizing stylus after which lesion severity
is calculated by computer.[17] Manual edge tracking is subject to
inter-observer and intra-observer variability due to the subjective process
of locating the vessel edge within the penumbra appearing on the film.[2] For
computerized image processing, selected frames from the cinefilm are
digitized with a video camera and computer programs are used to locate the
vessel edges and estimate the extent of lesions.[1,6,18-22] Published estimates indicate that the precision of the automatic edge tracking method is
about twice that of manual tracing.[6,7,21,23] However, human performance
factors influence results from the most advanced automated edge tracking
procedures in current use because humans must select lesions or vessel
segments for processing.

When film reading conditions are optimized, two member panels of human
readers are quite adequate in obtaining comprehensive lesion counts which are
important in studies of new lesion formation but difficult to obtain by
computer because current programs do not track vessels well at branch
junctions. Humans also outperform computers for integration of change in

several parts of the coronary circulation into single grade for the patient.

Clinical trials which test atherosclerosis therapy typically take 3-7 years to complete and so deterioration of the x-ray source with continued use, as well as change in the control of film development, are factors of importance. A study evaluating both long- and short-term factors influencing angiographic performance was conducted by Selzer and co-workers.[5] Twenty coronary angiograms were drawn at random from the Cholesterol Lowering Atherosclerosis Study (CLAS),[24] a trial which took over six years to complete, and three vessel edge measures D(3), D(90), and DAVG were computed for each frame in two complete cardiac cycles. D(3), the 3rd percentile diameter (97% of diameters in the profile are larger), was used as an estimate of the narrowest point in the segment. D(90), the 90th percentile diameter (only 10% of the diameters in the segment are larger), was used as an estimate of the normal appearing reference diameter of the segment. The average diameter, DAVG, was defined as the sum of all diameters divided by the total number of scanlines per segment. Percent stenosis was defined as: STEN = 100{1 - D(3)/D(90)}.

It was found that sampling DAVG in 3 sequential frames in end diastole produced the most precise measurements within a single cardiac cycle and reproducibility of DAVG was better than for D(3), D(90), or % STEN. DAVG provides an integrated measure of arterial dimensions within a vessel segment, while D(3) and D(90) are determined by a small subset of these diameters.

Frame averaging was recommended as a means to reduce the number of subjects required for angiographic trials planned to test a predetermined therapy effect. For example, Selzer[5] estimated that with angiograms spaced at intervals typical of current trials, a differential treatment effect of 2% in DAVG could be detected with 114 patients per study group when measurements were made on one frame. This number was reduced to 39 patients per study group if three sequential frames were averaged. Similar trials including 39 subjects per study group could detect differential effects of 7% and 12% respectively for D(3) and % STEN. In angiographic trials where the number of subjects is set by other considerations, frame averaging can allow smaller therapy effects to be detected.

Three angiographic trials have shown that atherosclerosis can be stabilized,[14,25,26] three that atherosclerosis is reversible,[24,27,28] and three that new lesion formation can be reduced.[24,29,30] The majority have tested blood lipid lowering therapy. In CLAS,[2] 16.2% of Colestipol/niacin treated subjects vs 3.6% of control (p <0.007) showed perceptible evidence of regression. In the Familial Atherosclerosis Treatment Study (FATS),[27] 15 among 32 Colestipol/niacin treated and 13 among 34 Colestipol/Lovastatin treated subjects showed regression as compared to 4 among 37 control subjects. Reduced formation of new lesions has been reported with lipid lowering,[24] aspirin/Dipyridamole therapy,[29] and Nifedipine.[30]

A concept useful in pooling results from different angiographic studies is based on findings from atherosclerosis studied at autopsy. Arterial lesions detected by angiography are those which intrude on the vessel lumen; they are equivalent to raised lesions recorded in population-wide autopsy surveys such as the International Atherosclerosis Project (IAP)[31] and the World Health Organization (WHO) studies.[32]. The extent of coronary luminal surface covered by visibly raised lesions is a major determinant of risk of death from myocardial infarction.[31]. In 1969, Gofman noticed that in data from the IAP there were vast differences in the prevalence of atherosclerosis and myocardial infarction in the disparate populations studied, but subjects who died of myocardial infarction had virtually the same degree of severity of coronary atherosclerosis. He analyzed risk for myocardial infarction as a function of severity of coronary atherosclerosis by comparing risk relationships in IAP populations with very little atherosclerosis and those in which atherosclerosis was quite common.[33] Gofman found that the best explanation of IAP data came from a sigmoid relationship between degree of coronary atherosclerosis and risk of myocardial infarction where the risk of myocardial infarction varies according to the degree of disease present as new lesions are added - Figure 2.

Early in the disease - at the bottom of the curve - when accumulation of more atherosclerosis brings about small increases in risk (which is low), the degree of regression seen in angiographic trials may not have measurable effects on risk of myocardial infarction. After lesions are far advanced the second inflection in a sigmoid curve has been reached and myocardial infarction risk is high. Regression at this stage also may not reduce risk of myocardial infarction greatly. Regression becomes critical in mid-portion of the curve where addition of new lesions imparts a steep increase in risk. Data from the IAP[31] and the WHO Study[32] indicate that the linear mid-portion of the sigmoid curve has been reached when 60% of the coronary surface is covered with raised lesions.

Implications for Primary Atherosclerosis Prevention

Of course, the optimal approach to prevention of myocardial infarction is to avoid the mid-portion of the curve by lesion suppression early in the disease when risk is low. In CLAS it was shown that new lesion formation in native ungrafted coronary arteries could be reduced by vigorous lipid lowering in men whose pre-treatment cholesterol levels averaged 246 mg%.[24] It also seems important that reduction of cholesterol level, plus reduction of both systolic and diastolic blood pressures, reduced new native lesion formation in the CLAS control group.[34]

An early case finding and treatment strategy (possibly modeled on tuberculosis control with case finding by chest x-ray) could be applied to

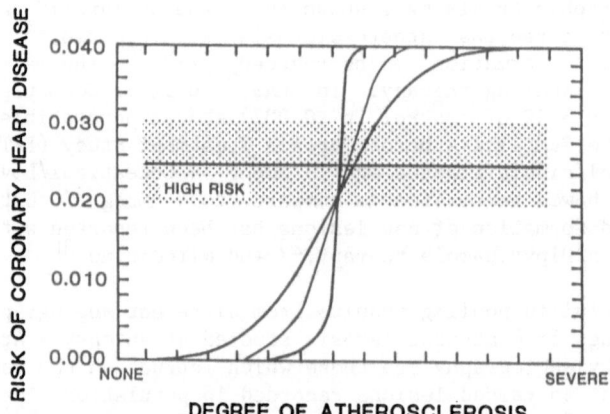

Fig. 2. Gofman's interpretation of the International Atherosclerosis Project data by Sigmoid curves explaining best the relationship between degree of atherosclerosis and myocardial infarction risk. Risk varies according to the degree of disease present as new lesions are added.

prevention of coronary atherosclerosis and myocardial infarction with non-invasive coronary imaging. Coronary atherosclerosis is ubiquitous, but we know that some individuals develop more severe coronary atherosclerosis than their peers at an early age. A case finding and treatment strategy based on coronary imaging would benefit those with premature atherosclerosis who are not recognized with current risk factor screening until they develop symptoms, such as angina pectoris, and are on the steep mid-portion of Gofman's sigmoid curve. Early case finding could also expand our ability to investigate atherogenic disease mechanisms. Two non-invasive imaging procedures with potential for application in case finding are Magnetic Resonance Imaging and Ultrafast Computed Tomography. Recent results with Ultrafast Tomography for identification of very small areas of coronary artery calcium mineral deposition are quite promising. Patients identified by such screening as being at high risk then could be treated vigorously early by diet and, if needed, drugs. The results of two trials are noteworthy with regard to the importance of treatment by diet.

Observational analyses of diet effects from the Leiden Intervention Trial which tested diet therapy but did not have a control group are relevant to population-wide dietary measures for primary prevention of atherosclerosis. The Leiden Intervention Trial,[14] a two-year test of vegetarian diet with P/S ratio greater than 2 and cholesterol intake less than 100 mg/day, included 39 patients with angiograms separated by two years. Eighteen patients showed no progression in coronary angiograms analyzed both by visual assessment and computerized image processing. Lesion progression was strongly related to the total cholesterol/HDL-cholesterol ratio and no coronary lesion progression occurred in patients with a total cholesterol/ HDL-cholesterol less than 6.9 or in those who had reduced a high ratio at baseline to less than 6.9. An important finding of the Leiden study was the indication that lesion progression can be reduced by dietary modification without weight loss. Atherosclerotic lesions have long been known to decrease with war-related severe dietary deprivation, as summarized by Schettler,[35] but the Leiden diet was not a hardship diet.

Additional observational analyses from the control group of CLAS indicate that new coronary lesion formation can be influenced by conventional diets that are self-selected and do not cause weight loss.[34] Standardized diet recall records obtained during CLAS were used for a conventional epidemiologic evaluation of risk factors and the appearance or absence of new lesions. Eighteen CLAS treated subjects who developed new coronary lesions in two years with compared with 64 who did not. Subjects who did not develop new lesions substituted low fat for high fat meat and dairy products and showed significant reductions in total plasma cholesterol and LDL-cholesterol levels. It is important to note that these dietary effects were seen in subjects who had reduced saturated fat intake below the average intake of Americans to levels close to the National Cholesterol Education Program recommendations.

References

1. W. J. Sanders, E. L. Alderman, and D. C. Harrison, Coronary artery quantification using digital imaging processing techniques, in: "Computers in Cardiology," K. L. Ripley and H. G. Ostrow, eds., IEEE Comp Soc, New York (1979).
2. J. R. Spears, Quantitation of anatomic coronary stenosis severity: limitations of accuracy, in: "State of the Art in Quantitative Coronary Arteriography," J. H. C. Reiber and P. W. Serruys, eds., Martinus Nijhoff, Dordrecht, Netherlands (1986).
3. R. H. Selzer, A second look at quantitative coronary angiography: some unexpected problems, in: "State of the Art in Quantitative Coronary

Arteriography, J. H. C. Reiber and W. P. Serruys, eds., Martinus Nijhoff, Dordrecht, Netherlands (1986).

4. J. R. Spears and D. W. Crawford, A catheterization technique for reproduction of a human atherosclerotic lumen within the dog coronary artery in vivo, Cath Cardiovasc Diag 9:19 (1983).

5. R. H. Selzer, C. Hagerty, S. P. Azen, M. Siebes, P. Lee, A. Shircore, D. H. Blankenhorn, and the Cholesterol Lowering Atherosclerosis Study Investigators and Staff, Precision and reproducibility of quantitative coronary angiography with applications to controlled clinical trials, J Clin Invest 83:520 (1989).

6. J. R. Spears, T. Sandor, A. V. Als, M. Malagold, J. E. Markis, W. Grossman, J. R. Serur, and S. Paulin, Computerized image analysis for quantitative measurement of vessel diameter from cineangiograms, Circulation 68:453 (1983).

7. J. H. C. Reiber, C. J. Kooijman, C. J. Slager, J. J. Gerbrands, J. C. H. Schuurbiers, A. den Boer, W. Wijns, P. W. Serruys, and P. G. Hugenholtz, Coronary artery dimensions from cineangiograms - methodology and validation of a computer-assisted analysis procedure, IEEE Transactions in Medical Imaging MI-3:131 (1984).

8. D. W. Crawford, E. S. Beckenbach, D. H. Blankenhorn, and S. H. Brooks, Grading of coronary atherosclerosis: Comparison of a modified IAP visual grading method and a new quantitative angiographic technique, Atherosclerosis 19:231 (1974).

9. P. Jaques, F. DiBianca, S. Pizer, F. Kohout, L. Lifshitz, and D. Delany, Quantitative coronary fluorography: Computer vs human estimation of vascular stenoses, Inves Radiol 20:45 (1985).

10. M. Siebes, M. Gottwik, and M. Schlepper, Quanlitative and quantitative experimental studies on the evaluation of model coronary arteries from angiograms, in: "Computers in Cardiology," IEEE Comp Soc, New York (1982).

11. T. Sandor, J. R. Spears, and S. Paulin, Densitometric determination of changes in the dimensions of coronary arteries, Spie Digital Radiography 314:263 (1981).

12. H. Tomoike, H. Ootsubo, K. Sakai, Y. Kikuchi, and M. Nakamura, Continuous measurement of coronary artery diameter in situ, Am J Physiol 240:H73 (1981).

13. S. F. Vatner, A. Pasipoularides, and I. Mirsmy, Measurement of arterial pressure-dimension relationships in conscious animals, Ann Biomed Eng 12:521 (1984).

14. A. C. Arntzenius, D. Kromhout, J. D. Barth, J. H. C. Reiber, A. V. G. Bruschke, B. Buis, C. M. van Gent, N. Kempen-Voogd, S. Strikwerda, and E. A. van der Velde, Diet, lipoproteins, and the progression of coronary atherosclerosis. The Leiden Intervention Trial, New Eng J Med 312:805 (1985).

15. W. L. Cashin, S. H. Brooks, D. H. Blankenhorn, R. H. Selzer, M. E. Sanmarco, and B. Benjauthrit, Computerized edge tracking and lesion measurement in coronary angiograms, Atherosclerosis 52:295 (1984).

16. S. Glagov, E. Weisenberg, C. K. Zarins, R. Stankunavicius, and G. J. Kolettis, Compensatory enlargement of human atherosclerotic coronary arteries, N Eng J Med 316:1371 (1987).

17. B. H. Brown, E. Bolson, M. Frimer, and H. T. Dodge, Quantitative coronary arteriography. Estimation of dimensions, hemodynamic resistance, and atheroma mass of coronary artery lesions using the arteriogram and digital computation, Circulation 55:329 (1977).

18. K. L. Gould, Quantification of coronary artery stenosis in vivo, Circ Res 57:341, (1985).

19. R. L. Kirkeeide, B. Wuesten, and M. Gottwik, Computer assisted evaluation of angiographic findings, in: "Thrombose und Atherogenese," K. Breddin, ed., Gerhard Witzstrock Verlag, Baden-Baden (1981).

20. F. Booman, J. H. C. Reiber, J. J. Gerbrands, C. J. Slager, J. C. H.

Schuurbiers, and G. T. Meester, Quantitative analysis of coronary occlusions from coronary cineangiograms, in: "Computers in Cardiology," R. L. Ripley and H. G. Ostrow, eds., IEEE Comp Soc, New York (1979).

21. R. L. Kirkeeide, P. Fung, R. W. Smalling, and K. L. Gould, Automated evaluation of vessel diameter from arteriograms, in: "Computers in Cardiology," IEEE Comp Soc, New York (1982).

22. D. C. Ledbetter, R. H. Selzer, R. M. Gordon, D. H. Blankenhorn, and M. E. Sanmarco, Computer quantitation of coronary angiograms, Noninv Cardiovasc Meas 167:27 (1982).

23. J. R. Spears, T. Sandor, T. A. Als, M. Malagold, J. Markis, and S. Paulin, Accuracy of computer vs. visual measurement of vessel diameter from cine angiograms, Circulation 64 (supp IV):130 (1981).

24. D. H. Blankenhorn, S. A. Nessim, R. L. Johnson, M. E. Sanmarco, S. P. Azen, and L. Cashin-Hemphill, Beneficial effects of combined colestipol-niacin therapy on coronary atherosclerosis and coronary venous bypass grafts, JAMA 257-3233 (1987).

25. J. F. Brensike, R. I. Levy, S. F. Kelsey, E. R. Passamani, M. J. Richardson, I. K. Loh, N. J. Stone, R. F. Aldrich, J. W. Battaglini, D. J. Moriarty, M. R. Fisher, L. Friedman, W. Friedewald, K. M. Detre, and S. E. Epstein, Effects of therapy with cholestyramine on progression of coronary arteriosclerosis: Results of the NHLBI Type II Coronary Intervention Study, Circulation 69:313 (1984).

26. R. G. Duffield, N. E. Miller, C. W. Jamieson, and B. Lewis, A controlled trial of plasma lipid reduction in peripheral atherosclerosis--an interim report, Br J Surg 69: Suppl:S3 (1982).

27. B. G. Brown, J. T. Lin, S. M. Schaefer, C. A. Kaplan, H. T. Dodge, and J. J. Albers, Niacin or lovastatin, combined with colestipol, regress coronary atherosclerosis and prevent clinical events in men with elevated apolipoprotein B, Circulation 80:II-266 (1989).

28. D. M. Ornish, L. W. Scherwitz, S. E. Brown, J. H. Billings, W. T. Armstrong, T. A. Ports, R. L. Kirkeeide, and K. L. Gould, Adherence to lifestyle changes and reversal of coronary atherosclerosis, Circulation 80:II-57 (1989).

29. J. H. Chesebro, M. W. I. Webster, H. C. Smith, R. I. Frye, D. R. Holmes, G. S. Reeder, D. R. Bresnahan, and R. A. Nishimura, Antiplatelet therapy in coronary disease progression, reduced infarction and new lesion formation, Circulation 80:II-266 (1989).

30. P. R. Lichtlen, P. Hugenholtz, W. Rafflenbeaul, S. Jost, and H. Hecker, Retardation of the progression of coronary artery disease with Nifedipine. Results of INTACT, Circulation 80:II-382 (1989).

31. R. H. Deupree, R. I. Fields, C. A. McMahan, and J. P. Strong, Atherosclerotic lesions and coronary heart disease. Key relationships in necropsied cases. Lab Invest 28:252 (1973).

32. Atherosclerosis of the aorta and coronary arteries in five towns. Bull World Health Organization 53:485 (1976).

33. J. W. Gofman, The quantitative nature of the relationship of coronary artery atherosclerosis and coronary heart disease risk, Cardiol Digest 4:28 (1969).

34. D. H. Blankenhorn, R. L. Johnson, W. J. Mack, H. A. El Zein, and L. I. Vailas, The influence of diet on the appearance of new lesions in human coronary arteries, JAMA 263:1646 (1990).

35. G. Schettler, Cardiovascular diseases during and after World War II: A comparison of the Federal Republic of Germany with other European countries, Prev Med 8:581 (1979).

B-MODE IMAGING TO MEASURE CAROTID ARTERY WALL THICKNESS AND ITS

RELATIONSHIP WITH SOME RISK FACTORS FOR ATHEROSCLEROSIS

A. Poli, E. Tremoli, P. Werba, D. Baldassarre

Institute of Pharmacological Sciences, E.G. Paoletti
Center for Atherosclerosis Research, University of Milan,
Italy; Turati Foundation, Gavinana (PT) Italy

INTRODUCTION

In vivo imaging of the extracranial carotid arteries can be
obtained using high resolution real-time echotomographic systems. This
technique is noninvasive, and provides real-time information on both
lumen and vessel wall characteristics.

Using this methodological approach, the arterial wall further from
the probe is visualized in normal vessels as a pair of roughly parallel
echogenic lines: the external line is generated by the media-adventitia
transition, while the internal one is generated by the blood-intima
interface (1).

In this study we have evaluated the association between the
presence of known risk factors for atherosclerosis (hyperlipidemia,
cigarette smoking) and the magnitude of the thickness of the intimal
medial complex in living human subjects.

PATIENTS AND METHODS

Thirty-six hypercholesterolemic patients with a diagnosis of type
IIa hyperlipoproteinemia were recruited in our Lipid Clinic (E. Grossi
Paoletti Center); thirty-one normolipidemic subjects, of similar age and
with similar smoker/non smoker and male/female ratios were selected as
controls.

Diabetic, obese and hypertensive patients and patients with a
clinical history suggesting atherosclerosis of the carotid arteries were
excluded. Patients with positive history for coronary artery disease
(n=5), or ischemic arterial disease of the lower limbs (n=2) were
admitted to the study.

Carotid ultrasound imaging was performed with a Bio-Sound
echotomographic system, model Phase-one (Bio Dynamycs, Indianapolis, IN,
USA).

Scanning of the extracranial carotid arteries in the neck was performed in three different projections (anterior and posterior: patient lying on his back; lateral: head turned 45 degrees contralateral to the carotid artery under examination).

The thickness of the intimal medial complex of the common carotid arteries was determined in patients starting with a standardized scan. The technique of the scan has been fully described elsewhere (2). Briefly, the common carotid artery is identified at the level of the bifurcation, and scanned in cranio-caudal direction. In each image, photographed under controlled conditions, the area between the luminal and the deeper echoes and the length of the segment of interest are measured using the graphic tablet of a personal computer. The "average thickness" of each projection of the artery is then obtained as the ratio between the total surface of the area limited by the echoes and its length (Fig.1). Values for the different projections and for right and left arteries are then averaged.

Plaques are defined as localized lesions of thickness $\geq$2.0 mm.

The reproducibility of the procedure, tested as inter-observer variability ratio in blinded experiments, was 4.6% (range: 0.1-12.1%). An intra-observer reproducibility experiment yielded similar results.

Total and HDL plasma cholesterol and plasma triglycerides were determined by standard laboratory enzymatic tecniques. Student's t test and Fisher's exact test (Yates modification) were used for statistical analyses.

RESULTS

The mean values of the Intimal Medial Complex Thickness (IMCT) of common carotid arteries of the studied hyperlipoproteinemic patients and of control subjects are shown in Table 1. The IMCT of the common carotid artery of type IIa is significantly greater than that of control subjects (p $<$0.001).

When the thickness values of control subjects and of hyperlipidemic patients were analyzed, controlling for smoking status, a significant difference was demonstrated between smokers and non-smokers in hyperlipidemic but not in normolipidemic subjects (Table 2). In normolipidemic patients, but not in the hypercholesterolemics, on the other hand, a significant correlation between IMCT and age could be shown (r=0.46 p $<$0.01).

The mean IMCT values of the common carotid arteries in hypercholesterolemic patients with plaques in the extracranial carotid bed were significantly different from corresponding values of patients whose carotid arteries did not shown the presence of such lesions (mean ± SD: 0.754 mm ± 0.141 mm and 0.647 ± 0.105 mm respectively, p $<$0.05). However, the mean thickness of carotid arteries of hypercholesterolemic patients not presenting focal atherosclerotic lesions was still significantly different from the corresponding parameter evaluated in normolipidemic subjects (p $<$0.01).

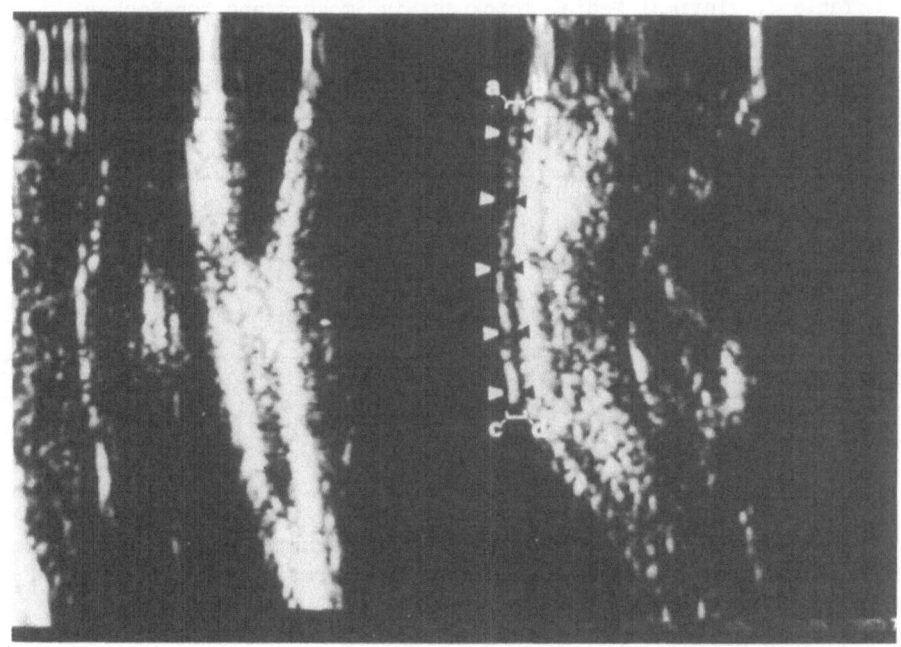

Fig.1. Picture of the carotid artery of a hypercholesterolemic patient,
showing the area (abcd), and the length (ad) of interest for
the determination of the average intimal complex thickness (see
text).

Table 1. Localization of Atherosclerotic Lesions of Common Carotid
Arteries of Type IIa Patients and Control Subjects

Values are expressed as means ± SD. ICA: internal carotid artery; ECA:
external carotid artery.

Parameter	Controls	Type IIa	Significance
Intimal-medial thickness (mm)	0.548±0.65	0.674±0.124	<0.01
Number of lesions ($\geq$2.0mm)			
bulb:	1	9	
ICA:	−	4	
ECA:	−	1	
total:	1	14	<0.05[a]

a: Fisher exact test.

Table 2. Intimal Medial Thickness in Smokers and Non-Smokers

	Intimal medial thickness (mm)		
	All subjects	Controls	IIa
Smokers(n)	0.665±156(19)	0.560±76(9)	0.760±150
Non-Smokers(n)	0.601± 92(40)	0.547±54(18)	0.646± 94(22)
P	0.1	ns	0.05

Values are expressed as means = SD

The prevalence of focal lesions was significantly higher in the hypercholesterolemic group as compared to the normolipidemic cohort (14 vs 1: p <0.05, Fisher exact test).

DISCUSSION

B-mode imaging of the extracranial carotid arteries of human subjects with different plasma cholesterol concentrations indicates that increased plasma lipoprotein levels are associated, in this arterial tree, with elevated values of IMCT and with an increased prevalence of small plaques.

If the different subgroups of subjects in which the IMCT was determined are independently analyzed, it is possible to consider specific aspects of the relationship between this parameter and some risk factors for the atherosclerotic disease.

In control subjects only, a positive correlation between age and IMCT (r=0.46) was found. On the basis of our data, arterial thickness apparently increases by about 1% per year. Such an association is not found in hypercholesterolemic patients indicating that the risk factor "cholesterol" may be outweighed by effect of age or other influences on IMCT. A correlation between cholesterol plasma levels and intimal medial thickness, on the other hand, was not found. This probably underlines the fact that other factors may actively partecipate in the process of wall thickening.

When the hypercholesterolemic patients who had lesions at the level of the bulb and/or of the first part of the internal carotid artery are independently considered, and are compared to patients without atherosclerotic lesions in the same location, or to normolipidemic controls, it appears that IMTC is highest among hypercholesterolemic patients with plaques, intermediate in hypercholesterolemic patients without plaques, and lowest in control subjects. Even if the absolute differences are rather small, these data could suggest that the first evidence of atherosclerotic involvement of the carotid artery is represented by an isolated intimal medial thickening, and that subsequently, while the intimal medial complex thickness further increases, localized lesions develop.

In conclusion, the reported data, although collected in a small sample of patients, suggest that the measurement of the IMCT of the carotid arteries may represent an index of preclinical atherosclerotic involvement.

This view is supported by the identification of a positive association between the magnitude of the parameter and recognized risk factors for atherosclerotic disease (hyperlipidemia, cigarette smoking, age), and with the presence of lesions definitely documenting an atherosclerotic involvement of the carotid artery under evaluation (plaques). Unfortunately, no correlation between this echotomographic parameter and known histological or anatomical pattern of the disease was possible in our study, since all the data were collected in living human subjects.

We believe that the determination of IMCT, and monitoring this parameter over time, using inexpensive, non-invasive, and safe B-mode ultrasound, represents a powerful model to study spontaneous or induced progression or regression of atherosclerosis.

REFERENCES

1. P. Pignoli, E. Tremoli, A. Poli, P.L. Oreste, R. Paoletti, Intimal plus medial thickness of the arterial wall: a direct measurement with ultrasound imaging, Circulation 74:1399 (1986).
2. A. Poli, A. Colombo, E. Tremoli, P. Pignoli, Spontaneous progression of a small carotid atheroma detected by echotomography, Lancet ii: 559 (1985).

QUANTITATIVE ULTRASONIC IMAGING OF THE ATHEROSCLEROTIC PLAQUE: IN VITRO AND PRELIMINARY IN VIVO FINDINGS

*Luigi Landini, Eugenio Picano, Pio Urbani, Marco Paterni,
*Maria Filomena Santarelli, Gualtiero Pelosi, Alessandro
Mazzarisi, and Antonio Benassi

*Institute of Electronics and Telecommunications, University
of Pisa, Via Diotisalvi, 2, Pisa - Italy. C.N.R. Institute of
Clinical Physiology, Via Savi, 8, Pisa - Italy

INTRODUCTION

Ultrasonic tissue characterization of atherosclerosis has been attempted in several studies in vitro[1-6]. Conventional ultrasound offers morphologic information, and some clue to the identification of plaque structure. However, there is greater potential in ultrasound for the characterization of plaque composition.

The hypothesis underlying ultrasonic tissue characterization of atherosclerosis is that pathologic changes occurring in atherosclerosis alter the physical properties of the tissue, and that these alterations can be quantified with indexes based on measurements of the ultrasonic attenuation and backscatter carried out over a range of frequencies.

Present research is designed to establish a correlation between ultrasonic measurements and tissue histology in order to broaden the diagnostic potential of ultrasound to detect arterial damage in patients. In this paper we will review the findings obtained in vitro with different ultrasonic parameters, based on ultrasonic attenuation and backscattering. The purpose of the in vitro studies has been twofold: to test new variables of potential diagnostic use, and to provide basic information for a better definition of limits and applicability of clinical echography. Finally, we will present preliminary in vivo results obtained in patients with carotid artery disease, by using a modified echographic apparatus.

REVIEW OF IN VITRO FINDINGS

The fundamental message of in vitro studies is that the main constituents of the atherosclerotic plaque (lipids, collagen, calcium) can be recognized in vitro by means of several ultrasound parameters of potential diagnostic use.

Attenuation measurements

Attenuation measurements are obtained by transmitting a short pulse of acoustic energy to the interrogated tissue and detecting the echo produced by a reflector placed behind the specimens.

Ultrasound attenuation is not suitable for in vivo applications, but identification of attenuation properties of normal and diseased arterial

Atherosclerotic Plaques, Edited by R.W. Wissler *et al.*
Plenum Press, New York, 1991

tissue can be helpful for a better understanding of the interaction between ultrasound and arterial tissue. Results obtained from ultrasonic attenuation and histological analyses[1] show that the attenuation is lowest in normal walls and progressively increases in fibrous, fibrofatty and calcific subsets (all intergroup differences were significant, except for the normal vs. fibrous comparison). Such alterations in ultrasonic attenuation may reflect intrinsic changes in biochemical and mechanical properties of atherosclerotic tissue. In fact, the biochemistry of the atheroma documents an increase in at least three structural components potentially responsible for increased attenuation of the plaque: i.e. collagen, lipids and calcium.

Backscatter measurements

Backscatter measurements are obtained by transmitting a short pulse of acoustic energy to the interrogated tissue and by detecting the backscatter signals directly from tissue. Therefore, in backscatter measurements, the reflected ultrasound is received directly from the target tissue, in a condition more like that in vivo. By using signal analysis, several different indexes can be extracted from the received signal: 1) the frequency dependence of ultrasonic backscatter; 2) the integrated backscatter index; 3) the angular dependence of ultrasonic backscatter; 4) the amplitude histogram of backscattered echoes.

Frequency dependence of ultrasonic backscatter: Ultrasonic backscatter represents a useful measure of the efficiency of the interrogated tissue volume over the frequency range determined by the transmitted pulse. For five groups of aortic specimens (normal and with different degrees of atherosclerosis) the ultrasonic backscatter coefficient was measured as a function of frequency in the range 4-14 MHz. The results of the study[5] are related to two classes of structures, i.e. connective and fatty tissue, as the main determinants of the scattering from arterial wall. The structure of connective tissue produces a typical low frequency power dependence of the backscatter coefficient typical which is significantly greater than the one obtained in fatty tissue.

Integrated backscatter: Since it is based on the evaluation of the backscattered energy from small tissue volume this index has potential for in vivo application, expecially when obtained with broadband signals. This approach utilizes a frequency domain averaging technique instead of a spatial average procedure, to measure the average scattering properties of a tissue, so that the index is not significantly affected by phase distortions. Therefore, measurements based on the integrated backscatter index can be correlated with the tissue histology. Based on this index a significant difference between five groups of normal and atherosclerotic specimens (normal, fatty, fibrofatty, fibrotic, calcific) was found[2]. Of the three major constituents of the plaque, fibrosis and calcium increase the reflectivity value, while fatty tissue tends to lower it.

Angular dependence: This technique makes it possible to determine whether or not a scatterer is of a "specular type" (i.e. angular dependent). This is a major limitation to any application based on a quantitative diagnostic approach in vivo, since specular reflectors give rise to a signal whose amplitude is highly dependent on the angle of incidence of the ultrasonic beam to the tissue target. Angular scattering measurements performed on normal and atherosclerotic specimens[2] identified two patterns: 1) a "directive" pattern, characterized by a strongly angle-dependent backscattering which falls abruptly when the beam is moved slightly away from normal incidence. This pattern was typical of calcified, fibrous, and less markedly, fibrofatty and normal specimen; 2) a "nondirective" pattern, characterized by a backscatter that is not significantly angle dependent and fluctuates throughout the entire angular range. This was typical of fatty samples. A directive angular response may be due to single planar organization of the targets within the tissue.Scatterers in the normal wall might be physically identified in the thin elastic membranes present within the normal media layer and perpendicular to the beam axis. In fibrous and calcified specimens, the scatterers might be physically identified in thick collagen bundles and calcium laminae, which are, like elastic membranes, oriented perpendicular to the beam. This might explain the very high directivity of these plaques. The absence of a spatial orientation and the small size of the scatterers both contribute to the nondirective type of angular scattering as in fatty plaques. In fatty plaques, lipids accumulate in the intima, mainly in the amorphous state but also as cholesterol crystals. In the fibrofatty plaque the markedly directive response is probably due to the fibrous cap; however, the coexistence within the scattering volume of a non-directive structure (the fatty core, absent in the purely fibrous plaques) partially blunts the directivity of the angular response which is substantially less than in the fibrous samples.

Amplitude histogram of ultrasonic backscatter: A statistical analysis of regional two-dimensional echographic gray level distributions may be used to successfully discriminate normal from pathological conditions in measurements in vivo. In fact, the gray-level histogram, is probably less dependent on potential sources of artifact that may be present in the clinical setting, such as an improper transducer angulation, selective attenuation from various tissues interposed between the transducer and the target organ, electronic setting. The amplitude distribution of the integrated backscatter was analyzed by calculating the following statistical parameters: mean value, standard deviation, skewness and kurtosis[3]. Such statistical parameters evaluated in normal and atherosclerotic segments, effectively differentiated between the two groups. Atherosclerotic disease is not characterized by a unique trend toward increased reflectivity. When atherosclerotic specimen with mostly fatty and fibrofatty sites were considered, it was still possible to distinguish normal from atherosclerotic regions based on statistical parameters, but not on integrated backscatter values. By quantitative analysis of integrated backscatter distribution, it might also be possible to identify ultrasonically "silent" lesions which cannot be recognized with the integrated backscatter amplitude.

PRELIMINARY IN VIVO RESULTS

The effective potentialities of the technique in characterizing atherosclerosis in vivo, have been assessed by using a modified commercial echographic apparatus. Such apparatus allows both conventional and quantitative tissue characterization imaging to be built into the same basic hardware.

Study design

In order to have a comparison with histologic findings, we selected patients who were scheduled for a vascular carotid surgery procedure. In all analyzed patients the carotid region imaged by ultrasound preoperatively was also excised during the surgical procedure and histologically evaluated in a blinded fashion. In this way, it was possible to establish a correlation between ultrasonic findings and histological features of the atherosclerotic plaque.

A diagram of the ultrasonic data acquisition system is shown in Fig. 1. It consists of an AU420 (ESAOTE Biomedica) B-mode echographic apparatus interfaced with a radiofrequency processing unit. The echographic apparatus is based on a mechanically focused ultrasonic transducer (1.3 cm diameter, focal distance 3 cm) operating in a frequency range of 5 to 10 MHz. The radiofrequency processing unit is fed by the native R.F. signal fetched before the processing chain of the B-mode instrument, so that it undergoes preamplification, bypassing the receiving circuits of the ultrasonic equipment. The amplification allows the full utilization of the input dynamic range of the analog to digital converter (AD). Only digitized signals corresponding to a two dimensional window selected by the operator on the B-mode screen, are AD converted (8 bits of amplitude resolution, 40 MHz of sampling rate) and analyzed both in real time and also transferred to a personal computer for additional analyses. The two dimensional window is visualized on the B-mode screen (Fig. 2), in order to ensure proper

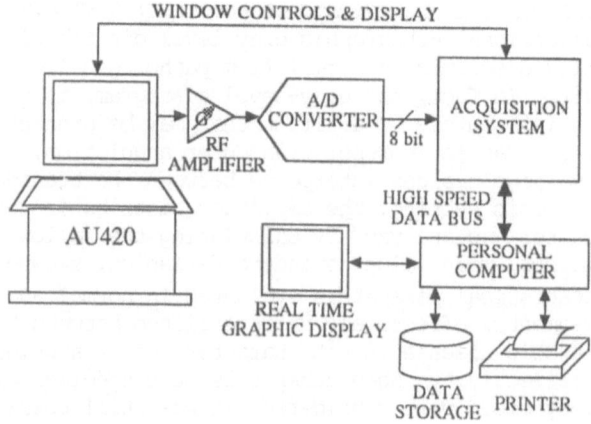

Fig. 1   Diagram of the ultrasonic data acquisition system.

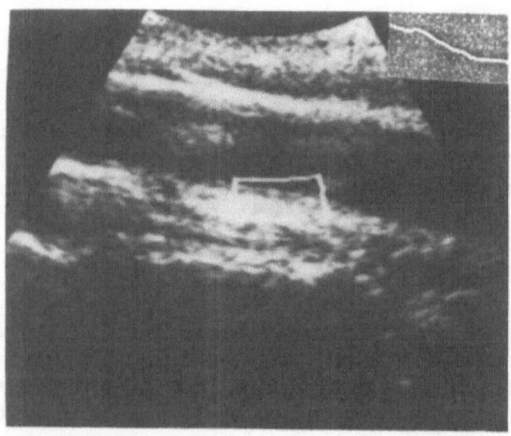

Fig. 2   Conventional B-mode image with superimposed   two dimensional window and IB profile.

positioning and size over the structure to be analyzed. On the same screen, the real time representation of the integrated backscatter index (IB) evaluated over the arterial profile, is shown.

<u>Ultrasonic data analysis</u>

In order to separate the wall input from that of the lumen, a masking operation was performed on each ultrasonic image under computer control. When the analysis was extended to the arterial wall, a thickness normalization procedure was carried out so that the measurement was independent of biological variability in wall thickness. A more sophisticated analysis was also performed on the stored data, including the radiofrequency signal demodulation and representation in pseudo-color display; the evaluations of the integrated backscatter and the amplitude histograms corresponding to areas selected on the two dimensional image; the radiofrequency signal representation (time domain) corresponding to a selected line of view. Ultrasonic results have been supported by histology (Masson-Goldner, trichromatic method) in order to confirm their validity.

RESULTS

The preliminary results obtained in vivo seem to fit the in vitro trend. In Fig. 3 and 4 typical patterns are shown for a normal and atherosclerotic arterial wall respectively. As expected, the tissue characterization pattern of a normal carotid artery wall is represented (Fig. 3) by a relatively low and uniform gray-level image, a low IB profile and a time domain echo pattern characterized by a relatively low amplitude at the blood intima and intima-media layers. The histogram analysis shows sharp amplitude distribution with low mean value. On the other hand, a more heterogeneous gray-level image as shown in Fig. 4 represents an atherosclerotic arterial wall, characterized by a non-unique trend in reflectivity as confirmed by the histogram analysis and an increase of the IB with respect to the normal wall. From these preliminary results it seems also possible to distinguish the plaque according to prevalence of fibrous or fatty tissue. Fig. 5a and b show a transverse section of two fibrofatty carotid arteries respectively characterized by a prevalence of fatty and fibrous tissue. Figs. 6a and b show two typical histological views of carotid arteries which can be related to ultrasonic data of Fig. 6.

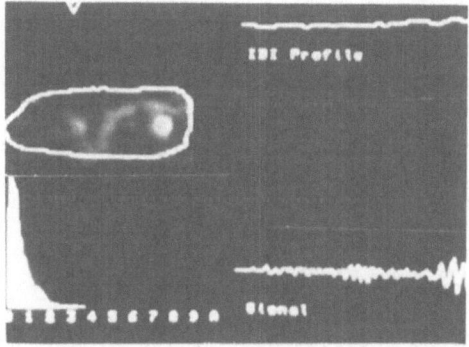

Fig. 3 Typical patterns of normal arterial wall: gray-level representation, IB profile, histogram, time domain echo pattern.

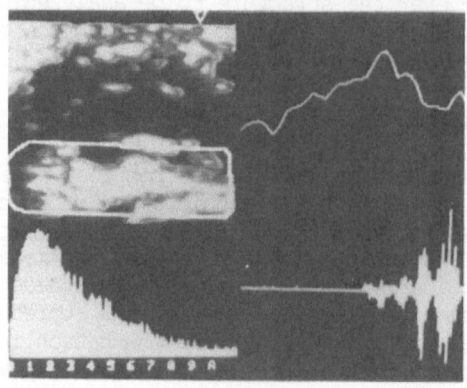

Fig. 4 The same representation as in Fig.3, for an atherosclerotic arterial wall.

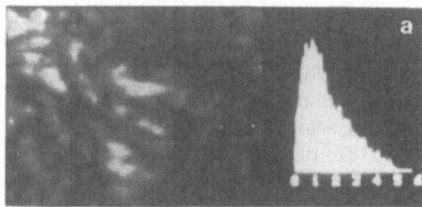 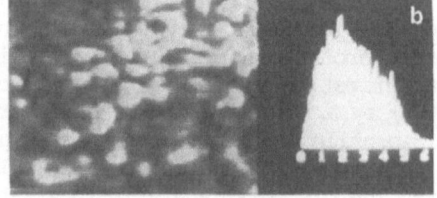

Fig. 5 Gray-level representation of a transverse section of a fibrofatty plaque with (a) prevalence of fatty (Fa+) and (b) fibrous (Fi+) tissue.

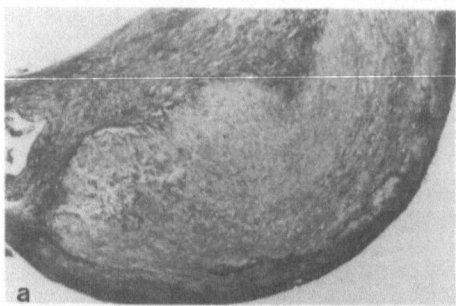 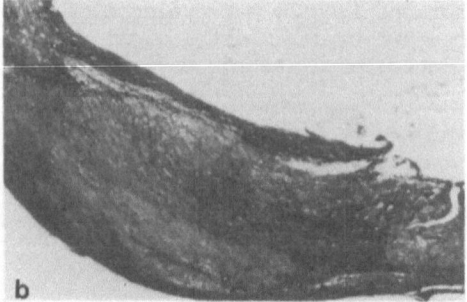

Fig. 6 Typical histological views of carotid arteries corresponding to data of Fig. 5: (a) fibrofatty plaque (Fa+); (b) fibrous plaque (Fi+).

CONCLUSIONS

The clinical arena theoretically limits in many ways the tissue characterization studies on the atherosclerotic plaque. The target tissue is pulsating, and a gated acquisition of the signal is required. A narrow frequency band (in our study, 5 MHz) is used, instead of a large broadband frequency (in our in vitro studies, 4 to 14 MHz) allowing more intense backscatter phenomena and a reduction of phase cancellation artifacts with frequency averaging. Subcutaneous and muscular tissue, of variable thickness and composition, is interposed between the transducer and the artery, giving rise to erratic diffraction and attenuation phenomena. Nevertheless, the clinically useful information on the histologic composition of the plaque is easily extracted with a radiofrequency - based quantitative ultrasonic imaging of the carotid. It is of the utmost importance that the fundamental tissue "library" recognizes in vivo basically the same gradient in echo reflectivity described in vitro[1-6]; the lipid tissue is relatively hypoechoic; the fibrofatty plaque has an increased echoreflectivity which increases with the relative contribution of fibrous tissue; the calcific plaque has the highest echogenicity. This relatively simple, quantitatively displayed information can represent the fundamental prerequisite for future studies on the biochemical remodeling of the atherosclerotic plaques following dietary, pharmacological and mechanical interventions. These interventions will be monitored and evaluated on the basis of their effects not only on plaque geometry but also on plaque composition. By radiofrequency analysis we hope to have resolution information on the differential diagnosis between lipidic plaque and fresh thrombus, as well as being able to identify the age of the thrombus, particularly for the "fresh" one that is very similar to blood echogenicity.

Finally, we have the possibility for a direct measurement and for an immediate imaging ("on-line," with an adequate gray-level or color-coding broad spectrum echoic-backscatter dependent) of the "elastic modulus of Young" of organic structure, static or moving. Perhaps, it will be possible (with an adequate gating dynamic acquisition, compatible with ultrasound limits) to obtain a direct measure in vivo of elastic modulus of the arterial wall, an expression of the integrity of large vessels which are age, sex and pressure dependent, and as a marker of prognostic value in atherosclerosis. At present, in vivo techniques provide only an indirect measurement of the elastic modulus of the artery wall.

REFERENCES

1) E. Picano, L. Landini, A. Distante, Fibrosis, lipids and calcium in human atherosclerotic plaque; in vitro differentiation from normal aortic walls by ultrasonic attenuation. Circ. Res., 56:556 (1985).
2) E. Picano, L. Landini, A. Distante, Angle dependence of backscatter in arterial tissues: a study in vitro. Circulation, 72:572 (1985).
3) E. Picano, L. Landini, F. Lattanzi, The use of frequency histograms of ultrasonic backscatter amplitudes for detection of atherosclerosis in vitro. Circulation, 74:10093 (1986).
4) L. Landini, R. Sarnelli, E. Picano, Evaluation of frequency dependence of backscatter coefficient in normal and atherosclerotic aortic walls. Ultrasound Med. Biol., 12:397 (1986).
5) B. Barzilai, J.E. Saffitz, J.G. Miller, Quantitative ultrasonic characterization of the nature of atherosclerotic plaques in human aorta. Circ Res., 60:459 (1987).
6) E. Picano, L. Landini, F. Lattanzi, Time domain echo pattern evaluations from normal and atherosclerotic arterial walls: a study in vitro. Circulation, 77:654 (1988).

PET AND SPECT FOR THE STUDY OF ATHEROSCLEROTIC DISEASES IN HUMANS

P. Pantano, C. Laudani*, V. Di Piero, R. Casati*,
M. Ricci, R.M. Moresco*, F. Fazio*, and G.L. Lenzi

Department of Neurological Sciences, V.le
dell'Universita, Rome, Italy
*Department of Biomedical Technologies, University of
Milan, S. Raffaele Institute, Italy

INTRODUCTION

Emission Tomography (ET) investigates physiological parameters and biochemical reactions in vivo in humans. Positron Emission Tomography (PET) is based on x-ray computerized tomography (CT) principles and provides a tomographic representation of tissue radioactivity due to positrons, such as carbon (C-11), oxygen (O-15), nitrogen (N-13),and fluorine (F-18).

PET allows a quantitative assessment of several physiological parameters related to cerebral functions, such as cerebral blood flow (CBF) and metabolic rates for both oxygen and glucose, extraction of nutrients, cerebral blood volume, and, more recently, receptor density and neurotransmitter distribution.

Single Photon Emission Computerized Tomography (SPECT) utilizes a signal produced by the excitation of a gamma-ray detector by photon emitter radioisotopes.

In regard to SPECT, the most studied physiological parameter has been the CBF by means of rotating gamma-cameras and labeled amines, such as I-123 IMP, I-123 HIPDM, and TC-99m HM-PAO. Furthermore, quantitative CBF studies may be performed by using the Xenon-1333 inhalation method with dedicated designed equipment.

PET AND SPECT IN CEREBROVASCULAR DISEASES

One of the major contributions of the ET techniques has been an increased knowledge of the pathophysiology of human cerebral ischemia.

The immediate consequence of acute arterial occlusion is the fall of distal blood pressure. The distal blood pressure level therefore becomes dependent on the possibility of compensation through collateral circulation.

Two major cerebral homeostatic mechanisms are aimed at preserving cerebral metabolism and, in turn, neuronal function. The first is due to cerebral autoregulation and consists of a local vasodilatation of distal resistance vessels induced by the reduced perfusion pressure. Because of this vasodilatation the CBF remains normal at rest. Through the application of an additional vasodilator stimulus, such as carbon dioxide or acetazolamide (Diamox), it is possible to demonstrate a reduced perfusion reserve (Di Piero et al., 1989; Chollet et al., 1989).

Below the autoregulation threshold at mean distal arterial pressure values lower than 60mmHg a constant and passive reduction of CBF occurs in normotensive subjects (pressure dependent). Thus the second compensatory mechanism comes into play through the extraction of arterial oxygen. Normally the brain uses only about 50% of the oxygen carried by the blood. As CBF decreases, and as cerebral extraction of arterial oxygen increases, cerebral oxidative metabolism is maintained. This condition is called "critical perfusion" and indicates a state of severe reversible hypoperfusion (Ackerman et al., 1981; Lenzi et al., 1982).

"Criticial perfusion" has been demonstrated in patients with atherosclerotic stenosis or occlusion of the internal carotid artery. PET and SPECT studies have shown that these patients, although asymptomatic, had reduced cerebral blood flow and increased oxygen extraction ratio (Baron et al., 1981a; Gibbs et al., 1984). Several studies have been performed to evaluate CBF and metabolism before and after external-internal carotid bypass surgery (Tanahashy et al., 1985; Carter et al., 1984). These studies demonstrated that there was an improvement of the CBF in the affected hemisphere during the first months after the EC-IC bypass which did not persist over time (Meyer et al., 1982; Di Piero et al., 1987).

Experimental data suggested that CBF may vary from the normal value of 60-50ml/100gr/min to 23ml/100gr/min without causing any clinical symptoms. Also, further CBF reductions are no longer compensated and clinical symptoms may occur. Therefore at CBF levels between 23ml/100gr/min and 10ml/100gr/min, although neuronal activity is impaired, tissue is still viable and function may recover following blood supply restoration. This clinical and pathophysiological state is called the "ischemic penumbra." Below the threshold of 10ml/100gr/min neuronal damage is irreversible (Astrup et al., 1977). Experimental studies have shown that the development of the ischemic damage is a function not only of CBF severity reduction, but also of arterial occlusion duration (Jones et al., 1981; Weistein et al., 1986). This indicates that there is a time interval during which therapy may be successful in preventing final ischemic tissue damage, namely the "therapeutic window."

The treatment of ischemic stroke must take into account both the "ischemic penumbra" and the "therapeutic window" concepts (Fieschi et al., 1988). In evaluating pathophysiologic features of the early phase of stroke, PET and SPECT studies may provide useful clinical data. Our group has recently demonstrated that CBF in the early phase of stroke was highly correlated with the final prognosis, both in terms of tissue lesion and patient outcome (Giubilei et al., 1990).

A further pathophysiologic aspect demonstrated by PET and SPECT studies is the decrease of CBF (and metabolism) in anatomically intact areas far from the ischemic lesion. This phenomenon, called diaschisis, is probably due to the decrease of the synaptic input causing a decrease of neuronal firing of the target structures. These remote effects have been observed in the cerebellar hemisphere contralateral to a supratentorial infarct (Baron et al., 1981; Pantano et al., 1986) and in the cortex ipsilateral to thalamic damage (Baron et al., 1986; Perani et al., 1988). Metabolic cerebral cortex damage in an otherwise normal CT scan may better explain such symptoms as cognitive function impairment, frequently observed in patients with subcortical lesion.

PET AND SPECT IN CARDIAC DISEASES

PET provides assessment of regional myocardial perfusion and metabolism. Myocardial perfusion is conventionally assessed by using Thallium-201 (201-Tl), 13N-ammonia ($^{13}NH_3$), H_2-^{15}O or Rubidium-82 (^{82}Rb). All these tracers point out hypoperfused myocardial areas, but are not able to define whether the hypo-perfused myocardium is necrotic or still viable (the so-called "hybernated" or "stuporous" myocardium). The assessment of myocardial metabolism by (^{18}F) fluorodeoxyglucose (18-FDG) is the only examination which allows a determination of the viability of the hypoperfused myocardium (Phelps et al., 1983). 18-FDG, an analogue of glucose which undergoes glucose phosphorylation, is not further metabolized and thus remains trapped in proportion to glucose consumption. In physiologic conditions and in fasting subjects the metabolic substrates used by the heart are mainly fatty acids, which are metabolized by beta-oxidation. On the contrary, in ischemic conditions, the heart can also use anaerobic glycolysis. As a consequence, 18-FDG selectively accumulates only in ischemic areas since normal areas do not use glucose, and necrotic areas cannot metabolize any substrates. Therefore, it is possible to detect myocardial ischemic areas by combined studies on perfusion and metabolism. This is clinically relevant both for the diagnosis and the prognosis. It has been observed that 50% of the areas that are considered necrotic only on the basis of 201-Tl still appear viable at the 18-FDG scan. Also, it has been demonstrated that regional myocardial function improves in 85% of the myocardial segments identified as viable by 18-FDG, after coronary artery bypass graft (CABG), whereas it does not improve in 96% of the segments identified as necrotic by 18-FDG. PET studies are, therefore, extremely useful for the evaluation of patients with coronary artery disease.

PET should be considered necessary in those patients with ejection fraction below 40%, where the surgery risk is high, in patients who are candidates to aneurysmectomy, and in patients where a choice should be made between CABG and heart transplant.

REFERENCES

Ackerman, R. H., Correia, J. A., Alpert, N. M., Naron, J. C., Gouliamos, A., Grotta, J. C., Borownell, G. L., and Taveras, J. M., 1981, Positron imaging in ischemic stroke disease using compounds labeled with oxygen 15. Initial results of clinicophysiologic correlation, Arc. Neurol., 38:537.

Astrup, J., Symon, L., Braston, N. M., and Lassen, N., 1977, Cortical evoked and extracellular K^+ and H^+ at critical levels of brain ischemica, Stroke, 8:51.

Baron, J. C., Bousser, M. G., Guillard, A., Comar, D., and Castaigne, P., 1981a, Reversal of focal misery perfusion syndrome by EC-IC arterial bypass in hemodynamic cerebral ischemica: A case study with 15-0 positron tomography, Stroke, 12:454.

Baron, J. C., Bousser, M. G., Comar, D., Dusquenoy, N., Sastre, J., and Castaigne, P., 1981b, Crossed cerebellar diaschisis: a remote functional depression secondary to supratentorial brain infarction in man, J. Cereb. Blood Flow Metab., 1(Suppl):500.

Carter, L., Crowell, R. M., Sonntag, V. K. H., and Spetzler, R. F., 1984, Cortical blood flow during extracranial-intracranial bypass surgery, Stroke, (Suppl 5):836.

Chollet, F., Celsis, P., Clanet, M., Guiraud-Chaumeil, B., Rascol, A., and Marc-Vergnes, J. P., 1989, SPECT study of cerebral blood flow reactivity after acetazolamide in patients with transient ischemic attacks, Stroke, 20:458.

Di Piero, V., Lenzi, G. L., Collice, M., Triulzi, F., Gerundini, P., Savi, A., Fieschi, C., and Fazio, F., 1987, Long-term noninvasive SPECT monitoring of perfusional changes after EC-IC bypass surgery, J. Neurol. Neurosurg. Psychiat., 50:988.

Di Piero, V., Pozzilli, C., Pantano, P., Grasso, M. G., and Fieschi, C., Acetazolamide efffects on cerebral blood flow in acute reversible ischemia, Acta. Nerol. Scand., 80:988.

Fieschi, C., Argentino, C., and Lenzi, G. L., 1988, Therapeutic window for pharmacological treatment in acute focal cerbral ischemica: Calcium antagonist pharmacology and clinical research, Ann. NY Acad. Sci., 522.

Gibbs, J. M., Wise, R. J. S., Leenders, K. L., and Jones, T., 1984, Evaluation of cerebral perfusion reserve in patients with carotid artery occlusion, Lancet, 1:310.

Giubilei, F., Lenzi, G. L., Di Piero, V., Pozzilli, C., Pantano, P., Bastianello, S., Argentino, C., and Fieschi, C., 1990, Predictive value of brain perfusion single photon emission computed tomography in acute ischemic stroke, Stroke, 12:895.

Jones, T. H., Morawetz, R. B., Crowell, R. M., Marcoux, F. W., Fitzgibbon, S. J., De Girolami, U., and Opemann, R. G., 1981, Threshold of focal cerebral ischemica in awake monkeys, J. Nerurosurg., 54:773.

Lenzi, G. L., Frackowiak, R. S. J., and Jones, T., 1982, Cerebral oxygen metabolism and blood flow in human cerebral ischemic infarction, J. Cerebr. Blood Flow Metab., 2:321.

Meyer, J. S., Nakajima, S., and Okabe, T., 1982, Redistribution of cerebral blood flow following STA-MCA by-pass in patients with hemispheric ischemia, Stroke, 13:774.

Pantano, P., Baron, J. C., Samson, Y., Boussen, M. G., Derouesne C., and Comar, D., 1986, Crossed cerebellar diaschisis: further studies, Brain, 109:677.

Perani, D., Di Piero, V., Lucignani, G., Gilardi, M. G., Pantano, P., Rossetti, C., Pozzilli, C., Gerundini, P., Fazio, F., and Lenzi, G. L., 1988, Remote effects of subcortical cerebrovascular lesions: a SPECT cerebral perfusion study, J. Cereb. Blood Flow Metab., 8:560.

Phelps, M. E., Schelbert, H. R., and Mazziotta, J. C., 1983, Positron computed tomography for studies of myocardial and cerebral function, Ann Int. Med., 98:339.

Tanahashy, N., Meyer, J. S., Rogers, L., Kitagawa, Y., Mortel, K. F., Kandula, P., Levinthal, R., and Rose, J., 1985, Long-term assessment of cerebral perfusion following STA-MCA bypass in patients, Stroke, 16:85.

Weistein, P. R., Anderson, G. G., and Telles, D. A., 1986, Neurological deficit and cerebral infarction after temporary middle cerebral artery occlusion in anesthetized cats, Stroke, 17:318.

WHAT HAVE WE LEARNED ABOUT THE ATHEROSCLEROTIC PLAQUE USING LASER

RADIATION?

Enrico Barbieri

Institute of Cardiology
University of Verona
Verona, Italy

INTRODUCTION

The development of percutaneous transluminal angioplasty has been
a milestone in the treatment of peripheral vascular disease (1).
Nevertheless the procedure has some major limitations: 1) Inability to
cross severe occlusion; 2) a 25% - 50% restenosis rate at two years
(2); 3) scant success in diffuse atherosclerotic arteries. The ability
to ablate atherosclerotic plaques without damaging the vessel wall was
the "dream" of the first pioneers who first used laser radiation in the
cardiovascular field. Extensive experimental and human clinical studies
have been performed in the last ten years to evaluate the effect of
laser radiation on the plaque. As a consequence our knowledge of the
optical, thermal and several other properties of the normal and
diseased vessel wall has increased greatly. Some of these new
developments are considered in order to understand better the behavior
of atherosclerotic plaque during laser application and to begin to
evaluate the possible uses of this powerful tool to alter and to
measure components of the artery wall lesions using exogenous
fluorescence.

LIGHT DISTRIBUTION

Laser radiation is a monochromatic, coherent and highly
directional light beam. Hitting a tissue the light can be: reflected,
transmitted through the tissue, without producing any effect, absorbed,
with heat production or scattered from the surface or inside the
tissue. The effect of laser radiation is due to the combined action of
these factors. The tissue components which absorb light are called
chromophores and are responsible for the variability of absorbance at

different wavelengths (ua, m^{-1} is the absorption coefficient). Proteins absorb the ultraviolet wavelengths (<300 nanometers, nm); hemoglobin, carotenoids absorb the visible and near infrared (300 - 1200 nm) and water strongly absorbs in the infrared region (>1200 nm). While the absorption coefficient varies with the endogenous chromophores, the scattering of light inside the tissue (us, m^{-1}, is the scattering coefficient) decreases with the increasing wavelength. The net light tissue distribution, which follows an exponential curve, is determined by the ratio: scattering coefficient/absorption coefficient, therefore the depth of light penetration is defined as 1/ua + us (3). Among the wavelengths used in humans, excimer and CO2 wavelengths have a high absorption coefficient and a short penetration depth, while Nd: Yag penetrates deeply.

LASER RADIATION DELIVERY AND THERMAL PROPERTIES OF TISSUE

Laser parameters involved in the tissue effect are the amount of power delivered (W), the length of time of its application (sec) and the area irradiated (cm^2): energy (Joules)= W x sec., power density = W/cm^2. Laser energy can be applied in a continuous or in a pulsed way.

Continuous Wave Delivery

When the laser exposure time is longer than a few milliseconds the energy delivered is absorbed and heat production starts. The local temperature increases and tissue changes appear: enzymatic damage at 45° - 60°, coagulation necrosis at 60°- 65°, drying at 90°- 100°, carbonization at 150°and vaporization at 300°. The result is a central crater of vaporization surrounded by a thin rim of carbonization, a zone of vacuolization (polimorphous lacunae) and a zone of coagulation. Charring and vacuolization are the histologic marks of thermal damage. Evaluation of the thermal response, by an infrared camera, has allowed a better understanding of the plaque property compared to normal vessel wall. In a diseased vessel wall after argon laser delivery in a continuous wave the temperature reached by a fatty plaque is greater than that of normal artery and fibrous plaque. The reason is due to the lower thermal conductivity and diffusivity of the fatty plaque (4). The plaque acts as an insulator (5) allowing a selective ablation.

Pulsed Wave Delivery

The major disadvantage of continuous laser delivery is the thermal damage to the tissue surrounding the crater of vaporization. If the exposure is reduced below the thermal tissue diffusion time (<1 usec) with an energy per pulse above the ablation threshold (pulsed laser) and a repetition rate adequate for thermal relaxation of the tissue, the thermal damage can be reduced or eliminated. In recent years research has concentrated on the clinical application of pulsed lasers and several wavelengths can be applied in this way. The energy/photon (E) of laser radiation is higher at a short wavelength (E = h/wavelength) and some ultraviolet lasers (<350 um) have a photon/energy

higher than the peptide bond in tissue (3.6 eV). As a consequence each
pulse of an excimer laser deposits a large amount of energy (megawatts)
in tissue over a short time, breaking the intramolecular bonds
(photoablative ablation) without thermal effect.

IDENTIFICATION OF ATHEROMA. IS LASER USEFUL?

Optical Properties of Atheroma

     In an effort to ablate the atherosclerotic plaque selectively
without damaging the surrounding tissue, research on the optical
property of the arterial wall and atherosclerotic plaque has been
intensified. Optical transmission (ratio of light intensity transmitted
through tissue to saline), correlated to the sample thickness, varies
directly with wavelength. From 450 nm to 800 nm (visible wavelength
area) the optical transmission of the atherosclerotic tissue is lower
than normal vessel wall per unit thickness. The ratio of normal tissue
optical transmission to atherosclerotic plaque at the same sample
thickness as a function of wavelength in the visible range yields
valuable data. The ratio changes from 10 (at 600 - 800 nm) to 1.5 at
500 nm (6), indicating a reduction of transmission at this wavelength.
This is due to a stronger absorption by the atheroma in the region of
420 - 530 nm. The ratio of atheroma to normal aorta absorption is
largest at 470 nm, ranging from 1.5 to 3.8 (7). The explanation can be
found in the presence of chromophores (mainly carotenoids) in the fibro
fatty plaque, which preferentially absorb light at 450 - 500 nm
wavelength.

     These data are very important for several reasons: 1) A prefe-
rential absorption at 450 - 500 nm means that a selective ablation
could be obtained using a laser operating at this wavelength. The argon
laser emits at 488 - 514 nm, but can be tuned to its 488 nm line. 2)
The plaque specificity for light absorption can be increased if the
carotenoid chromophores can be enhanced, making laser ablation safer
and more effective. Human studies have shown that the administration of
180 mg beta carotene/day for one month causes a 50 - fold increase in
plaque beta carotene (8) which doubles the plaque absorption of 450 -
500 nm radiation. 3) When we deliver laser energy in vivo, the vessel
wall is in contact with blood. Hemoglobin has a typical optical
transmission spectrum with high absorbance at 410 nm (900 OD/cm), and
smaller peaks at 520 and 580 nm (9). At the argon laser wavelength the
hemoglobin absorption is lower (60 OD/cm), which means that at this
wavelength there is a window in the hemoglobin transmission property.
As a consequence argon laser radiation is poorly absorbed by the blood
and can reach the vessel wall. A result of the different absorbing
properties between normal intima and atherosclerotic plaque is the
selectivity of ablation which is several times more pronounced for
fibrofatty plaque using the 480 - 490 nm radiation at a pulse width < 50
usec. At this wavelength the ablation threshold is more than twice that
for normal intima as compared to fibrofatty plaque (10).

Fluorescence Spectroscopy

One of the more exciting areas disclosed by laser research is the ability of low power laser radiation to induce arterial fluorescence, making diagnostic fluorescence spectroscopy feasible. Fluorescence is the property of some molecules called fluorophores to be exited by the absorbed light. The excited electron returns to the ground state emitting photons of longer wavelength relative to the absorption. Several fluorophores are present in arteries: proteins, nucleic acid, coenzymes, porphyrins, carotenoids. The difference in the quantity and character of the fluorophores gives a characteristic fluorescence emission which allows the discrimination between normal and atherosclerotic vessel wall and the three layers of the artery. The low power laser induced fluorescence can be transmitted to a spectral analyzer. If the fluorescence spectrum received is compatible to plaque a computer emits, through the same fiber, a pulse of high power laser energy to ablate the target. The identification of a fluorescence spectrum compatible with the media inhibits the delivery of a subsequent pulse (11).

After several experiments performed in vitro, a dual laser system, incorporating a 325 nm laser for fluorescence spectroscopy and a 480 nm dye laser for ablation, the latter operating at 2 usec pulse width, 15 - 35 mJ/pulse, 5 pulses/sec., was used in peripheral artery human occlusions (12). The plaque showed a 30 - 50% reduction in fluorescence intesity compared to normal artery and a shift of the peak intensity from 450 nm to 470 - 475 nm. Ablation of plaque and nearness to vessel media were identified by a sudden increase of the fluorescence intensity and normal shape. Because the emitted fluorescence arises from a tissue zone of 150 um the ablation speed of the catheter should be less than this distance to avoid wall perforation, mainly in small vessels like coronary arteries. Although cost, complexity and the unsolved perforation problem make fluorescence guided laser angioplasty an experimental technique, many exciting data have been obtained on the property of the vessel wall.

Exogenous Arterial Fluorescence

Besides carotenoids other compounds, such as hematoporphyrin derivatives (13) and tetracycline, can preferentially accumulate in plaque (exogenous chromophores). After i.v. administration a 2.3 - fold increase in porphyrin was found in plaque in the aorta, when compared with normal aorta in animals. Since skin phototoxicity of hematoporphyrin derivatives is a major problem in humans, other compounds were investigated. Tetracycline preferentially binds to atherosclerotic plaque with a 4 - fold greater concentration than in normal vessel. The absorption spectrophotometry showed a peak at 355 nm, which should increase the ability of laser irradiation at a wavelength near the chromophore absorption peak to ablate the plaque with little damage to the normal artery (14). Hematoporphyrin derivatives (HPD) and tetracycline fluoresce when irradiated with ultraviolet light (HPD at 625 and 690 nm, tetracycline at 550 nm). This can allow the identification and localization of atherosclerotic plaques using angioscopy. Both the substances can be photoactivated by a wavelength that penetrates into tissue (630 nm for HPD and 355 nm for tetracycline) inducing changes in atherosclerotic plaque. The in vitro plaque ablation caused by ultraviolet radiation was 2.2. $\pm$ .25 nm in tetracycline treated plaques vs 1.3 $\pm$ .55 mm in untreated plaques. However more studies are required to allow definite statements regarding the selectivity and safety of photodynamic therapy for the treatment of atherosclerotic disease (15).

Properties of Calcified Plaque

The inability of thermal laser to ablate calcified plaque has given a major impetus to a precise identification of calcium deposits and evaluation of their optical and thermal properties.
A) Fluorescence spectroscopy of calcified artery shows a characteristic change with an autofluorescence intensity four times that of non - calcified regions (16).
B) The thermal behaviour of calcified plaque is very different from fatty plaque for several reasons: 1) the ablation process is a very slow one (the vaporization temperature for calcium is 1200 °C) 2). The thermal conductivity and thermal diffusivity of calcium are high. During continuous lasing of a calcified plaque with argon and Nd Yag the temperature rises quickly, and subsequently remains stable for several seconds till plaque disintegration. Due to the long exposure time required and the high thermal conductivity and diffusivity of calcium deposits the heat generated diffuses largely to the surrounding tissues causing extensive charring before calcium ablation. As a consequence the thermal laser systems do not work on calcified plaques. They produce severe thermal damage to the surrounding area which modifies the mechanical property of tissue, making vessel perforation easier.
Calcium salts have a broad spectrophotometric absorbance band in the range of 2.9 - 3.3 um (17) and experimental studies on bone have shown that a pulsed laser at this wavelength (2.94 um: Erb : Yag) ablates calcium precisely with minimal thermal damage. Erbium Yag laser causes a strong increase of bone internal pressure till a microexplosion occurs. The histologic aspect resembles that produced by excimer laser. But the excimer laser with its high energy ultraviolet photons causes a photodecomposition without thermal damage (18). The major problem of the Erbium laser is the fragility of the zirconium fluoride fibers required for the transmission of this wavelength.
Trying to answer the initial question about the ability of laser to identify atheroma we can say that absorbance and fluorescence spectroscopy, using a monochromatic, coherent light (laser), allow a precise identification of plaque and have given the rationale for its selective ablation.

THE LAST QUESTION TO BE ANSWERED IS: WHAT HAVE WE LEARNED FROM THE APPLICATION OF LASER RADIATION TO THE HUMAN ATHEROMA?

In the last five years several lasers have been used in humans for the treatment of atherosclerotic artery disease mainly of the lower limbs. The systems used can be divided into two groups according to the capability to ablate plaque by a photothermal or photochemical process; the majority vaporizes tissue by a thermal effect and includes all the lasers working in a continuous way (Argon, Nd Yag) coupled to bare optical fiber, optical fiber with a sapphire lens or a metal cap on its distal end (hot tip). Recent technological development of optical fiber has made the use of excimer laser in human circulation possible. The excimer laser causes a photochemical ablation with minimal or absent thermal damage.

Thermal Systems

Among the thermal systems the one most commonly used has been the "hot tip", which is really a pure thermal, and not a laser system, because laser energy is only applied to increase the temperature of the metal cap until tissue vaporization occurs. Clinical experience (19, 20, 21) has shown the ability of hot tip to recanalize occluded arteries, through a combined mechanical and thermal action. The major limitations are: 1) inability to ablate calcified plaque because of inadequate temperature, 2) severe thermal damage to surrounding area (22), mainly when calcium is present, with change of tissue mechanical property and perforation and 3) a high restenosis rate (fig. 1).

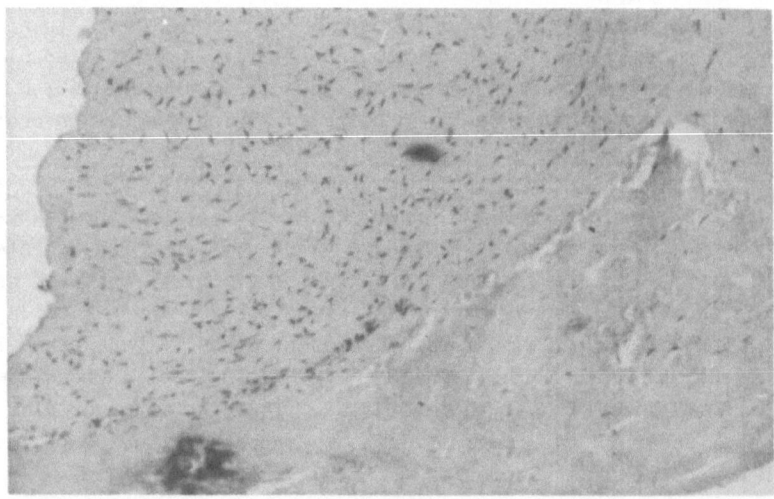

Fig. 1. Restenosis after laser thermal angioplasty.
Histology (hematoxylin eosin stain) of a sample removed by atherectomy, from site of restenosis, in a patient previously treated by hot tip laser angioplasty. On the right the atherosclerotic plaque with few cells, above it hyperplasia within a connective mixoid matrix. (by E. Barbieri).

Regarding quantification of ablation the amount of atheroma vaporized in vivo is very small. Our experience at the University of Verona in more than one hundred patients has shown that the recanalization channel obtained after lasing is very small and irregular requiring a balloon dilatation to maintain the patency of the artery.

Excimer Laser

The ability to ablate plaque using ultraviolet wavelength without thermal damage has been encouraging, due to higher safety of the system and consequently the theoretically reduced risk of perforation. Our and other experiences (23, 24, 25) in humans have shown a larger recanalization channel after lasing with the excimer laser (308 nm) , compared to the hot tip, and a lower restenosis rate, probably related to the minimal thermal damage and a more extensive plaque ablation. It is our impression that the creation of a larger channel (mean channel 1.5 - 2 mm) is mainly due to the development of a multifiber catheter. The multifiber catheter is made of several (12 - 19) small optical fibers (100 - 250 nm) concentrically arranged around a central lumen. The fibers fire at the same time delivering 12 - 20 mJ/pulse at a repetition rate of 20 - 40 Hertz. The development of larger catheters (9F) will make recanalization possible in the peripheral arteries using laser radiation without balloon dilatation.

To conclude we believe that human application of laser has shown that atheroma can be ablated, but even with all these improvements the major limit of laser therapy remains; the vessel wall perforation problem has not been solved yet. Only a precise device for identification and quantification of atheroma combined with a sophisticated delivery system, with feed-back mechanism, could allow safe and complete vaporization of the plaque without damaging normal vessel wall.

ACKNOWLEDGEMENT

I am grateful to Piero Tanganelli for his assistance in evaluating atherectomy samples.

REFERENCES

1. A. Gruntzig, D.A. Kumpe, Technique of percutaneous transluminal angioplasty with the Gruntzig balloon catheter, AJR 132:574 (1979).
2. D. M. Widlus, F. A. Osterman, Evaluation and percutaneous management of atherosclerotic peripheral vascular disease, JAMA 261:3148 (1989).
3. A. J. Welch, J. W. Valvano, J. A. Pearce, L. J. Hayes, M. Motamedi, Effect of laser radiation on tissue during laser angioplasty, Lasers Surg Med 5:251 (1985).
4. A. J. Welch, The thermal response of laser irradiated tissue, J Quantum Elec QE 20:1471 (1984).

5. J. W. Valvano, L. Hayes, A. J. Welch, S. Bajekal, D. Colvin, H. Hussein, Thermal properties of plaque and vessel wall, Lasers Surg Med 3:318 (1984).

6. T. J. Bowker , P. Edwards, T. A. Hall, M. Regel, S. G. Bown, K. M. Fox, P. Poole Wilson, A. F. Rickards, Optical transmission of normal and atheromatous arterial wall: a spectral analysis, Cardiovasc Res 20: 393 (1986).

7. M. R. Prince, T. F. Deutsch, M. M. Mathews Roth, R. Margolis, J. A. Parrish, A. R. Oseroff, Preferential light absorption in atheromas in vitro, J Clin Invest 78:295 (1986).

8. M. R. Prince, G. M. La Muraglia, E. F. MacNichol, Increased preferential absorption in human atherosclerotic plaque with oral beta carotene, Circulation 78:338 (1988).

9. I. P. Kaminow, J. M. Wiesenfeld, D. Choy: Argon laser disintegration of thrombus and atherosclerotic plaque, Appl. Optics 23:1301 (1984).

10. F. M. La Muraglia, S. Murray , R. R. Anderson, M. R. Prince, Effect of pulse duration on selective ablation of atherosclerotic plaque by 480 - to 490 nanometer laser radiation, Lasers Surg Med 8:18 (1988).

11. C. C. Hoyt, R. R. Richards Kortum, B. Costello, B. A. Sacks, C. Kitrell, N. B. Ratliff, J. R. Kramer, M. S. Feld, Remote biomedical spectroscopic imaging of human artery wall, Lasers Surg Med 8:1 (1988).

12. M. B. Leon, Y. Almagor, A. L. Bartorelli, L. G. Prevosti, P. S. Teirstein, R. Chang, D. L. Miller, P.D. Smith, R. F. Bonner, Fluorescence guided laser assisted balloon angioplasty in patients with femoropopliteal occlusions, Circulation 81:143 (1990).

13. J. R.Spears, J. Serur, D. Shropshir, S. Paulin, Fluorescence of experimental atheromathous plaques with hematoporphyrin derivate, J Clin Invest 78:395 (1986).

14. D. Murphy - Chutorian, J. Kosek, W. Mok, S. Quay, W. Huestis, J. Mehigan, D. Profitt, R. Ginsburg, Selective absorption of ultraviolet laser energy by human atherosclerotic plaque treated with tetracycline, Am J Cardiol 55:1293 (1985).

15. G. M. Vincent, G. S. Abela and E. Barbieri, Photosensitizer - enhanced laser angioplasty. In Lasers in cardiovascular medicine and surgery: fundamentals and techniques, GS Abela ed., Kluwer Academic Press, Boston (1990).

16. M Sartori, R. Sauerbrey, S. Kubodera, F. K. Tittel, R. Roberts, P.D. Henry, Autofluorescence maps of atherosclerotic human arteries. A new technique in medical imaging, J Quantum Elec QE 23:1794 (1987).

17. J. S. Nelson JS, L. Yow, L. H. Liaw, L. Macleay, R. B. Zavar, A. Orenstein, W. H. Wright, J. J. Andrews, M. W. Berns, Ablation of bone and methracrylate by a prototype mid - infrared Erbium: Yag laser. Lasers Surg Med 8:494 (1988).

18. R. C. Nuss, R. L. Fabian, R. Sarkar, C. A. Puliafito, Infrared laser bone ablation, Lasers Surg Med 8:381 (1988).

19. G. S. Abela, J. M. Seeger, E. Barbieri, D. Franzini, A. Fenech, C. J. Pepine, C. R. Conti, Laser angioplasty with angioscopic guidance in humans, J Am Coll Cardiol 8:184 (1986).

20. T. A. Sanborn, D. C. Cumberland, A. J. Greenfield, C. L. Welsh, J. K. Guben, Percutaneous laser thermal angioplasty: initial results and 1 - year follow up in 129 femoropopliteal lesions, Radiology 168:21 (1988).

21. A. Perbellini, E. Barbieri G. Taddei, A. Scuro, G. Mazzilli, S. Imperio, M. Lino, G. Destro, L. Lucchese, Recanalization of occluded peripheral arteries by "Hot tip" laser system, Vasc Surg 23:371 (1989).

22. E. Barbieri, G. S. Abela, A. I. Khoury, C. R. Conti, Temperature characteristics of laser thermal probes in the coronary circulation of dogs, Circulation 76:IV-47 (1987).

23. E. Barbieri, A. Perbellini, A. Scuro, G. Taddei, G. Mansueto, G. Bau, P. Ghini, G. Destro, Excimer laser in the treatment of peripheral artery disease: acute and short term results, 37th Meeting American College of Angiology 20, Atlanta (1990).

24. G. Biamino, G. Stefan, H. Bottcher, U. Flesch, U. Kar, K. Dorschel, P. Skarabis, M. Gross, H. Witt, G. Muller, Excimer laser revascularization: clinical results. Cardiovascular and Interventional Radiological Society of Europe, Annual Meeting 182, Brussel (1990).

25. D. Rothbaum, F. Litvach, J. Margolis, "Stand alone" percutaneous excimer laser coronary angioplasty, J Am Coll Cardiol 15:26A (1990).

NEW TECHNIQUES IN ASSESSING THE ANATOMY AND FUNCTION OF

ATHEROSCLEROSIS: PROMISES AND PITFALLS

Peter Liu

University of Toronto
Toronto, Ontario, CANADA

Diseases that are the consequences of vascular atherosclerotic process still constitute the most important cause of mortality and morbidity in the Western world. Despite advances in the understanding of the disease process [1,2], our ability to assess the early presence, the anatomical extent and functional impact of atherosclerosis is still limited. The availability of new and better tools to assess atherosclerosis will provide us with means to monitor the effectiveness of preventive and therapeutic strategies. With the recent rapid advances in technology, many modalities are now available to permit us to assess atherosclerosis with different approaches. This paper will outline these general approaches, and will concentrate on two areas of endovascular ultrasound and new myocardial perfusion agents.

PRINCIPLES OF IMAGING TECHNIQUES IN ATHEROSCLEROSIS

Assessment of The Anatomical Extent of Atherosclerotic Lesions

To examine the extent of atherosclerotic surface that impinges on the vessel lumen, the most traditional technique is *quantitative angiography*, which still constitutes the gold standard of evaluating coronary atherosclerosis. Angiography provides a high resolution longitudinal silhouette of vascular lumen, and can detect irregular atherosclerotic surfaces that impinges on the smooth outline of the vascular blood column. By using various quantitative threshold techniques, we may assess the degree of coronary stenosis in terms of diameter reduction from a single view, and percent area reduction on multiple views. However this technique markedly underestimates the anatomical extent of atherosclerosis when compared to pathological evaluation or intra-operative ultrasound studies [3,4]. Quantitative angiography also becomes extremely complex when dealing with multiple lesions that have irregular surfaces. Despite these limitations, arteriography has been successful in demonstrating the regression of atherosclerosis in major secondary prevention trials [5-7].

To better assess the in vivo lumenal surface of atherosclerosis, the advances in fiberoptic technology provided us with *coronary angioscopy*. The introduction of a flexible angioscope into the coronary arteries for the first time permitted direct visualization of arterial surface activities in patients with coronary artery atherosclerosis [8,9]. In addition to confirming the extent of atherosclerosis underestimated by angiography, this technique also identified plaque ulceration and thrombus as part of the complex atherosclerotic plaques. The precise correlation of these findings with various clinical syndromes has permitted the reconstruction of the pathogenesis of unstable angina and myocardial infarction.

Unfortunately, the disadvantage of image distortion, inability to quantitate dimensions, the requirement of a continuously flushed field in current generation of angioscopes will probably limit the use of angioscopy as a means to assess progression of disease.

Assessment of Tissue Components of Atherosclerotic Lesions

The pathology of atherosclerotic lesions is usually complex, and consists of a heterogeneous collection of lipids, fibrous and nonfibrous connective tissues, and calcified matrix [1], with cellular proliferation and thrombus formation. The contents of these components are related to the age and activity of the individual plaque. Realizing the limitations of surface sensitive techniques, newer methods that can assess the full thickness of the lesions with the ability to characterize tissue components constitute a major promise. Examples of these techniques include ultrasound and nuclear magnetic resonance (NMR).

Ultrasound images are formed from reflections of sound waves at interfaces of tissues with different acoustic-impedance. Because the various components of the atherosclerotic lesions have different acoustic properties, ultrasound can provide a clue to the location and composition of the plaques in addition to the degree of lumenal narrowing. Ultrasound has been applied to both epicardial coronary vessels during open heart operations [4], as well as intravascularly through percutaneous catheterization [10]. The latter will constitute the second major component of this discussion.

Another technique that may show significant promise is *nuclear magnetic resonance* (NMR) imaging/spectroscopy. NMR imaging is sensitive to both the quantity of hydrogen nuclei and its chemical environment of hydrogen nuclei. NMR imaging has high discriminatory powers amongst calcium, fat, and water components in the tissues. Imaging of atherosclerosis in the aorta has already shown significant promise in identifying various components of atherosclerosis. The evolving capability of combining imaging with spectroscopy adds further potential to this technique. However, its use in smaller peripheral vessels such as the carotid or coronary arteries is limited by spatial resolution. Many technical challenges will need to be met before wider applications to this very important field can be carried out.

Assessment of Metabolic Activities of Lesions

One of the visionary goals in the assessment of atherosclerosis is a means to define the metabolic activity of individual lesions, and to predict their potential biological behavior. In recent pathology studies, macrophages have been shown to play a major role in the transformation of the fatty streaks, as well as lymphocyte infiltration. Using immunohistochemical techniques, various specific antigenic components of the atherosclerotic lesions have been identified, and their role in its pathogenesis clarified. Imaging approaches in this area are very preliminary, although some studies have demonstrated the feasibility of using *labeled LDL* as a tracer to identify atherosclerotic lesions and the active sites of LDL metabolism [11]. *Monoclonal antibodies* against components of the atherosclerotic plaque have also been used, such as antibodies to LDL or other components. Furthermore, *labelling blood components* such as platelets using In-111 oxime has been attempted in the carotid and peripheral arteries to localize the site of early platelet adhesion and potential sites of thrombus formation. The success of these techniques will depend on the specificity of the label, and the ability to provide high enough target to background activity. Significant progress will need to be made in this area before clinical applications become feasible.

Assessment of Functional Consequences of Atherosclerotic Lesions

The imaging techniques discussed thus far offer assessment of morphology of individual atherosclerotic plaques, but do not offer information on the functional consequences of the presence of the lesion. Ultimately, it is the compromise of blood flow that results in morbidity and mortality. Techniques which assess the functional consequences of atherosclerotic narrowing confer a more global picture of the total atherosclerotic burden, while reflecting on the extent and severity of the underlying disease process. Techniques of assessment generally are all based on the principle that vessels involved with atherosclerosis will lose their normal endothelially mediated vasodilatory function. Under situations of increased demand in blood flow, these vessels will fail to dilate adequately. This is termed "decreased vasodilator reserve." This concept can be assessed in the cardiac catheterization laboratory by selective infusion of *intracoronary acetylcholine* and assessing the degree of vasodilatation following infusion [12]. Severely atherosclerotic vessels with destruction of normal endothelial will paradoxically constrict on exposure to acetylcholine.

Vasodilator reserve can also be assessed by placing a *Doppler coronary flow catheter* in the proximal portions of the artery, and produce vasodilatation using smooth muscle vasodilators such as papaverine or dipyridamole. However, to assess these processes non-invasively, the use of *regional myocardial perfusion tracers* in combination with stress has become the major clinical technique of detecting the presence of coronary artery disease. Myocardial perfusion tracers currently used include thallium, sestamibi (Dupont) and teboroxime (Squibb).

ENDOVASCULAR ULTRASOUND IN CORONARY ARTERIES

Significant progress has been made over the past few years in the development of ultrasound catheters that can be introduced percutaneously to assess atherosclerotic plaques. This technique combines the advantages of anatomic assessment of coronary atherosclerosis, with the ability to detect the components of atherosclerotic plaque below the surface. The image information is provided by this method in real time, and can be interfaced easily with interventional procedures. The tomographic sections of the vessel wall can also be integrated to provide a 3-D representation of the atherosclerotic segment.

Principles of Endovascular Ultrasound

Ultrasound images are formed by reflection and refraction of high frequency sound waves meeting tissues of differing acoustic impedances. Endovascular ultrasound devices are constructed as miniature ultrasound probes located at the end of a catheter. Typically, the ultrasound frequency of these instruments is in the range of 20-40 MHz with a resolution of 0.25 mm. The penetration of the sound waves into the vessel wall is limited to distances immediately below the surface, and therefore is ideally suited for small vessels such as the coronary arteries. All existing catheters emit sound at 90° from the catheter perpendicular to the vessel wall. Thus the images are representations of the 360° section immediately surrounding the tip of the catheter. Current devices can only offer cross-sectional anatomy without forward viewing capabilities.

Currently available devices generally fall into two major design categories. The first is a mechanical system composed of rotating ceramic crystals at the tip of the catheter or stationary crystals with rotating mirrors operating at speeds of 700-1800 rpm (figure 1). Due the presence of a motor, these catheters tend to be larger in size (minimum 5.5F). The second is a phased array system with electronic sequential multi-crystal activation, such that the crystals are fired in prescribed a sequence to collect information circumferentially (figure 2). The advantage of this type of system is that it has few moving parts, and can be further miniaturized. Currently, the ultrasound catheters are independent systems that are flexible enough to be introduced into coronary arteries. They can be introduced either directly, through a guiding sheath or advanced over a guidewire through a central lumen. Several centers have successfully obtained images from human coronary arteries, and has established the safety of this imaging device in the clinical realm [13].

Endovascular Ultrasound Development to Date

The development of endovascular ultrasound arose from a need to define accurately the characteristics of atheroma. Assessment of primary and secondary prevention strategies requires an accurate delineation of atherosclerosis severity. Ultrasound characterization of atherosclerotic plaques has been carried out previously. The most notable work has been done in the operating room where high frequency ultrasound probes are placed on the epicardial arteries to assess characteristics of the atheroma [4].

These landmark studies have established a relationship between the ultrasound and the angiographic measurements. It has also demonstrated ability for ultrasound techniques to assess the entire vascular thickness from intima to adventitia. In addition, they have provided further striking in vivo evidence that the degree of atherosclerosis is always more diffuse and advanced than that depicted on angiography. In fact in areas of "normal vessels" on the angiogram, there may be very extensive atherosclerotic disease. These studies also highlighted the observation that eccentric lesions may in fact have preserved vasoactivity in the normal wall segment, and that progressing lesions remodel the artery to increase its lumenal area to accommodate this growth as previously noted [14].

Image Characteristics in Normal Arteries

As shown in excised pathological samples and now confirmed in patients, normal coronary arteries are represented on endovascular ultrasound as bright circular vessel wall with a three layered appearance. The lumen is usually signal free, and the catheter itself appears as a small circular ring as a reference. Controversy still exists regarding the exact cause of the three layer appearance. However, it does appear that the inner layer represents the blood interface with intima with the majority of the echoes arising from the internal elastic lamina. The middle layer is usually hypoechoic and represents the muscular media. Finally, the outer layer represents the combination of external elastic lamina and adventitia. Thus far, studies of anatomic specimens have found excellent correlation of endovascular ultrasound dimensional measurements with anatomical standards [10,15]. Resulting data can be expressed as lumen diameter, lumen area, wall thickness and percent area stenosis. This has also now been validated in patients when compared to coronary angiography [15].

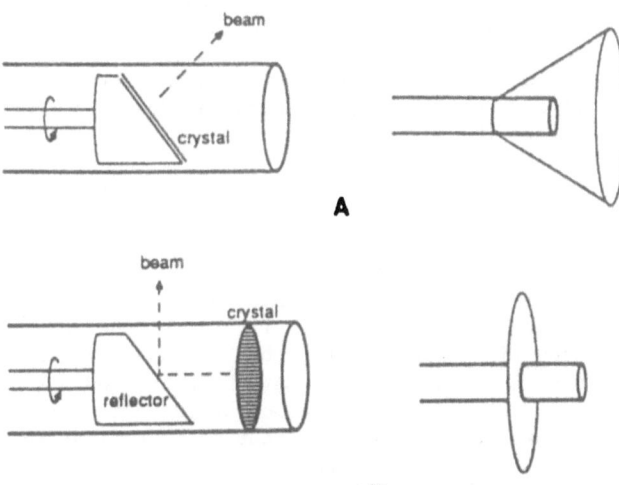

Figure 1.   Diagram of a currently available mechanical system of delivering
intravascular ultrasound. The system consists of either rotating
crystals attached to a high speed motor, or fixed crystals with
rotating mirror. These systems have the advantage of simpler
mechanics and high sample rates.

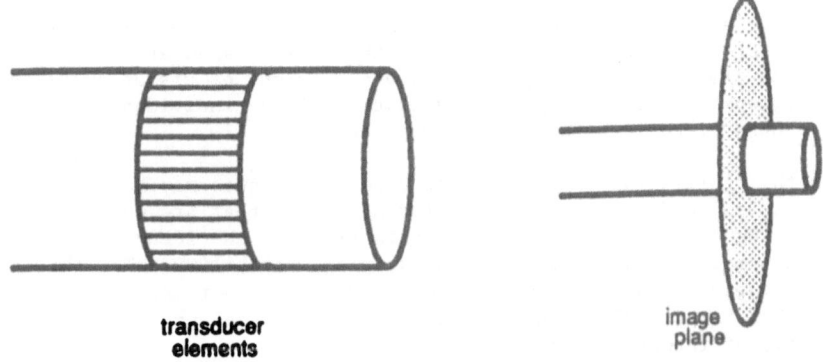

Figure 2. Diagram of the currently available phased array system for intravascular ultrasound. The transducer elements are aligned radially on
the shaft, and the order of crystal emission is electronically
controlled. The advantage is the lack of moving parts and the
potential for miniaturization.

Image Characteristics of Atherosclerotic Coronary Arteries

Endovascular ultrasound has also been successful in assessing the plaque morphology. Ultrasound can detect the proliferating intima by an increase in intimal thickness (figure 3), fibrosis and calcification, as these generally have more echogenic characteristics than the surrounding structures. It can also detect necrotic lipid tissue lakes, which can be found as zones devoid of echoes in the medial layer [10,13,15].

A further strength of ultrasound may lie in its ability to characterize tissue. In terms of the degree of echo reflectance and the acoustic shadow it casts, one may distinguish calcified plaques from fibrous or lipid laden tissues. In terms of the three tissue types, calcified plaques give the most intensive echoes with significant acoustic shadowing or attenuation of the signal distal to the plaque (figure 4). Both fibrous tissue and lipid structures show much less acoustic shadowing, but the fibrous tissue component is much more echogenic than is lipid. Studies have been carried out to assess the predicted accuracy for plaque identification based on these ultrasound tissue characterization criteria. From one group of investigators, the accuracy of plaque identification which compared to pathology was 96% [15]. The only errors occurred in areas beyond calcified plaques, where acoustic shadowing led to erroneous conclusions.

Another potential area of application for endovascular ultrasound is the assessment of interventional procedures. Studies have thus far demonstrated the ability for ultrasound to detect and quantitate the presence of coronary thrombus, exhibited as granular echoes. Therefore, it offers major promise in the ability to assess acute coronary thrombosis, as well as thrombus formation following interventions such as laser or balloon angioplasty. Furthermore, models of intimal tear and intimal flap formation have also demonstrated the accuracy with which ultrasound can detect these common complications following angioplasty. This is especially useful in situations where this procedure can be combined with interventional techniques. The accuracy of assessing these complications is comparable to although does not exceed that of angioscopy.

Advantages of Endovascular Ultrasound

The major advantages of ultrasound compared to other modalities that can assess atherosclerosis are visualization of the entire vascular wall thickness, accurate dimensional measurements, and assessment of tissue characteristics. These capabilities will permit evaluation of the individual lesions and the total atherosclerotic burden in a given patient.

With the realization that different types of plaques may have different natural histories, and that it is lipid-laden lesions that are more likely to rupture, leading to acute coronary thrombosis [16,17], the identification of this type of lesion may allow estimations of plaque stability. The ability of real time vascular measurements can be combined with either mechanical or pharmacological interventions, to assess underlying vessel physiology as a research tool, or interventions as a therapeutic maneuver.

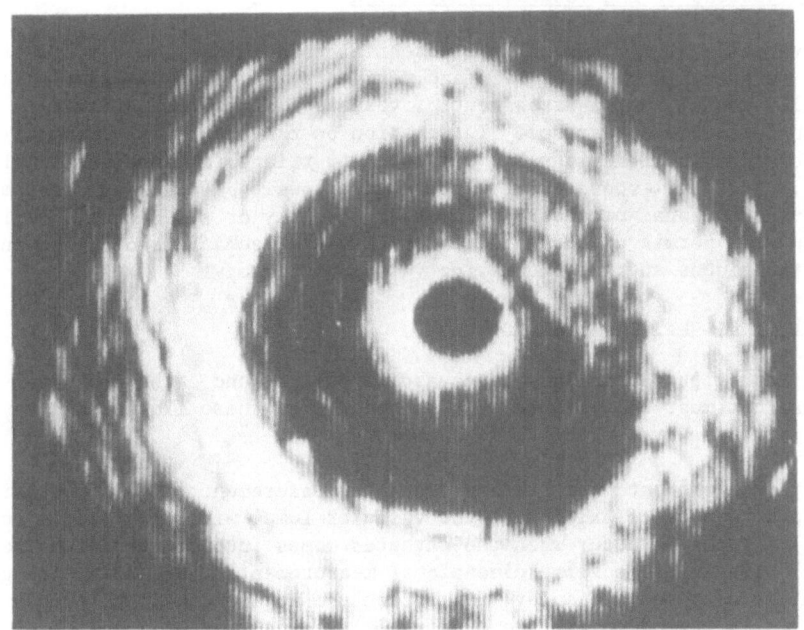

Figure 3.   *Example of intravascular ultrasound image from human coronary with fibrous plaque present. The vessel has the typical 3 layer appearance with intimal thickening and bright internal elastic lamina, while the atherosclerotic plaque is more echogenic and localized to one portion of vessel.*

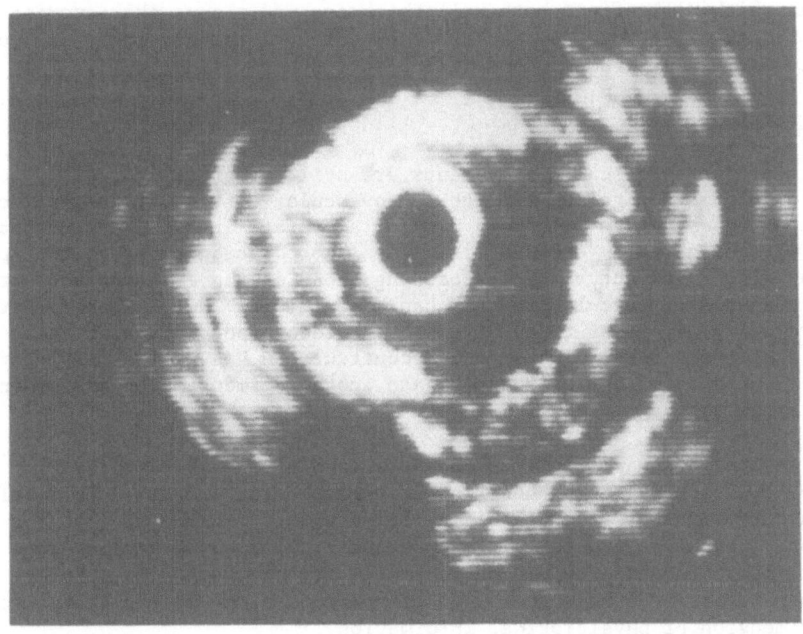

Figure 4.   *Example of a severely calcified plaque with extremely bright echoes accompanied by acoustic shadowing beyond the calcium. Otherwise the large lipid lakes and fibrous tissues are as noted previously.*

Current Indications of Endovascular Ultrasound

Endovascular ultrasound has the potential to document atherosclerotic extent and severity in both coronary and peripheral vascular diseases. This is especially useful in the assessment of vessels that have apparently "normal" angiographic appearance. Information on the exact tissue characteristics of individual lesions may allow better triage for interventional procedures. Finally, endovascular ultrasound allows the follow-up assessment after an interventional procedure such as angioplasty or atherectomy. This information will permit us to better understand the mechanisms of these interventional techniques and the underlying vessel physiology.

Potential Limitations of Ultrasound

Despite obvious advantages, endovascular ultrasound catheters have limitations that must be realized. It is hoped that these limitations may be overcome in future versions of these catheters.

First and foremost, for achieve accurate measurement, it is imperative that the catheters be co-axial with the vascular lumen without adhering to the vessel wall. Problems occur when the catheter comes into contact with the vessel wall, leading to a false dimensional measurements. Secondly, the gain setting on the ultrasound display will affect the apparent wall thickness and may artificially introduce extraneous signals arising from adjacent structures. This is especially a problem in large vessels where high gain settings are necessary to penetrate the vessel.

Currently available catheters are of large size (minimum 3.5 French), confining them to only proximal large coronary vessels. However, modifications in the future may further miniaturize the catheter assembly. As previously mentioned, calcified plaques do have significant acoustic shadow beyond the plaque which will affect both wall thickness and tissue characterization. Finally, the exact structures that are echogenic are not precisely nor quantitatively defined at present, and will need further validation.

Future Directions

Significant technical improvements are still progressing rapidly to increase the information gained from the endovascular ultrasound examination. Forward-looking catheters will have a major advantage in assessing coronary stenosis without actually crossing it. The incorporation of synthetic aperture array will allow actual depth focusing ahead of the catheter to further increase the area of vasculature that can be examined. Multiplane catheter probes are being developed to observe along a second perpendicular short axis plane to facilitate three-dimensional reconstruction, as well as examination along the long axis of the catheter to add another dimension of assessment to stenotic areas.

To enhance plaque definition, computerized tissue characterization will add to the decision-making process in the treatment of plaques. This will allow ultrasound catheters the capability to precisely monitor progression or regression of atherosclerosis. Incorporation of ultrasound devices into angioplasty, laser and atherectomy devices will further facilitate these ultrasound studies. Perhaps these can be combined with Doppler probes to add another dimension of physiological information.

The assessment of regional myocardial perfusion using radiolabeled tracers provides information on functional consequences of atherosclerosis. This still forms the cornerstone of clinical decision making in atherosclerotic coronary disease, even in this era of interventional cardiology [18,19].

General Principles of Myocardial Perfusion Tracers

To be useful as a myocardial perfusion tracer, the tracer must distribute linearly with myocardial blood flow, but also have adequate residency time in the myocardium to allow proper image acquisition. Myocardial perfusion will in addition, reflect the degree of atherosclerosis, the vascular tone, vasomotion, presence of collaterals and other factors affecting coronary flow. To increase the sensitivity of detecting coronary atherosclerosis, it is routine to combine myocardial perfusion assessment with stress (e.g. exercise, dipyridamole, or adenosine) to maximally exhibit the differences in myocardial flow reserve.

New Myocardial Tracers to Assess Myocardial Perfusion

Traditionally, thallium-201 has been the myocardial tracer of choice. However thallium has several major drawbacks in assessing the degree of coronary atherosclerosis with high precision. Due to its relatively low energy emission (68-80 Kev) and poor dosimetry, the resolution is relatively poor. Therefore, thallium is only useful in detecting large areas of myocardial hypoperfusion.

With the advent of improvements in radiochemistry, newer technetium labeled myocardial perfusion agents are now available. The advantage of technetium is that it is a high energy isotope (140 Kev), and more ideally suited to the current generation of gamma cameras. Furthermore, because of the shorter half-life of technetium, large doses of the tracer can be given, thus vastly improving the target to background ratio in addition to better resolution.

New myocardial perfusion agents of this category include technetium-99m (Tc-99m) sestamibi (methoxy-isobutyl-isonitrile) and technetium-99m teboroxime; both of these compounds are complexed ligands of technetium and are myocardial seeking agents. However, their myocardial kinetics are completely different. Tc-sestamibi is taken up by the myocardium with a first pass extraction fraction of 65% [20]. Once it is taken up by the viable myocardium, it binds avidly to an intracellular binding site, and remains stable in the myocardium for a significant duration of time [21]. Therefore, once sestamibi has been injected, it "locks in" the myocardial perfusion pattern, and does not change significantly with time, having an extremely slow clearance. This has the advantage that myocardial image can be carried out with time flexibility, and excellent tomographic images can be obtained due to the stability of the images.

Technetium-99m teboroxime is an extremely lipophylic compound that is extracted by the myocardium about 90% of a given dose on first pass extraction [22]. However, it has an extremely short myocardial residence with the first component half life of only 9 1/2 minutes [23]. Therefore, seconds after the agent is given, it localizes to the myocardium initially, and begins to clear quickly. This necessitates rapid imaging techniques to capture the myocardial perfusion. This substance has the advantage of allowing repeat studies to monitor changes in coronary blood flow [24].

To further enhance the ability to detect coronary artery stenosis, the use of positron-emitting isotopes have come to the forefront. They have the advantage of higher emitting energy with little tissue attenuation. Absolute tracer quantitation can be theoretically obtained. With the availability of generator derived isotopes such as Rubidium-82, it is now possible to obtain positron images of myocardial perfusion with relative ease [25,26]. Recent studies from several PET centers have demonstrated the superiority of rubidium over traditional gamma-based radiotracers. Despite these advantages, PET scanners are still limited in resolution to about 5 mm, and the cost of PET facilities will prohibit this method from becoming a widespread tool to assess atherosclerosis.

Advantages of Using Myocardial Perfusion Tracers

Compared to other modalities used in the assessment of atherosclerosis, myocardial perfusion studies have the advantage of being non-invasive, reproducible and have excellent correlations with invasive studies such as angiography. In addition, it combines anatomic information with functional assessment of the impact of coronary atherosclerosis on overall myocardial perfusion. Clinically myocardial perfusion has been useful as a screening tool to determine who needs angiography, and to assess the physiological impact of a given anatomical lesion, once the patient has had angiography. Also it can be used to follow patients serially, and to reflect the impact of treatment on atherosclerosis.

Limitations of Using New Myocardial Perfusion Tracers

Despite better imaging characteristics, the radionuclide perfusion tracers still lack resolution in terms of localizing coronary lesions. Furthermore they generally detect only hemodynamically important lesions, typically exceeding 50% in anatomic stenosis diameter. This would exclude perfusion techniques from detecting extremely early atherosclerosis, but will be useful in monitoring relatively severe disease. Another limitation in the assessment of diffuse atherosclerosis is that perfusion physiology can be intrinsically variable with influence from drugs, blood pressure changes, circadian rhythm, etc., and these factors must be controlled if serial studies are to be carried out.

Examples of Use of Perfusion Tracers to Detect Complications of Coronary Disease

Many reports have been published on the accuracy of myocardial perfusion studies in detecting coronary disease [27,28]. We and others have used these techniques to detect patients with silent ischemia [29], and to screen for early restenosis following angioplasty [30,31]. The availability of the new tracers will allow better detection of coronary disease, and better follow-up of complications from interventional procedures.

These tracers can also be used to assess complications of atherosclerosis such as acute coronary occlusions and the effect of thrombolytic therapy on reperfusion [32,33]. With the improvement of future tracers in terms of myocardial kinetic properties, better non-invasive information on the effect from intervention can be assessed.

CONCLUSIONS

We are at an exciting juncture in time where rapid advances in imaging technology combined with new understandings of physiology and pathology allow us opportunities to better assess coronary atherosclerosis. The anatomic modalities combined with tissue characterization will have significant long-term impact in research in interventional studies and ultimately on clinical practice. Functional and metabolic assessment will be important in determining the physiological impact of the atherosclerotic disease, and in clinical outcome. Understanding the advantages and limitations of these techniques will provide the investigator and clinician

REFERENCES

1. R. Ross, The pathogenesis of atherosclerosis - An update, N Engl J Med. 314:488-500 (1986).
2. D. Steinberg, S. Parthasarathy, T.E. Carew, J.C. Khoo, and J.L. Witztum, Beyond cholesterol: Modifications of low-density lipoprotein that increase its atherogenicity. N Engl J Med. 320:915-924 (1989).
3. C.M. Gondin, I. Dydra, A. Pasternac, L. Campeau, M.G. Bourassa, and J. Lesperance. Discrepancies between cineangiographic and postmortem findings in patients with coronary artery disease and recent myocardial revascularization. Circulation 49:703-713 (1974).
4. D. D. McPherson, L.F. Hiratzka, W.C. Lamberth, B. Brandt, M. Hunt, R.A. Kieso, M.L. Marcus, and R.E. Kerber, Delineation of the extent of coronary atherosclerosis by high frequency epicardial echocardiography, N Engl J Med. 316:304-309 (1987).
5. D.H. Blankenhorn, S.A. Nessim, R.L. Johnson, M.E. Sanmarco, S.P. Azen, and L. Cashin-Hemphill, Beneficial effects of combined colestipol-niacin therapy on coronary atherosclerosis and coronary venous bypass grafts, JAMA. 257:3233-3240 (1987).
6. B.G. Brown, J.T. Lin, S.M. Schaefer, C.A. Kaplan, H.T. Dodge, and J.J. Albers, Niacin or lovastatin, combined with colestipol, regress coronary atherosclerosis and prevent clinical events in men with elevated apolipoprotein, Circulation 80(II):266 (1989).
7. A. Loaldi, A. Polese, P. Montorsi, N. De Cesare, F. Fabbiocchi, P. Ravagnani, and M.D. Guazzi, Comparison of nifedipine, propranolol and isosorbide dinitrate on angiographic progression and regression of coronary arterial narrowings in angina pectoris, Am J Cardiol. 64:433-43 (1989).
8. J.S. Forrester, F. Litvack, W. Grundfest, and A. Hickey, A perspective of coronary disease seen through the arteries of living man. Circulation 3:505-513 (1987).
9. C.T. Sherman, F. Litvack, W.S. Grundfest, M. Lee, A. Hickey, A. Chaux, R. Kass, C. Blanche, J. Matloff, L. Morgenstern, W. Ganz, H.J.C. Swan, and J. Forrester. Demonstration of thrombus and complex atheroma by in-vivo angioscopy in patients with unstable angina pectoris, N Engl J Med. 315:913 (1986).
10. N.G. Pandian, A. Kreis, B. Brockway, J.M. Isner, A. Sacharoff, E. Boleza, R. Caro, and D. Muller, Ultrasound angioscopy: Real-time two-dimensional, intraluminal ultrasound imaging of blood vessel, Am J Cardiol 62:493-494 (1988).
11. A.M. Lees, R.S. Lees, and F.J. Schoen, Imaging human atherosclerosis with Tc-99m-labeled low density lipoproteins. Arteriosclerosis 8:461-470 (1988).
12. P.L. Ludmer, A.P. Selwyn, T.L. Shook, R.R. Wayne, G.H. Mudge, R.W. Alexander, and P. Ganz, Paradoxical vasoconstriction induced by acetylcholine in atherosclerotic coronary arteries, N Engl J Med. 315:1046-1051 (1986).
13. N.G. Pandian, Intravascular and intracardiac ultrasound imaging: An old concept, now on the road to reality, Circulation 80:1091-1094 (1989).
14. S. Glagov, E. Weisenberg, C.K. Zarins, R. Stankunavicius, and G.J. Kolettis, Compensatory enlargement of human atherosclerotic coronary arteries, N Engl J Med. 316:1371-1375 (1987).

15. B.N. Potkin, A.L. Bartorelli, J.M. Gessert, R.F. Neville, Y. Almagor, W.C. Roberts, and M.B. Leon, Coronary artery imaging with intravascular high-frequency ultrasound, Circulation 81:1575-1585 (1990).

16. J.A. Ambrose, S.L. Winters, and A. Stern, Angiographic morphology and the pathogenesis of unstable angina pectoris, J Am Coll Cardiol. 5:609-616 (1985).

17. M.J. Davies, N. Woolf, P.M. Rowles, and J. Pepper, Morphology of the endothelium over atherosclerotic plaques in human coronary arteries, Br Heart J. 60:459-464 (1988).

18. D.S. Berman, H. Kiat, J. Maddahi, and P.K. Shah, Radionuclide imaging of myocardial perfusion and viability in assessment of acute myocardial infarction, Am J Cardiol. 64:9B-16B (1989).

19. G.A. Beller, Noninvasive assessment of myocardial salvage after coronary reperfusion: a perpetual quest of nuclear cardiology, J Am Coll Cardiol. 14:874-876 (1989).

20. J.A. Leppo, and D.J. Meerdink, Comparison of the myocardial uptake of a technetium-labeled isonitrile analogue and thallium, Circ Res. 65:632-639 (1989).

21. R. Beanlands, F. Dawood, W.H. Wen, P.R. McLaughlin, J. Butany, and P. Liu, Are the kinetics of technetium 99m-methoxy isobutyl isonitrile affected by cell metabolism and viability? Circulation (in press) (1990).

22. J.A. Leppo, and D.J. Meerdink, Comparative myocardial extraction of two technetium-laeled BATO derivatives (SQ30217,SQ32014) and thallium, J Nucl Med. 31:67-74 (1990).

23. R.K. Narra, A.D. Nunn, B.L. Kuczynski, T. Feld, P. Wedeking, and W.C. Eckelman, A neutral technetium-99m complex for myocardial imaging, J Nucl Med. 30:1830-1837 (1989).

24. D.W. Seldin, L.L. Johnson, D.K. Blood, M.J. Muschel, K.F. Smith, R.M. Wall, and P.J. Cannon, Myocardial perfusion imaging with technetium-99m SQ30217: Comparison with thallium-201 and coronary anatomy, J Nucl Med. 30:312-319 (1989).

25. A.P. Selwyn, K.M. Allen, A. L'Abbate, P. Horlock, P. Camici, J. Clark, H.A. O'Brien, and P.M. Grant, Relationship between regional myocardial uptake of Rb-82 and perfusion: Absolute reduction of cation uptake in ischemia, Am J Cardiol 50:112 (1982).

26. H.R. Schelbert, M.E. Phelps, S.C. Huang, N.S. MacDonald, H. Husen, C. Selin, and D.E. Kuld, N-13 ammonia as an indicator of muyocardial blood flow, Circulation 63:1259 (1981).

27. P.C. Albro, K.L. Gould, R.J. Westcott, G.W. Hamilton, J.L. Ritchie, and D.L. Williams, Noninvasive assessment of coronary stenoses by myocardial imaging during pharmacologic coronary vasodilatation. III. Clinical trial, Am J Cardiol. 42:751-760 (1978).

28. E. DePasquale, A. Nody, G. DePuey, E. Garcia, G. Pilcher, C. Bredleau, G. Roubin, A. Gober, A. Gruentzig, P. D'Amato, and H. Berger, Quantitative rotational thallium-201 tomography for identifying and localizing coronary artery disease, Circulation 77:316-327 (1988).

29. D. Fell, J. Goodman, P.R. McLaughlin, L. Harris, S. Houle, M. Chin, B. Ross, R. Holloway, and P. Liu, Modification of silent and exercise induced ischemia by diltiazem in stable coronary disease, Circulation 78:326 (1988).

30. D.D. Miller, P. Liu, P.C. Block, H.W. Strauss, C.A. Boucher, and R.D. Okada, Prognostic value of exercise thallium imaging early after percutaneous transluminal coronary angioplasty (PTCA): quantitative and qualitative analysis, J Am Coll Cardiol 5:532 (1985).

31. D.D. Miller, P. Liu, H.W. Strauss, P.C. Block, R.D. Okada, and C.A. Boucher, Prognostic value of computer-quantitated exercise thallium imaging early after percutaneous transluminal coronary angioplasty, J Am Coll Cardiol 10:275-283 (1987).

32. R.J. Gibbons, M.S. Verani, T. Behrenbeck, P.A. Pellikka, M.K. O'Connor, J.J. Mahmarian, J.H. Chesebro, and F.J. Wackers, Feasibility of tomographic 99mTc-hexakis-2-methoxy-2-methylpropyl-isonitrile imaging for the assessment of myocardial area at risk and the effect of treatment in acute myocardial infarction, _Circulation_ 80:1277-1286 (1989).

33. F.J. Wackers, R.J. Gibbons, M.S. Verani, D.S. Kayden, P.A. Pellikka, T. Behrenbeck, J.J. Mahmarian, and B.L. Zaret, Serial quantitative planar technetium-99m isonitrile imaging in acute myocardial infarction: efficacy for noninvasive assessment of thrombolytic therapy, _J Am Coll Cardiol_ 14:861-873 (1989).

Summary of Discussion following Session 3

Rubba in discussing Poli's paper indicated that he was puzzled about the relationship between wall thickness in the carotid artery and its function as an indirect marker of disease. Poli pointed out that up to the present time he could not be sure that wall thickness reflects atherosclerotic involvement of the artery. He pointed out that attempts are being made to correlate these measurements with atherosclerotic thickening at the histopathological level. He also pointed out that the system he is using is known as Biosound; he and his colleagues perform their quantitative measurements from a video print of the ultrasound images which have been recorded and then enlarged by means of a photographic technique. This makes it easier to establish precise points and exact edges from which surfaces and length determinations can be made.

The discussion then turned to Kramsch's paper and he was asked to give the specific criteria for defining a new lesion and for determining what happens in the case of two neighboring lesions with a small valley between them. Kramsch pointed out that they really do not have the means of defining a new lesion with certainty by arteriography under these circumstances and that when these lesions appear at branch points, the computer cannot be utilized very effectively to define the development of new plaques. He also pointed out that in the systems they are using they have not counted the number of lesions so that they confine their analyses to a subjective decision as to when new lesions develop. Lenzi indicated that many workers in the field believe that one has to have a certain position of the neck in order to make valid interpretations of the carotid artery images. Kramsch stated that the arteriography had not been utilized successfully so far for quantitative studies of the carotid artery, popliteal artery, and the brachial arteries, and that studies at the University of Southern California are utilizing angiography only for coronaries. Paulin indicated his doubts that the angiographic findings reported thus far really indicated regression of atherosclerotic lesions. Kramsch pointed out that the progressive nature of regression between two and four years helped add confidence that these favorable changes were occurring. He pointed out that several groups have now reported angiographic evidence of regression so that at least it appears as if the early results are being confirmed.

The discussion then turned to Landini's presentation and Mercuri inquired about Landini's instrumentation and whether the system of analysis that he is using would be applicable for clinical purposes. Landini pointed out that in their studies thus far they have performed an amplification that is controlled and directed by the operator as the signal is transferred to the computer. Therefore, their results are independent of the setting of the machine. They avoid logarithmic, i.e., non-linear amplifications, and this gives a satisfactory representation of the image. The instrumentation that Landini employs also makes it possible to develop analyses which are much more sophisticated than those which have been obtained with the conventional instrument. Their major problem at present is with signal to noise ratio and certain artifacts which are not easy to avoid. Wissler pointed out that he admires the types of exploration that Landini is pursuing because it should lead to a greater understanding of the nature of the lesions that one images with B-mode ultrasound. He encouraged the use of both chemical analyses and histological and histochemical examinations of the lesions, which are imaged when the opportunity presents itself, in order to verify the types of fibro-fatty or fatty-fibro interpretations which are being made. He also indicated that it is important to understand that one is dealing with a spectrum and not with separate stages, a truth that is revealed if one studies a succession of lesions with fat stains. He outlined the methods being used in the PDAY studies. These make it possible to define the lesions histologically and at the same time have high resolution fat stains and a quantitative analysis of the components of both fibrous and fatty components of the developing plaque such as the quantitative assessment of the types of cells present and the amounts of intra and extracellular lipid. Landini responded that he hoped that with time he would be able to develop these kinds of quantitative tissue characterizations to aid in the understanding of the ultrasound images. Paulin indicated that if the tissue analysis by means of radiofrequency signals is hampered by the distance of the object to the transducer, the same kinds of analyses should be possible in the femoral artery with no more problems than one experiences in the carotid studies. Landini indicated that he believed there would be more artifacts and problems with the femoral artery than with the carotid.

Following the presentations by Lenzi and Pontano there was a brief question and answer period, initiated first by Rubba. He discussed the advantages of the transcranial doppler for evaluating flow from the middle cerebral artery, and Lenzi responded by indicating that many patients cannot be studied with the transcranial doppler. Although the transcranial doppler is an excellent technique in the hands of very experienced physicians, there are major problems when one tries to compare the results from the same laboratory at two different times or from different laboratories. Finally, he said that the quantification of data is much better with SPECT.

Following Barbieri's presentation, Wissler asked him to describe a little more fully the diagnostic laser and how it might compare, as it continues to be developed, with other diagnostic devices such as the ones involving ultrasound or various forms of angiographic imaging of contrast media. Barbieri responded that he thought that at the present time it was very difficult to compare the various established methods of imaging with the diagnostic laser but that it was important to note that with the optical fiber one can go along the circulatory system. Theoretically, with a very small optical fiber, one could go almost anywhere that atherosclerosis might occur. He indicated that the circulating blood could pose problems because the optical fiber might read the blood instead of the artery wall. He also pointed out that because the spectra of blood are quite different from the vessel wall and from the atheroma, one can certainly identify when blood is interfering.

Wissler went on to inquire about the guidance systems for the diagnostic laser and Barbieri said it is still a major problem because fluoroscopy is not an adequate guiding system and angioscopy clearly has great problems, especially when one works with the smaller branches of the coronary artery. He agreed that intravascular ultrasound is probably the best developing method at the present time, but even here one has problems because when there is severe stenosis or occlusion, it is almost impossible to get adequate data. Cornhill complimented Barbieri on his studies of the stenosis problem and indicated that these are among the first in the world that have been presented using the results after thermal treatment of the stenosis.

Cornhill asked two questions: One, concerning the hot tip from Cumberland and Sanborn, and one concerning the indications that the Excimer laser might be the method of choice. Barbieri responded that he thought the hot tip was likely not to be used very frequently since it is very difficult to control if one works in an area where thermal damage is likely to be a very serious consequence. He pointed out that the Excimer, while not yet completely developed, has an excellent background in theory and that one should be able to ablate the obstruction without tissue damage. There is still the problem of avoiding perforation because one needs a guiding system to be sure that it is not producing mechanical damage to the artery wall. Furthermore, it appears that the Excimer laser does not have the ideal wave length to ablate calcium; calcium mainly absorbs energy at about 2,900 nanometers. Theoretically, then, the Erbium laser would be the best. The development needed for the Erbium laser is the production of a less fragile optical fiber so that one would not have the problem of breakage of the fiber during the examination.

The discussion then turned to the pulsed-Holmium laser and Barbieri indicated that the Holmium laser was a second choice after the Erbium laser. The Holmium laser is a 2,100 nanometer wave length, and that means that the action is in the infrared region where water absorbance is very high. Therefore, these wavelengths are very well absorbed, but the main problem with Holmium is, from what we know today, that tissue is ablated mainly through shock waves, and these shock waves can probably create some problems that need further study.

Bonnet then entered the discussion and asked what Barbieri thought about the chemical photoactivation of the atherosclerotic plaque by the laser. Barbieri pointed out that the application of these methods to render atherosclerotic plaque visible through an orange fluorescence has not been applied to human subjects because of problems with phototoxicity. The use of tetracycline as a method for identifying plaques has also been explored and was followed by the measurement of ultraviolet radiation which localizes in the plaque and has, thus far, yielded promising results in vitro.

Kramsch then closed the discussion by asking Barbieri about the application of the laser, both diagnostically and therapeutically, in the carotid arteries. Barbieri described the limited experience at his center as well as elsewhere with treating carotid artery lesions with laser approaches and indicated that many cardiovascular scientists are cautious about using this system in the carotid arteries because of the possibility of distal embolization to the brain.

Liu's presentation was followed by an active discussion including a number of relevant questions. Bini led off the discussions by requesting more information about the technetium ligand called sestamibi (cardiolite). Liu explained that this is a compound in which technetium is incorporated in a hexamethoxy-isobutyl-isonitrile complex consisting of six molecules of isonitrile surrounding a technetium center. It mainly localizes intracellularly according to viability and membrane charge. It localizes in the heart muscle cells and stays there for a prolonged period of time so that if one is studying the effects of intervention then one can give a single dose prior to intervention, and afterwards the image will still represent the way the lesion was before intervention. One can then give a second dose and, using emission tomography, see what has happened because of the intervention.

Bini continued her questioning and asked whether, when this indicator is used on the myocardium, it is dependent on reperfusion and oxygenation of the tissue. Liu replied in the affirmative. Then Wissler turned to the endovascular approach that Liu had demonstrated and asked whether in the current state of development one could tell whether artery lesions had changed after several months of therapy. Wissler then noted that even though lesions are very densely calcified, that does not mean that this is irreversible because even densely calcified lesions frequently have a large cholesteryl ester and necrotic core component. Even these lesions, then, can get smaller, since it is the lipid that is most labile and is most likely to be lost during the currently used regression regimens. He also noted that studies in several centers have indicated that the more severe the lesions, and the more severe the lipid abnormalities, the more likely one is to observe regression when effective lipid lowering therapies are used. Kramsch pointed out that the system should also be useful for determining compensatory vasodilatation. Liu responded that the intervascular ultrasound system had not been clinically available for more than a few months and that these kinds of measurements for the most part have not yet been attempted. Compensatory dilatation has been observed with epicardial ultrasound systems. He indicated that sequential studies should definitely be possible and that one should be able to gain information regarding the vessel wall composition beyond the lumen of the artery. The major challenge in technical development is a precise system that will allow one to go back to exactly the same spot in the artery to make the measurements. He believes that this will be possible with a multiplane system in which three-dimensional information can be obtained and a computerized integration system helps to reconstruct the information on line. Bond then commented that the dark areas in the slides that Liu had shown could consist of many different elements including accumulations of smooth muscle or hemorrhage. Under these circumstances, the impression of regression might be mistaken because there are many elements in the arterial wall and the arterial lesions that can cause dark shadowing. This means that those who examine arteries microscopically are going to need to be much more specific regarding the form in which the various lesion components are present. Kramsch asked Liu whether he thought that the sequential imaging would soon be developed to the point where one could examine the same spot after one year, two years, four years, etc. Liu pointed out that this had not yet been attempted since this approach was only about six months old in clinical use, but approaches involving three dimensional measurements and longitudinal as well as transverse orientation should make it possible to get back to the same precise area for rexamination. He also pointed out that it is possible at present to test the replication of measurements on two or three closely spaced occasions so that reproducibility can be obtained. At the present time this appears to be in the range of 5%, with considerable possible improvement with further experience of the endovascular system.

The session then continued as a general discussion and the first question was asked by Rubba, who requested that Kramsch give more information about the femoral and carotid parts of the CLAS study. The response from Kramsch made it clear that both femoral arteries and carotid arteries are being quantitatively evaluated in the CLAS study, and the problems with the computer assisted measurements have been overcome so that a paper is to be sent for publication very soon. There is definite evidence of regression of atherosclerotic lesions in these two areas, just as has been reported in some detail in the coronary arteries of the same patients. The problems of curvature of the femoral arteries have been solved and the study of the carotid arteries, which was mostly carried out by means of ultrasound, are being gathered together for publication, which will include some comparison with what was found by ultrasound and by carotid contrast media arteriography. Poli asked Kramsch about the results of CLAS II, i.e., observations made after four years of therapy and whether the same trends that Brown had shown for clinical events were demonstrated by the CLAS II results. Kramsch indicated that there were very definite beneficial results of this type in the CLASS II study in regard to the need for further medical or surgical intervention or regarding untoward clinical effects. These results were in the same direction as those being reported by Brown for the FATS study. He cautioned that one has to remember that Brown was using an entirely different selection process to choose the patients who were being treated and that, in general, the patients involved in the FATS study had a much stronger genetic background to their hyperlipidemia than those patients being treated in the CLAS study. In response to a question from Bond, who pointed out that the enlargements of the lumens of the arteries in the CLAS study might really be due to dilatation rather than regression, he stated that it was only possible to measure the lumen with the radio-opaque angiographic methods that they are using in Los Angeles at the present time for the CLAS study.

Bond pointed out in discussing Kramsch's presentation that he was impressed with the data that had been presented by Glagov at the University of Chicago and Armstrong at the University of Iowa and several other investigators who have pointed out that on a basis of cross sectional data, arteries compensate for atherosclerotic plaques by enlargement. Kramsch indicated that he felt that compensatory dilatation was not a very important factor in their measurements since the placebo groups should have shown that that reaction was not present. He also pointed out that the difference between the placebo and the blood related group's response was much greater than the potential errors of measurement that are an integral part of the panel method of grading angiograms which they have employed.

There was further discussion by Heistad pointing out that the absolute changes in artery lumen were relatively small as far as lumen diameter was concerned, but of course this represents a rather substantial change in lumen circumference. Kramsch pointed out that the possibilities for improvement in blood flow might very well be involved since the patients with angina pectoris generally showed improvement in their signs and symptoms. Heistad went on to indicate that he thought that some of the changes in the lumen size might be a function of factors related to the endothelium. Wissler pointed out that in the studies which he and Weber had carried out on regression of atherosclerosis in rhesus monkeys, one of the first things that happen when blood lipids are lowered is that the endothelium shows evidence of healing of the multiple small ulcers that are present over the surface of the advanced plaques in these species and which also have been demonstrated over advanced plaques in people. He indicated that one should not be too concerned as to whether one is seeing a plaque that is getting a lot smaller or if one is seeing a much more functional vessel with a much better lining. Liu pointed out that one of the aspects of Brown's study is that there is sometimes progression in one lesion and regression in another; this really points out that one needs to understand that this is a very complicated field and that the mechanisms may not apply to all of the lesions.

Kramsch referred to experiments by Lees at MIT and the Massachusetts General Hospital which indicate that some plaques are much more active than others in taking up labeled low density lipoproteins. The general goal is to produce a favorable response so that further progression of the disease is kept at a minimum, and that those parts of the family of plaques in the coronary arteries which are susceptible to regression have every opportunity for that to take place. He said that the results of CLAS at four years certainly indicate that the therapy is having a very important impact on the prevention of further progression and upon the clinical aspects of the ischemic heart disease. He also indicated that it is the reason that their group has used a global score, which considers the entire heart. Wissler then indicated that he needed more help in understanding why the PET and SPECT results appeared to show a rather low resolution and whether this is likely to be improved as more work is done with the technology. Pantano pointed out that the resolution of the PET machine was now below 10 mm and that there will be further progress in this field. She did not believe, however, that it would be possible to study the arteriosclerotic plaque directly using these approaches. They are much more useful to study the effects of the plaques, especially in the brain. <u>Lenzi</u> pointed out that in order to detect the activity with these approaches, one has to detect a photon that comes from a particular point. Positrons, when they are emitted from the particles, travel in the tissue until they find a normal negative electron and then they produce the signal. This distance of travel may be as long as 6 mm. It depends on the energy of the positron, so that at present we are uncertain as to how far this system can develop so that one can detect a single photon. He pointed out that he did not see any possibility of a major improvement in the resolution of this technique.

ULTRAFAST CARDIAC MRI: PRESENT STATUS

Sven Paulin, Dennis J. Atkinson, Deborah Burstein,
Robert R. Edelman, Eric T. Fossel, Warren J. Manning

Beth Israel Hospital
330 Brookline Avenue
Boston, MA   02215

Magnetic resonance imaging has made a spectacular appearance in clinical medicine within less than a decade. Although its major practical application is in imaging of the brain, it competes most favorably with CT scanning, it has already now found wider applications to other organ systems, including the heart.[1] In contrast to CT scanning, MRI benefited from two initially unexpected characteristics in its applicability to studies of the central cardiovascular system; firstly, there exists an intrinsic contrast between the organic cardiovascular structures and their blood-containing cavities and lumina; and secondly, it soon became apparent that it was relatively easy to gate the acquisition of images with the EKG and without any major time penalty. MRI using conventional spin-echo technique had, by the mideighties, provided the most detailed images of intracardiac anatomy, successfully rivaling other imaging methods used for cardiac examinations, including contrast angiography. When applied to the heart, synchronization with the mechanical events during the cardiac cycle eliminates, or at least decreases, the detrimental effect of cardiac motion. EKG-gating permits the accumulation of a large number of phase encoding steps over a relatively long period of time (up to several minutes for high spatial resolution). Speeding up the imaging process can be accomplished by either decreasing the number of excitations or reducing the matrix size of the image. Trade-offs are reduced signal-to-noise ratio, artifacts, and less image resolution.[2]

Although cardiac MRI examinations were relatively time consuming, the ability to apply multi-slice technique in almost unlimited different projections and their subsequent assembly resulted in a most impressive and reliable delineation of anatomic structures. Consequently, the technique has been proven most useful in the evaluation of cardiac abnormalities, including even the most complex congenital entities. Enlargements of different cardiac chambers and their interrelationship can be identified rather easily. Assessment of myocardial wall thickness is possible and permits important and relevant observations with regard to the diagnosis of valvular abnormalities, heart disease, or myopathies. Wall thickness measurements and application of geometric algorithms have led to myocardial mass determination which appears to be very reliable and reproducible. In addition, MRI has been shown to be very powerful in its ability to identify and delineate neoplastic growth within the heart.[3]

With regard to ischemic heart disease, the most important clinical cardiologic problem in the western world, MRI of the heart did not seem to play a major role as a diagnostic tool because of its limited spatial resolution power, estimated not to be significantly better than 1 mm. On occasion smaller anatomic structures, such as the proximal portions of the coronary arteries, had been demonstrated. In a prospectively performed study,[4] we explored the potentials of coronary artery visualization with spin-echo technique using a 1.5 Tesla field strength equipment. We examined seven patients who recently underwent coronary arteriography. With the benefit of prior knowledge of the existing anatomy, we directed the examinations so to obtain optimal planes and directions of the images. An initial coronal scan was performed in the recumbent position using eight 7mm thick slices with a 2.1 mm gap. After having identified the position of the aortic root from which the coronary arteries are known to arise (Fig. 1), we proceeded to take appropriate transverse scans with 5 or 3 mm thickness.

As we intercalated different runs obtained during different phases of the heart cycle, we accomplished for all practical purposes, a complete and continuous coverage of this anatomically crucial area by closely adjacent image slices. Additional examination planes directed at visualization of other major coronary branches were performed provided that we could accomplish these within a preset time limit of two hours. This is the maximum length of time we permitted for these patients with angina pectoris symptomatology. In fact, one of our patients developed claustrophobia shortly after being placed in the narrow apparatus and the examination had to be terminated prematurely.

Although identification of the proximal coronary arteries (Fig. 2) can be accomplished, we concluded from this study that the technical limitations and difficulties in image interpretation make this method impractical for a prospectively conducted diagnostic examination of the entire coronary arterial tree. We also observed in two cases that downstream arterial obliteration confirmed what we theoretically suspected. We found that the open proximal portion of the artery could not be detected with MRI because the signal drop out which results in the blackness of the vascular lumen is related to the rapid movement of the blood within it. We concluded, on the other hand, that conditions that result in significant coronary arterial dilatations, such as coronary arteriovenous fistulas or aneurysms secondary to arteritis, are likely to be identified readily by use of this technique.

The technique for fast MR movie sequences was described in 1976 by Haase and colleagues.[5] This method includes so-called gradient-echo techniques, which make use of a dramatically shortened repetition time. The gradient-echo-pulse sequence is a simplified version of the spin-echo sequence. It uses a reduced flip angle of less than 90°. This permits each excitation to be repeated rapidly; therefore, many more signals can be measured per second. For cardiac imaging purposes, these images can be reassembled in relation to their incidence during the heart cycle, so-called retrospective gating, or delivered so as to coincide

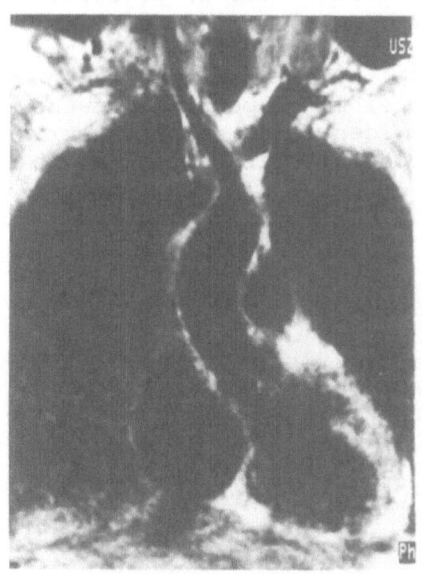

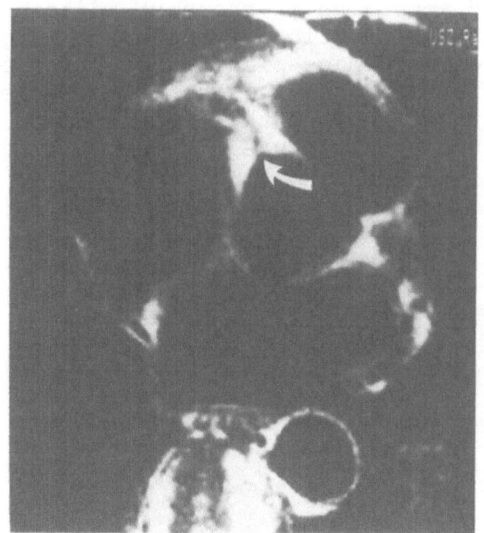

Fig. 1. MR examination performed with a 1.5-T
field strength equip-
ment using spin-echo-
sequences with ECG
gating. The 7-mm
thickness coronal
scan was out of ten
slices. It illus-
trates left ven-
tricular outflow,
aortic valve plane,
and the ascending
aorta. These scout
examinations were
used, together with
information from
coronary angiograms,
to identify optimal
location and angula-
tion of subsequent
transverse scans.

Fig. 2. Transverse scan shows
small right coronary
artery orifice origi-
nating from anterior
wall of the aortic root
(curved arrow). Several
centimeters of the
artery are visible. The
coronary angiogram
showed a small but
normal right coronary
artery with a maximum
diameter of less
than 2 mm.

after a predetermined interval in relation to the EKG, a method
which is called prospective gating.[2]

In contrast to spin-echo technique, the new method demonstrates flowing blood in the form of bright, signals, the intensity of which relates to the speed of flow.[6] We also recognized the advantage of having access to a great number of
images within the same plane during the heart cycle and we
were particularly impressed by the convenience with which the
sequential and cinematography-resembling display of images
obtained at eight different planes could be observed and analyzed
simultaneously on an image monitor (Fig. 3). For an experienced
observer, identification of the major portions of the large
coronary arteries did not pose any greater difficulty. Analysis

of several planes on the split monitor screen made it possible to observe certain arterial segments moving out from one plane and appearing in the next adjacent one in close relation to the intrinsic motion of the heart (Figs. 4). This also applied to sagittal image planes where, for example, major portions of the left main stem and the LAD are clearly identified, albeit not as impressively on this static image reproduction in comparison to the motion picture display.

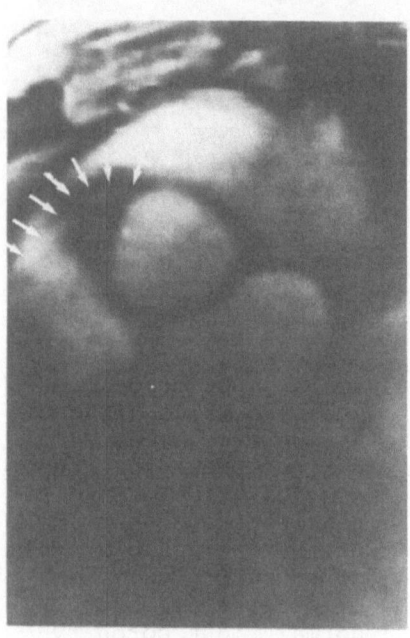

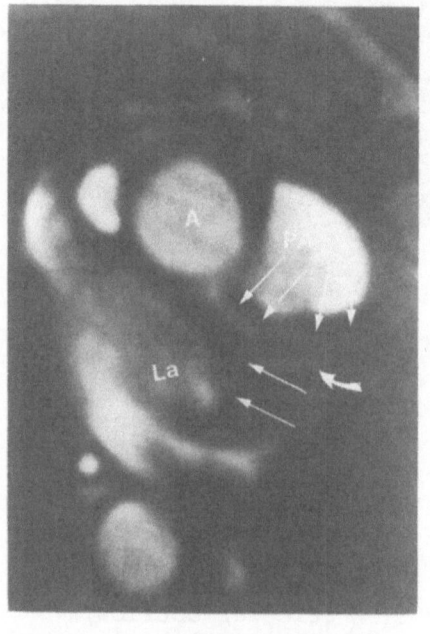

Fig. 3. Enlarged single image out of series of eight. Centrally located round structure represents aortic root. Anteriorly located very bright structure is a section through the outflow tract of the right ventricle. Linear bright band (arrows) indicates the right coronary artery arising from the anterior aspect of the aorta and curving laterally between the base of the pulmonary artery and right atrial appendage.

Fig. 4. Enlarged single Fig. 3 with increased angulation in order to align image plane with left coronary artery and its bifurcation. A=ascending aorta; PA=pulmonary artery; LA=left atrium. Long arrows indicate left main coronary artery arising from the left posterior aspect of the aortic root, bifurcating into proximal left anterior descending and left circumflex branch. Curved arrow points at broad, bright band running parallel behind left anterior descending artery and is most likely representing a segment of the great cardiac vein.

Ultrafast MR, so-called echo-planar technique,[7,8,9] will theoretically increase the speed of examination and thus make it less dependent on cardiac gating which may not be possible in the presence of cardiac arrhythmias. Since this technique will represent a further trade-off between spatial and temporal resolution, its advantages with regard to visualization of the coronary arteries is questionable.[10]

Ongoing MRI coronary angiography research efforts address the application of more advanced or innovative imaging sequences. Isolated heart preparation or other animal models are useful for this purpose as they eliminate, to some extent, the problems that are associated with respiratory or intrinsic cardiac motion. Once one has established optimal MRI sequences one may then hope that these can be applied successfully in the clinical situation.[11] Examples of such stepwise research efforts are presented Fig. 5 which demonstrates a standard MRI spin-echo image of an isovolumic perfused rat heart in long axis view. The aortic root, right ventricular and left ventricular cavities contrast as dark structures against the signal-generating myocardium and vascular walls. This heart is approximately 1.5 cm long and the images were obtained with cardiac gating in a 4.7 Tesla research instrument.

Figures 6a and 6b show a flow-compensated gradient-echo image of a similar isovolumic perfused rat heart utilizing presaturation of the stationary spin. In Fig.6a, a long axis

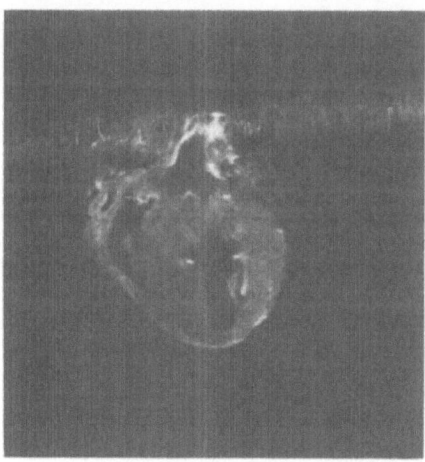

Fig. 5. Standard spin-echo (TE=34) image of an isovolumic perfused rat heart in long axis view. The aortic root, right ventricular and left ventricular cavity are contrasting as dark structures against signal generating myocardium and vascular walls. This heart is approximately 1.5 cm. The images were obtained with cardiac gating.

view, similar to Fig. 5, illustrates the bright flow from the aortic cannula into the aortic root. The visibility of linear structures representing major coronary artery branches indicates the superiority of this technique. In Fig. 6b the short axis view of the same heart demonstrates conclusively the aortic root with its three aortic valve cusps and the proximal portions of both coronary arteries. This image is zoomed by a factor of two (2) in each direction relative to the image in Fig. 6a.

Performing multiple, short axis cuts at equal distance in so-called "bread loaf" orientation through the length of the left ventricle, the bright signals from the mostly transversely imaged coronary arterial lumina are identified. These can then be assembled in a 3-D display.

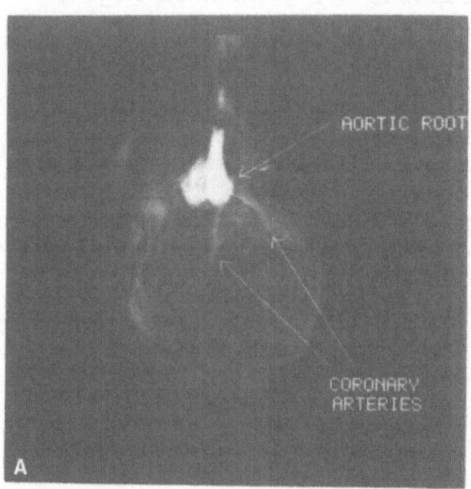 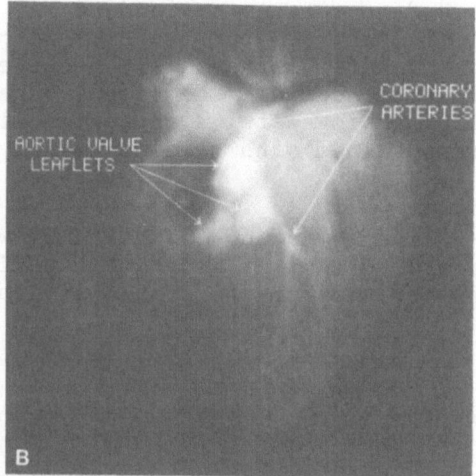

Fig. 6A&B. Flow compensated gradient echo (TE=2) images of an isovolumic perfused rat heart utilizing presaturation of the stationary spins. In Fig. 6A a long axis view shows the bright flow from the aortic cannula into the aortic root. In Fig. 6B, a short axis view through the aortic root demonstrates the region of the aortic valve leaflets and the proximal coronary arteries. This image is zoomed by a factor of 2 in each direction relative to the image in Fig. 6A.

The final illustration addressing these research efforts (Fig. 7) demonstrates a gradient-echo image of an in vivo rat heart dissecting the aortic root. The proximal left coronary artery can be identified. The field view of this image is 2 cm and the slice thickness 0.35 mm.

These results demonstrate that visualization of the coronary artery may be possible with MR imaging techniques. In order to make them feasible in clinical situations in which the heart rate may be more erratic, ultrafast imaging will need to be implemented. This might be possible by dividing the total number of phase encoding steps for an image into groups within the same portion of several cardiac cycles.

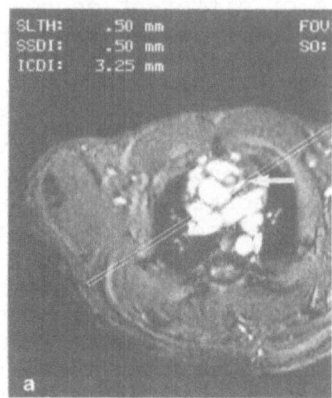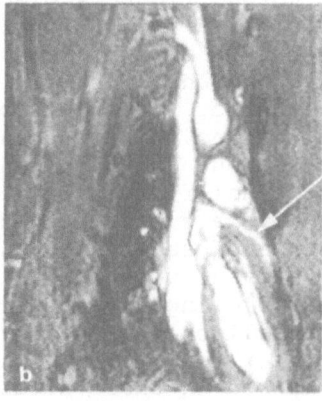

Fig. 7A&B. Fig. 7A demonstrates a gradient-echo image of an
in vivo rat heart at the level of the aortic root.
The proximal left coronary artery can be seen
(Arrow). Observe line traces on this transverse
section identifying the obliquity of the coronal
plane used in Fig. 7B, which shows rather well, a
large left-sided coronary artery branch. Other
bright appearing structures are the two cardiac
ventricles separated by the septum, the superior
vena cava and the aortic arch, as well as the main
stem of the pulmonary artery.

Obviously there is a difference between a mouse and a human
subject. From the coronary arterial images obtained with any
hitherto available MRI techniques, it is clear that subtle initial manifestation of atherosclerosis which occur in the arterial
walls are unlikely to be recognized. The inferiority in spatial
resolution will not permit us to make observations of rather mild
and non-obstructive wall irregularities that usually can be identified in a high quality cineangiogram.

Magnetic resonance imaging may be used similarly to other
non-invasive procedures to identify the effects of coronary
artery disease on the myocardium. An example of such a diagnostic approach is the widely used technique of radionuclide
scanning with thallium, preferentially performed both at rest
and exercise. Echocardiography may also be used for similar
purposes as it can depict regional wall motion abnormalities.
A PET scanner may even identify abnormalities in myocardial
metabolism and delineate its degree and extension. Magnetic
resonance imaging is just about to make similar diagnostic
approaches by combining fast imaging technology with the use of
MRI contrast agents which are practically free from adverse side
effects.[12]

For myocardial flow scanning, ultrafast images are acquired
within a given delay after the R-wave of the EKG, using so-called
turbo-flash technique. The acquisition of images occur when the
natural contrast of myocardium is close to zero. When the intravenously injected MRI contrast agent, gadolinium-DTPA, arrives in
the area to be studied, the MRI signals are increased in relation
to the contrast agent's local concentration. Repeating such image
acquisition with each second or third heartbeat, the intensity
of the bright signals can be plotted so as to present flow curve
for this within the area. We have studied healthy subjects and

patients with coronary artery disease of different degree and severity and compared the regional MRI flow values with the findings on the coronary arteriograms. On the short axis cuts through the left ventricle, the myocardial wall presents in the form of a ring and the anterior, lateral, posterior and septal portions can be readily identified. Windows can be placed by the observer in the different regions and a command is given to the computer to provide the regional flow curves of the contrast agent. Regionally decreased signals and delayed arrival correlated positively with the presence of severe coronary arterial stenosis or occlusions in the relevant vessels. In some patients, the examinations were repeated following revascularization procedures, either in the form of balloon angioplasty or bypass surgery. We were then able to observe a return of the regional peak intensity to normal, most marked in those areas that were severely depressed during the initial examination. These encouraging preliminary observations have to await confirmation. The test will achieve true clinical value when one can perform it in conjunction with cardiac stress, either in the form of physical exercise or pharmacologic intervention.[12]

Potentially, MRI cinematography can offer a very useful diagnostic method which can precisely evaluate regional myocardial wall motion abnormalities.[14] The myocardium can be labeled by radio frequency presaturation pulses which tag it in a grid pattern. Such a technique will allow the direct identification of myocardial contraction in a given area of injury. One should be able to identify precisely an akinetic segment by the absence of any change in the local grid pattern, thus identifying it correctly as not having any intrinsic contraction. Thus, it should eliminate the problem of passive motion in a given area which might be secondary to tethering from adjacent healthy myocardium, a problem inherent in practically all available imaging techniques for left ventricular mechanical function analysis.

NMR spectroscopy has, for some time, held the promise of providing important clinical information not available from any other source. A major example is the ability to distinguish stunned or hibernating myocardium from that which has suffered irreversible injury. Recent advances in localized spectroscopy techniques have made such clinical application available in many health care centers. Phosphor-31 NMR spectroscopy has been shown to be sensitive to ischemia, hypoxia, and work level.[15] The resonances, of inorganic phosphate, creatinine phosphate, and the three resonances of ATP--beta, alpha, and gamma can be identified and quantified separately. At the onset of ischemia, creatinine phosphate falls, followed by a fall in ATP. These are converted to inorganic phosphates and sugar phosphates which show a corresponding increased peak. As long as the phosphor-containing substrates remain within the cell, the ischemic injury is reversible. Once phosphate begins to leak out, irreversible injury occurs. Consequently, by measuring the intensity of the total phosphate signals from a volume of tissue, the myocardium is assumed to be stunned or hibernating and not dead as long as the total phosphor content does not decrease.

In conclusion, currently available methods and techniques using magnetic resonance imaging do not compete successfully with the radiographic contrast angiogram of the coronary arteries and thus will not be the method of choice for direct identification or quantitative analysis of atherosclerotic processes within the coronary arterial walls. Magnetic resonance techniques, however, hold great promise for indirect identification of coronary atherosclerosis of wall motion studies, including myocardial tagging technique and first pass perfusion studies with contrast agents, offers the potential for the most complete functional analysis of the heart and may prove especially useful when combined with NMR spectroscopy. This holds the potential key for a better understanding of difficult problems and complex situations in clinical cardiology that reach from transient ischemia, contractile depression, stunned and hibernating myocardium, to permnent injury in the form of myocardial scars, aneurysm formation or wall perforations.

REFERENCES

1. I. A. Simpson, R. W. Newman, J. F. Martin, and K. J. Chung, Cine MR imaging of the heart, in: "Clinical Magnetic Resonance Imaging," R. R. Edelman and W. P. Hesslink, eds, W. B. Saunders Company, Philadelphia (1990).

2. R. R. Edelman, J. Kleefield, K. U. Wents, and D. J. Atkinson, Basic principles of magnetic resonance imaging, in: "Clinical Magnetic Resonance Imaging," R. R. Edelman and W. P. Hesslink, eds, W. B. Saunders Company, Philadelphia (1990).

3. C. B. Higgins, Overview of MR of the Heart 1986, AJR 146:907-18 (1986).

4. S. Paulin, G. K. von Schulthess, E. T. Fossel, H. P. Krayenbuehl, MR imaging of the aortic root and proximal coronary arteries. AJR 148:665-70 (1987).

5. A. Haase, D. Matthaei, W. Hanicker, FLASH imaging: rapid NMR imaging using low-flip angle impulses, J. Magn. Res. 67:258-66 (1986).

6. R. Herfkens, J. Utz, G. Glover, E. Fram, A. Shimakawa, J. Heinsimer, Rapid dynamic NMR imaging of the heart: initial clinical experience (abstract), Society of Magn. Res. in Med. Bk. of Abstracts 1:347-8 (1986).

7. P. Mansfield, Multi-planar image formation using NMR spin-echoes, J. Phys C10:L55-L58 (1977).

8. R. R. Rzedzian, I. L. Pykett, Instant images of the human heart using a new, whole body MR imaging system, Amer. J. Roentgenol 149:245-50 (1987).

9. M. Stehling, A. Houseman, et al, Real time NMR imaging of coronary vessels, Lancet II 964-5 (1987).

10. D. J. Atkinson, D. Burstein, R. R. Edelman, Perfusion imaging of the heart using instant magnetic resonance imaging: preliminary observations, Radiology (in press 1990).

11. D. Burstein, MRI of coronary artery flow in isolated and in vivo hearts, unpublished manuscript (submitted 1990).

12. W. J. Manning, D. J. Atkinson, R. R. Edelman, W. Grossman, S. Paulin, First-pass cardiac studies using gadolinium-DTPA in subjects with coronary artery disease: preliminary results, unpublished manuscript (submitted 1990).

13. D. J. Arkinson, R. R. Edelman, Cineangiography of the heart is a single breath-hold segmented with a turbo-flash sequence, unpublished manuscript (submitted 1990).

14. E. A. Zerhouni, D. M. Parish, W. J. Rogers, et al., Jungenhod: tagging with MR imaging--a method for noninvasive assessment of myocardial motion, Radiology 169:59-63 (1988).

15. M. R. Goldman, G. M. Pohost, J. S. Ingwall, E. T. Fossel,
    Nuclear magnetic resonance imaging: potential cardiac
    applications, Am. J. Cardial 46:1278-83 (1980).

SYNCHROTRON ANGIOGRAPHY

GENERAL CONSIDERATIONS

W.-R. Dix(1), K. Engelke(2), W. Graeff(1), J. Heuer(1),
W. Kupper(3), M. Lohmann(1), B. Reime(1), R. Reumann(1)

(1) Hamburger Synchrotronstrahlungslabor HASYLAB at DESY
    Hamburg, FRG
(2) Orthopädische Klinik, Universitäts-Krankenhaus Eppendorf
    Hamburg, FRG
(3) Kardiologische Abt. der Medizinischen Klinik,
    Universitäts-Krankenhaus Eppendorf, Hamburg, FRG

INTRODUCTION

In the near future selective coronary angiography will still be the
only method to visualize the small branches of the coronary arteries.
This method gives excellent images but has a certain risk for the
patients with respect to morbidity (1.2 to 2.2%) and mortality (0.07 to
0.23%). That is why at different institutions worldwide[1,2,3,4] efforts
are being made to develop a non-invasive method for coronary angiography
in order to investigate ambulatory patients with mild symptoms of
coronary heart disease, and to monitor disease progression routinely.

All systems developed for non-invasive coronary angiography use
Digital Subtraction Angiography (DSA). In DSA two images with large
difference in iodine contrast and practically no difference in contrast
from all other structures, e.g. bone and soft tissue, are subtracted,
thus strongly enhancing the signal from iodine. In DSA methods used in
clinical studies the two images for subtraction are produced in time
subtraction mode. In this mode one image is taken before injection of
contrast material and one image after injection. Because of the time
difference between the two images this method is not suited for imaging
of coronary arteries. The fast motion of these arteries - up to 6 cm/s
in RAO 30° projection - leads to artifacts. Electrocardiographic
triggering cannot overcome this problem for structures which measure as
little as 1 mm because of the nonperiodic motion of the heart
(translation and rotation) even if the respiration is stopped.

New systems under development use a different mode of DSA, the
energy subtraction mode (dichromography). Using this method the two
images for subtraction are taken at the same time when the contrast
material (iodine) is present. The method uses the discontinuity of
absorption at the so-called K-edge (Fig.1) of the contrast material.
Iodine differs by a factor of 6 in absorption below and above the K-edge
at 33.17 keV. If the two images for subtraction are simultaneously taken
with two different monochromatic energies - one energy below and the
other energy above the K-edge - the contrast from iodine is strongly
enhanced after subtraction. For an energy separation of the two

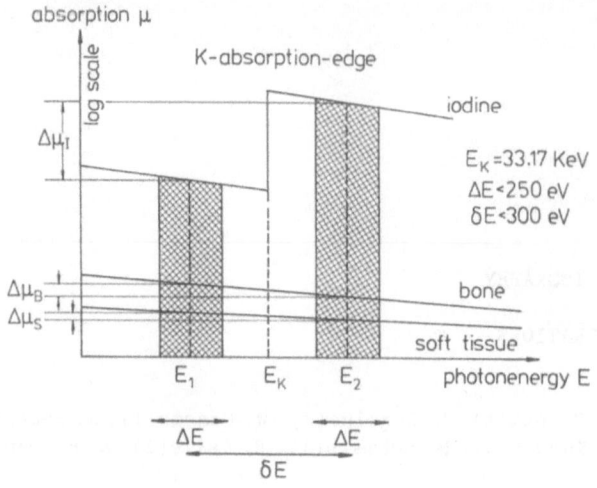

Figure 1. K-edge of iodine at E_K = 33.17 keV. E_1 and E_2 denote the two energies of the quasi-monochromatic beams for dichromography with bandwidth ΔE.

monochromatic energies of 300 eV the sensitivity to iodine is 10000 times higher than that to soft tissue. Since this method requires monochromatic X-rays with very high intensity all new systems are developed at synchrotron radiation facilities where these X-rays are available.

SYSTEM PARAMETERS

Because all systems for non-invasive coronary angiography under development use the same principle the following medical and physical requirements are valid for all designs.

Imaging Mode

From the physician's point of view two-dimensional image recording is most desirable. But tests with a commercially available area detector (image converter/TV-system Sirecon BV) showed that it is not suited for dichromography, mainly because of the following reasons:

- The dynamic range is too low. It was measured to be D = 85. This value was even reduced by K-edge yield variation in the iodine containing image converter and single frame exposure to D ≤ 30. The dynamic range should be at least D = 8400 (see below).
- Due to the TV-system the detector showed long afterglow. We measured 15% after 60 ms for a Saticon-tube and 50% after 100 ms for a Hivicon-tube.

- The presence of iodine in the input phosphor results in a decrease of 34% in yield for X-ray photons with energies below the K-edge of iodine.
- A large scatter fraction defined as

$$R = \frac{\text{detected scattered radiation}}{\text{total detected radiation}}$$

was measured behind a 17,5 cm thick water phantom, e.g. 8% for an area of 100x7 mm². Niklason et.al[5] showed that the scatter fraction amounted to 90% near lung tissue. These high values are not acceptable for dichromography because the signal/noise ratio decreases with increasing scatter fraction, thus reducing the contrast.

Even after major changes to the existing image converter/TV-systems, the high scatter fraction which is relevant for all area detectors, cannot be overcome. Using antiscatter grids as a precaution will result in increased dose. Therefore, line scan detectors are better suited, though their frame sequence is much slower. In line scan systems the scatter fraction is reduced to about 1.5%. In order to avoid fast moving mechanics like switching monochromators and beam switchers in the different systems, two-line detectors are used which simultaneously record the two lines with the energy above and below the K-edge, respectively. These detectors also have the advantage that they make better use of photon flux than a one-line detector. Only the Tsukuba group (Japan)[3] at present explores the possibilities of a two-dimensional image intensifier/TV-system.

Temporal Resolution

When using a line scan system one has to determine how fast the scan must be in order to avoid artifacts. By taking lines from subsequent images of an angiography sequence we composed new images which show the simulation of images with different line scan speed. The results showed that images have to be taken in the slow motion phase of the heart. Assuming the heart is 12.5 cm high, the spatial resolution is 0.5 mm (see below), and the duration of the slow motion phase of the heart is 250 ms, the exposure per time must not exceed 1 ms. Assuming a pixel size of 0.5x0.5 mm² and allowing a shift of the structures of interest from one energy image to the other of maximal 15% of pixel length, during the slow motion phase of the heart the time delay between exposures of the same pixel in the two energy images must not exceed 4 ms.

Spatial Resolution

In order to image arteries of 1 mm diameter a spatial resolution of at least 0.5 mm is necessary. Every increase in spatial resolution will increase quadratically the radiation dose and should be omitted if possible. Images from the same projection of 1 mm thick arteries, but with different resolution, show that a resolution of 0.5 mm is adequate to visualize stenosis of interest (70% and more) in the arteries. The group in Hamburg (FRG)[4] has decided to use 0.5 mm resolution, the group in Stanford (USA)[1] plans 0.25 mm resolution and the two-line detector developed in Siegen (FRG)[6], 0.4 mm resolution.

Contrast Material

In the clinical environment iodine is normally used as contrast material. Its K-edge is at 33.17 keV. Because photons of this energy in soft tissue have an absorption length of only 2.1 cm, one could use contrast materials with a higher Z and therefore a K-edge at higher energy, in order to minimize the radiation dose for patients. A good candidate is Gadolinium (K-edge at 50 keV) which is used in magnetic resonance imaging (MRI). Contrast material with an iodine concentration of 370 mg/ml is available. Calculations show that contrast material containing 370 mg/ml of Gadolinium would be better with respect to the radiation dose for the patients. Unfortunately, Gadolinium contrast material is only available in a concentration of 160 mg/ml. Therefore, it is only better suited than iodine for soft tissue of 25 cm and more. All existing systems use iodine as contrast material.

Mass Density

For non-invasive application of contrast material we aim at the application of 10 ml of contrast material within 1 s into a brachial vein. If the concentration of iodine in the contrast material is 370 mg/ml this results in 10mg/ml of iodine in the aorta and the coronary arteries. Assuming this concentration of iodine, its mass density in arteries of 1 mm diameter is about 1 mg/cm².

Dynamic Range

A structure with this mass density of iodine shows a 3% difference between the two images. If we assume a ratio of about 60 for the transmission through areas dominated by lung tissue and those dominated by bone tissue, calculations show that the dynamic range must be at least D = 8400.

Energy Bandwidth

Two contradictory requirements determine the bandwidth ΔE. From the flux point of view a high bandwidth is necessary. On the other hand energy separation ΔE (see Fig.1) larger than 300 eV yields a higher contrast for bone and soft tissue when compared to the contrast in the smallest artery. This means that ΔE must be less than 300 eV in order to avoid the overlap of the two energy bands.

Flux

Because a 1 mm thick vessel gives a 3%-signal and because a signal/noise ratio (SNR) of at least 3 is necessary, the quantum noise in the subtracted image must not exceed 1% or 0.7% in the unsubtracted image, and the electronic noise and other uncertainties in the system must not exceed 0.1%. In order to obtain a noise limit of 0.7% in the energy images, 20,000 photons per pixel must be registered. For a pixel size of 0.5x0.5 mm², 20 cm of soft tissue and an assumed detecting quantum efficiency (DQE) of the detector of 60%, this leads to $\Phi_o = 10^8$ photons/mm² in front of the patient. Therefore for an exposure time per line of 1 ms an intensity of 10^{11} photons/(mm²·s) must be available. If 2.5 cm of the 20 cm of soft tissue are replaced by bone tissue, the numbers for flux and intensity increase by a factor of 4 in order to maintain a SNR=3 for a 1 mm artery. If on the other hand the intensity is kept constant, behind 2.5 cm of bone and 17.5 cm of soft tissue a SNR=3 is achieved for 2 mm thick arteries. If the delivered intensity from the source is lower than the above stated values a longer exposure time per line must be used.

Radiation Dose

A flux of 10^8 photons/mm² corresponds to a skin dose of K = 1.1 rem. Such a dose would limit the resolution of arteries behind bones to 2 mm diameter if the DQE of the detector is 60%. Investigations of patients have to show whether the dose has to be increased to 4.5 rem per scan in order to resolve arteries of 1 mm size that are behind bone tissue. The aim is not to exceed a skin dose of 5 rem per investigation.

Projection Angles

After rapid intravenous bolus injection of 10 ml of contrast material the right heart and lungs are free of iodine when the left atrium, left ventricle, aorta and coronary arteries are opacified by iodine. However, important parts of the coronary arteries at that time are superimposed by other iodine containing structures such as the left heart chambers and aorta. To overcome this problem and to visualize all segments of the coronary arteries two methods can be used:

- Use of projection angles for the investigation of patients where the artery of interest is moved into a clear field.
- Use of image processing algorithms such as edge enhancement to visualize arteries that are superimposed on other opacified structures.

To examine the first possibility, 22 human hearts were excised in toto between 1 and 3 days after death[7]. Left chambers, ascending aorta and coronary arteries were filled with $BaSO_4$ in gelatine and examined using different viewing angles. This study demonstrated that it is possible to visualize the right coronary artery (best projection LAO-40° and CC-20°) and left anterior descending artery (best projection RAO-40° and CC-20°) completely without superimposition, but that it was difficult to visualize the left main artery and the proximal left circumflex coronary artery (Cx) because of superimposition of other iodine containing structures. In most cases the left main artery is superimposed on the aorta or left atrium and part of the left circumflex by the left atrium. We calculated the signal/noise ratio for these superimposed arteries and assumed there was a 1% noise on the average in the subtracted image. For example the left main artery (assumed thickness of 5 mm) superimposed on the aorta (assumed 50 mm) had a SNR of 7. If there was an additional 1.8 cm of bone, then the SNR decreased to 3.

Tests with image processing algorithms using simulated images with different noise levels showed that edge detection algorithms were accurate down to a SNR of 4. Improvement was also achieved with edge preserving smoothing to the same SNR. Theoretically then, it is possible to image all parts of the coronary arteries by selecting correct projection angles for 2 or 3 different scans, and by using image enhancement algorithms for those parts of the arteries which are superimposed on other structures. This procedure will not increase the skin dose because the entrance areas of the beam do not overlap.

SYSTEM NIKOS II

The existing systems for non-invasive coronary angiography have six main components:
- A synchrotron radiation source,

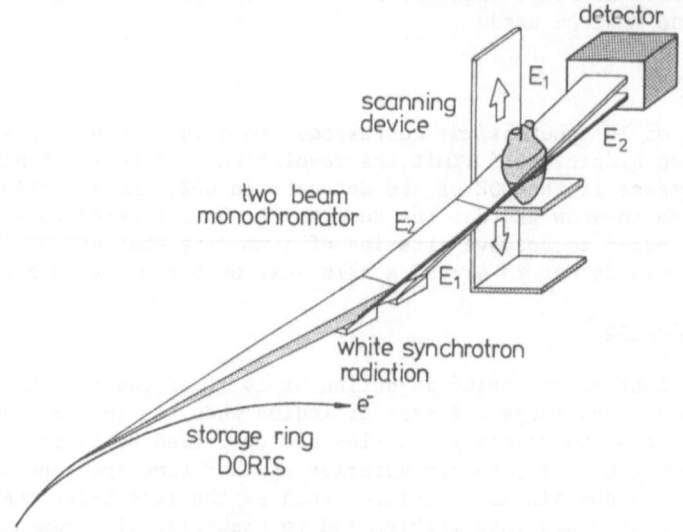

Figure 2. Schematic diagram of the system NIKOS II.

- a monochromator which filters two monochromatic X-ray beams out of the white synchrotron radiation beam,
- a scanning device (only in line-scan systems) which moves the patient through the two X-ray beams,
- a detector,
- a computer system,
- and a safety system.

As an example the system NIKOS II[4] is described in Fig.2.

Synchrotron Radiation Source

Synchrotron radiation is produced in the bending magnets of synchrotrons or storage rings for high energy physics. In the storage ring DORIS, which is used as a source for the system NIKOS, the spectrum of this electromagnetic radiation ranges from infrared to hard X-rays. The advantages of synchrotron radiation are its high intensity and small divergence. If a higher intensity than that produced by a bending magnet is necessary, then wigglers (Fig.3) are installed. These are magnetic structures in straight parts of the storage ring which force the electrons in the ring to follow a slalom-like path thus increasing the intensity of the synchrotron radiation corresponding to the number of curves along the path (poles in the wiggler). The system NIKOS II uses the wiggler HARWI[8] with 20 poles and a field of 1.0 T. It is constructed with permanent magnets ($Co_{17}Sm_2$) while the magnetic field of the wiggler in Stanford (8 poles, 1.8 T) is produced with electromagnetic coils.

Monochromator

Single crystals are used for filtering the quasi-monochromatic beams from the white synchrotron radiation beam. Following the Bragg formula

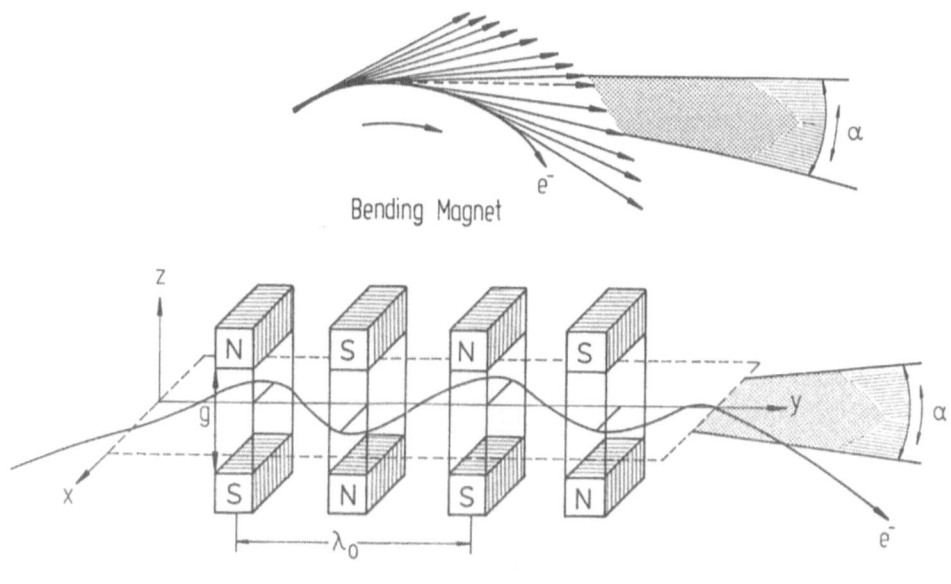

Bending Magnet

Multipole Wiggler

Figure 3. Schematic view of a multipole wiggler.

$$n \cdot \lambda = 2 \cdot d \cdot \sin \Theta$$

(d = lattice plane crystal spacing), under the angle Θ X-rays of
wavelength λ are reflected. With Ge(111) crystals under Θ = 3.28° X-rays
of λ = 0.373 Å corresponding 33.17 keV are produced. In the
monochromator of NIKOS II (Fig.4) two Ge(111) crystals are installed in
a He-filled tube. They vertically split the incident synchrotron
radiation beam into two parts with each crystal delivering one of two
monochromatic beams, 10 cm x 0.5 mm. The measured flux in the system
was $0.13 \cdot 10^{11}$ photons/(mm²·s). This type of monochromator has
disadvantages, e.g. it is sensitive to motions of the incident beam and
produces X-rays of 99.51 keV which lead to beam hardening effects.
Tests of monochromators with designs better suited for dichromography
were previously not successful.

The design of the monochromator used at Stanford is similar to that
of NIKOS however only one crystal is used in Tsukuba. In order to get
the two energies for the two images in the system, the Bragg angle must
be adjusted quickly, i.e. within 2 ms (at the moment within 125 ms).

Scanning Device

For the line scan mode used in the NIKOS system a scanning device is
needed. The maximum scan velocity is 50 cm/s and is kept constant over a
distance of 15-20 cm with a precision of 1%. The total lift of 40 cm in
the device includes an additional 20 cm for acceleration and
deceleration. The actual vertical position of the chair is determined by
a precise optical scale which triggers a new readout of the detector
every 0.5 mm. The velocity of the chair which determines the patient
exposure is monitored routinely by additional angle encoders (see safety
system below). The moving force of the scan device is generated in a
hydraulic system with proportional valves under computer control. The
chair allows for a patient rotation of ± 40° about a vertical axis and

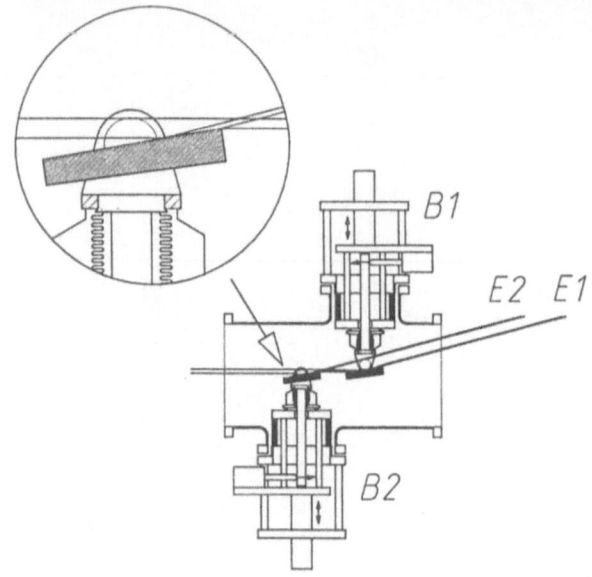

Figure 4. Schematic diagram of the monochromator installed in the system NIKOS II.

± 20° about a lateral axis in order to set the appropriate projection angles. The patient is scanned with raised arms which accelerates the flow of contrast material, and avoids overlap problems with the arms in extreme projection angles. The arms rest on pads where the cables and tubes for ECG and the injector can be fixed. For a precise positioning of the patient a light frame is projected on the patient's body which indicates the irradiated area. The scanning device is ECG-triggered by the computer.

Detector

In NIKOS II a two-line detector (Fig.5) is installed which registers the two beams simultaneously[9]. The detector is based on commercially available photodiode arrays which integrate the light generated in a phosphor and which is amplified through an image intensifier. At the entrance face two lines of scintillators (Gd_2O_2S:Tb powder) convert the incoming X-rays into visible light. Each line has 250 pixels (0.5 x 0.5 mm² each). The lines have a vertical spacing of 2 mm and the light is guided by special glass fiber optics through two two-stage proximity focussing image intensifiers onto the two photodiode arrays (1024 photodiodes each, 4 for each pixel). One photodiode array per line is needed and the readout of the two lines is controlled by a common digital control board triggered by the linear optical encoder of the scanning device. The maximum readout frequency of the detector is 0.5 kHz and corresponds to a scan velocity of 25 cm/s. For this frequency the DQE is 15% and the dynamic range is 1:3000. Two-line detectors for dichromography have also been developed in Stanford[1] (semiconductor) and in the University of Siegen[6] (position sensitive ionization chamber).

Computer System

The computer system in NIKOS II consists of a PDP 11/73 for system control and a MicroVAX-WSII/GPX for data acquisition and image

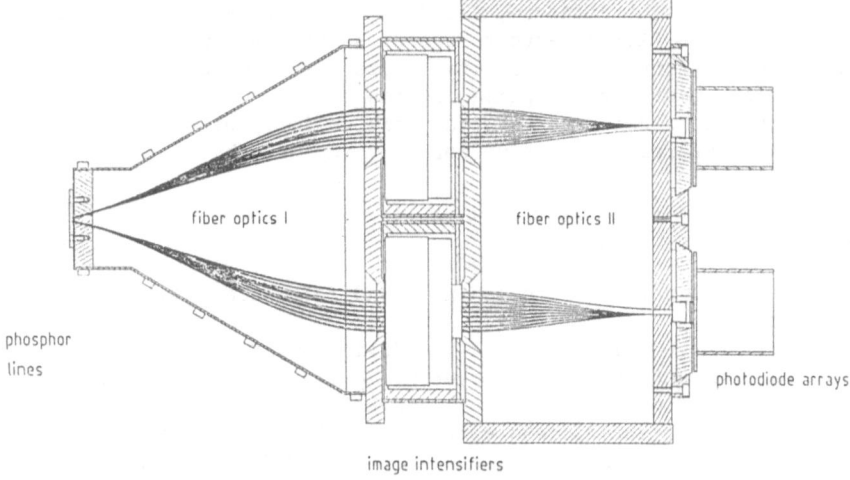

Figure 5. Vertical cut through the NIKOS detector.

processing. These two machines are interfaced with the DESY computer center. After data acquisition the data of the energy images are preprocessed for fast fluctuations in the incident beam, for irregularities in the scanning device and for beam hardening effects, dark current, fixed pattern noise, afterglow from line to line and crosstalk from pixel to pixel. The two images are then subtracted logarithmically. The resulting image is corrected for residual fixed pattern and grey level adjustment is made.

Safety System

For a standard scan, a radiation dose of 1 rem is necessary. With an exposure time of 1 ms per line the corresponding dose rate in each beam amounts to 500 rem/s. The sudden stop of the scanning device or a change of the scanning speed is the main disadvantage during the exposure of the patient. Therefore, the scanning device speed is permanently controlled by two independent angular encoders which are interfaced with the moving part of the scanning device by a cog wheel running on a cog rail. Malfunction of the scanning device or power failure or breakdown of electronic components in the safety system switch automatically off the beam using two very fast beam shutters. The beam is switched off also if the patient leaves the scanning device with the shutters closing within less than 10 ms.

SUMMARY

The development of systems for non-invasive coronary angiography using dichromography began 1979 at Stanford and Novosibirsk (USSR), in 1981 at Hamburg and in 1983 at Tsukuba. Four years after the beginning all groups started in-vivo investigations of animals. Currently, patients are investigated only at Stanford (1986) and at Hamburg (1990). The images from these initial studies as yet do not have the quality necessary for routine clinical use, but do demonstrate the potential of the method when the systems are optimized. In all systems used to date the intensity of the monochromatic beams is not yet adequate. New wigglers and monochromators will potentially overcome this problem. With the exception of Stanford, all detectors have a too low dynamic range and low DQE. All detectors regardless of the center, must demonstrate substantial reliability before they can be applied in a medical environment. After optimizing the system components, several patients must be studied to ascertain the validity of this method when compared to invasive coronary angiography.

REFERENCES

1. E. Rubenstein (these proceedings) and references mentioned therein.
2. E.N. Dementyev, E.Y. Dovga, G.N. Kulipanov, A.S. Medvedko, N.A. Mezentsev, V.F. Pindyurin, M.A. Sheromov, A.N. Skrinsky, A.S. Sokolov, V.A. Ushakov, and E.I. Zagorodnikov, First results of experiments with a medical one-coordinate X-ray detector on synchrotron radiation of VEPP-4, NIM, A246:702 (1986).
3. K. Nishimura, K. Hyodo, R. Hosaka, M. Ando, F. Toyofuku, A. Akisada, S. Hasegawa, and E. Takenaka, High Speed Image Acquisition System for Energy Subtraction Angiography, Rev. Sci. Instrum. 60:2260 (1989).
4. W.-R. Dix, K. Engelke, G. Heintze, J. Heuer, W. Graeff, W. Kupper, M. Lohmann, I. Makin, T. Möchel, R.Reumann, and K.-H. Stellmaschek, NIKOS II - a system for non-invasive imaging of coronary arteries, in: "Medical Imaging III: Image Formation", SPIE 1090:282 (1989).
5. L.T. Niklason, J.A. Sorenson, and J.A. Nelson, Scattered Radiation in Chest Radiography, Med. Phys. 8:677 (1981).
6. E. Hell, H.-J. Besch, L. Brabetz, P. Kuhn, and A.H. Walenta, Position Resolution, High Rate Behaviour and Space Charge Induced Image Distortions of a Multiwire X-Ray Detector for Digital Subtraction Angiography, NIM A269:404 (1988).
7. W. Kupper, W.-R. Dix, W. Graeff, P. Steiner, K. Engelke, C.-C. Glüer, and W. Bleifeld, Projection Angles for Intravenous Coronary Angiography, in: "Synchrotron Radiation Applications to Digital Subtraction Angiography (SYRDA)", E. Burattini and A. Rindi, eds., Italian Physical Society, Vol.10, Bologna (1987).
8. W. Graeff, L. Bittner, W. Brefeld, U. Hahn, G. Heintze, J. Heuer, J. Kouptsidis, J. Pflüger, M. Schwartz, E.W. Weiner, and T. Wroblewski, HARWI - A hard x-ray wiggler beam at DORIS, Rev. Sci. Instrum. 60:1457 (1989).
9. M. Lohmann, W.-R. Dix, K. Engelke, W. Graeff, J. Heuer, W. Kupper, T. Möchel, and R.Reumann, A Fast Line Scan X-Ray Detector for Medical Applications - a Status Report of the NIKOS II Detector -, in SPIE Vol. 1245 (in press).

TRANSVENOUS CORONARY ANGIOGRAPHY

WITH SYNCHROTRON RADIATION

E. Rubenstein
Stanford University School of Medicine
Stanford, California 94305, U.S.A.

X-ray-based angiography continues to be the standard method of
assessing the severity and the extent of coronary atherosclerosis. The
relative insensitivity of conventional X-ray imaging systems to
iodine-containing contrast agents necessitates that the images be acquired
with essentially undiluted contrast agent in the lumen of the vessels
being studied. This, in turn, requires arterial catheterization and the
insertion of the catheter tip in or near the ostia of the vessels and the
direct injection of the contrast agent. The health risks and monetary
costs of the procedure have limited its use to circumstances in which
there is a high probability of the presence of severe disease. Despite
these problems, coronary angiography has been employed in serial studies
to evaluate the effects of drug therapy and diet on coronary
atherosclerosis (1).

The deployment of synchrotron radiation as an illuminating source for
X-ray imaging systems offers the prospect of replacing intraarterial with
intravenous injections of the contrast agent, thereby eliminating the main
source of risk and cost of coronary angiography. The approach is based on
the principle of iodine dichromography, using monochromatic X-ray beams
whose energy closely brackets the K-edge of iodine (2,3). (Fig. 1) The
increase in sensitivity to the contrast agent that is achieved by this
method allows for the imaging of coronary arteries despite the 20- to
30-fold dilution of the contrast agent that takes place during its transit
from the venous to the arterial circulation. Because the X-ray dose is
modest compared with the arterially invasive procedure and the volume of
contrast agent required is similar, synchrotron radiation coronary
angiography appears to be well suited for the long-term, serial evaluation
of the effects of various interventions.

PRINCIPLE

The emission of electromagnetic radiation by ultrarelativistic charged
particles of low mass is characterized by a Lorentz transformation, which
results in the confinement of the beam of radiation within a
forward-directed cone (4). The small solid angle (θ) of the cone
is determined by the rest mass (mc^2) and the total energy (E) of
the emitting particle

$$\theta = mc^2/E$$

With electrons or positrons as the emitting particles ($mc^2 = 0.51$
MeV) and a particle beam energy of 3.0 GeV, the angle is < 1 milliradian
(4). The natural collimation of virtually all of the radiation provides

Atherosclerotic Plaques, Edited by R.W. Wissler *et al.*
Plenum Press, New York, 1991

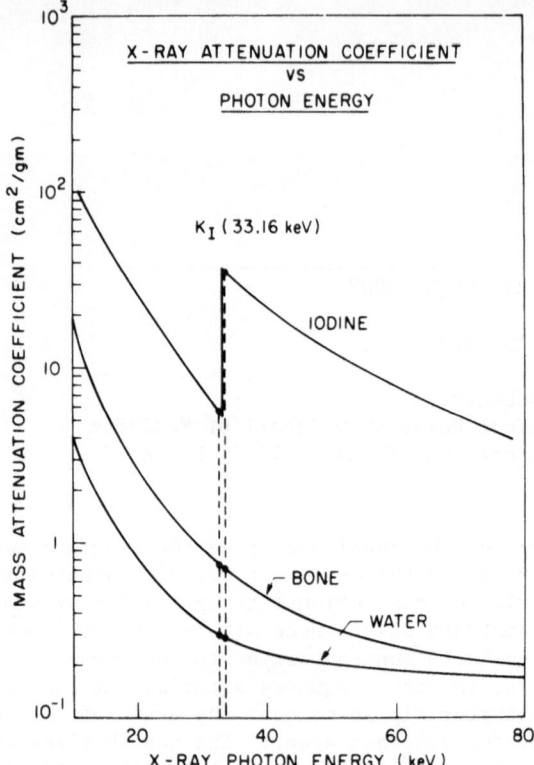

Figure 1   X-ray attenuation as a function
of energy. The upper curve shows the
attenuation by iodine, the middle curve the
attenuation by soft tissue, and the lower
curve the attenuation by bone. There is a
six-fold stepwise increase in attenuation by
iodine at 33.16 keV.

exceedingly high X-ray fluence in an essentially planar, fan-shaped beam,
which can be readily monochromatized by Bragg diffraction. The energy of
the diffracted beam can be selected by adjustment of the incident angle,
as given by the Bragg equation

$$n\lambda = 2d \sin \theta$$

The optical system has been designed so that two line images are
recorded simultaneously, one with an X-ray beam whose energy is slightly
above the K-edge of iodine, and the other with energy slightly below the
K-edge. The logarithmic difference of these images is an image in which
the signals arising from the photoelectric interaction with iodine are
preserved, and signals arising from soft tissue, bone, and Compton
scattering off iodine are essentially eliminated by the energy subtraction
process.

THE ELECTRON STORAGE RING AND THE BEAM LINE

Synchrotron radiation is generated within an accelerator known as an
electron storage ring, an evacuated annular pipe in which there are curved
sections and straight sections. The particles, usually electrons, are

preaccelerated in a linear accelerator or in a synchrotron, and then introduced into a straight section of the storage ring. The position and strength of the fields of a lattice of magnets surrounding the storage ring are adjusted so as to bend the trajectory of the electron beam into an orbital path which takes the shape of the ring. As the electrons accelerate through curved sections, they lose energy, which is emitted in the form of synchrotron radiation. The radiation leaves the storage ring through beryllium windows, which preserve the vacuum but are transparent to X-rays. The radiation propagates down a beam line, is monochromatized by diffracting elements, is continuously monitored for fluence and position by ionization chambers, passes through the subject and then impinges on a pair of segmented line detectors. The signals are amplified, computer-processed, and displayed electronically. (Fig. 2)

To maintain the electron beam at its original energy, it is necessary to restore the energy lost in the synchrotron radiation process. This is accomplished by applying Rf energy generated by klystrons. The need for precise timing of the Rf pulses with the passing bunches of electrons, which are traveling essentially at the speed of light, gave rise to the term synchrotron.

The intensity of the X-ray beam can be greatly increased by the use of an insertion device known as a wiggler. This consists of an array of magnets, with reversed polarity, positioned above and below a straight section of the ring. As electrons pass through the alternating fields of the wiggler they are compelled to execute tight sine-wave excursions, the

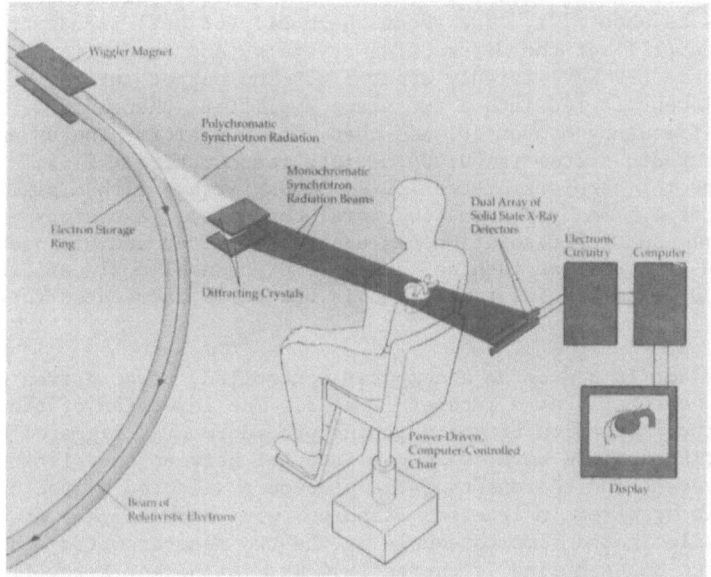

Figure 2   The optical system employing synchrotron radiation for transvenous coronary angiography. The polychromatic radiation is monochromatized by diffracting elements that provide two monochromatic beams with energy closely bracketing the K-edge of iodine. The beams cross at the position of the subject's heart, diverge and the impinge upon the dual detectors.

accelerations of which result in the emission of copious amounts of radiation downstream. The use of wigglers with high field strength makes it possible to generate intense beams of radiation with the critical energy needed for iodine K-edge coronary angiography.

THE STANFORD CORONARY ANGIOGRAPHY OPTICAL SYSTEM

The imaging system has been developed at the Stanford Synchrotron Radiation Laboratory (SSRL) in a collaborative effort involving members of the faculties of the Department of Physics, the Department of Applied Physics, and the Department of Medicine at Stanford University, together with staff from the Lawrence Berkeley Laboratory. The experiments began in 1979 (3). In the present dual-beam, dual-detector system the white synchrotron radiation is monochromatized off a pair of asymmetrically cut (1.9 off-plane) silicon (111) crystals. The crystals are positioned so that one intercepts the upper half of the transverse beam, and the other the lower half of the beam. The positioning of the two crystals must be precise because at their location the vertical dimension of the beam is only about 1.0 mm. The incident angle of each crystal is adjusted so that one provides a monochromatic beam with energy just above the K edge of iodine (33.16 keV), and the other provides a monochromatic beam with energy just below this threshold. The energy separation of the two beams is 300 eV and the bandwidth is 15-25 eV. The two beams cross at the position of the subject's heart, diverge and then impinge on the photosensitive elements of two solid-state line detectors.

These consist of lithium-drifted silicon. The photoelectric and scattering interactions of X-ray photons with the atoms of the detector crystal result in the production of electron-hole pairs. Each 33 keV photon generates about 11,000 of these. The detector efficiency for 33 keV photons is about 70%. The second harmonic (66 keV) is not transmitted by the plane (111) of the diffracting crystals, and the efficiency for the third harmonic (99 keV) is only about 5 %. The output current of each detector element is fed into a two-stage amplifier, then into a voltage-to-frequency converter, and then into a scaler. The dynamic range of the electronic system is 40,000:1, in a readout time < 2 ms. The present detector consists of two 150 mm linear arrays with a pixel resolution of 0.5 mm by 0.5 mm (600 total channels). A prototype detector with 0.25 mm spatial resolution has been constructed and has been shown to function in a similar fashion, and a 1,200-channel dual detector with 0.25 mm by 0.25 mm spatial resolution is now being fabricated for clinical use.

The subject is seated on a computer-controlled, power-driven chair and is scanned vertically at a rate of 12 cm/s. The injection of the contrast agent and the initiation of the scanning procedure are triggered by the electrocardiographic R wave, with the interval between the electrocardiographic event and the onset of the procedure selected by the operator. The image is acquired in line-scan fashion, with each segment of 0.5 mm thickness illuminated simultaneously by the two monochromatic beams. The exposure time of each line is currently 4 ms. At higher X-ray fluence, the scan rate can be increased to 24 cm/s, and the exposure time reduced to 2 ms. A full scan of the heart at 2 cm/s takes about 1 s, and therefore the vertical segments of the image are recorded at different stages during the cardiac cycle. The line-scan geometry minimizes background signals arising from scattered radiation.

The contrast agent is injected into the central venous circulation by means of a pervenous catheter. In experiments conducted to date, Renograffin-76 has been power-injected in boluses of 35-50 ml, given at a rate of 12 ml per s. The radiation exposure for each scan is about 0.5 rad.

The imaging system was developed in a stepwise series of experiments on phantoms, excised animal hearts, and anesthetized dogs (5-9). The first studies on human subjects were conducted in 1986, followed by a second set of experiments using the same imaging system during 1987 (10-11). These studies confirmed the feasibility of the approach and indicated that increased X-ray fluence was needed to reach a signal-to-noise ratio that would provide images of clinical quality (11). (Fig. 3, 4)

In 1988 the construction of a new dual-beam, dual detector optical imaging system was started, and completed in early 1989. This system eliminated the need for a rapid beam switcher, increased X-ray fluence by a factor of 2.5, and made possible for the first time the acquisition of high- and low-energy images simultaneously, thus eliminating artifacts arising from time subtraction. The system was used to image the coronary circulation of a human subject in March, 1989 (12), (Fig. 5, 6).

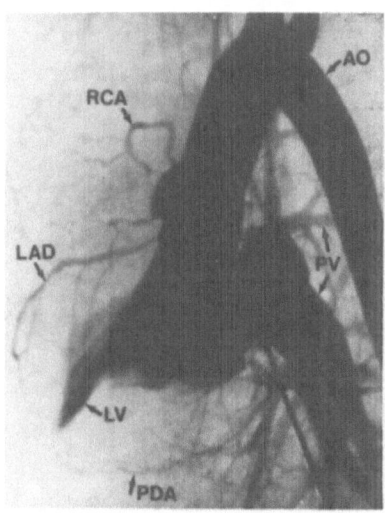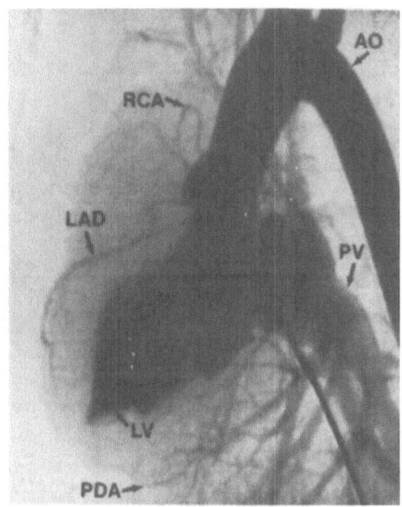

Figure 3   This is an in vivo coronary angiogram of an anesthetized dog recorded in May, 1986.
Asymmetrically-cut diffraction crystals were used, and the rapid beam switcher system was improved so that images were recorded at a scan speed of 12 cm/s. The contrast agent volume was 0.75 ml/kg, and the rate of administration was 15 ml/s. There is good visualization of the left ventricle (LV), the aorta (AO), the pulmonary veins (PV), the right coronary artery (RCA), the left anterior descending artery (LAD), and the posterior descending coronary artery (PDA). The image on the right was recorded 1.2 sec after the image on the left. The contrast agent has reached the capillary circulation in the later image and the myocardium is therefore opacified. The homogeneity of the myocardial opacification indicates that coronary perfusion is evenly distributed. Note the differences in the cardiac cycle. (SSRL)

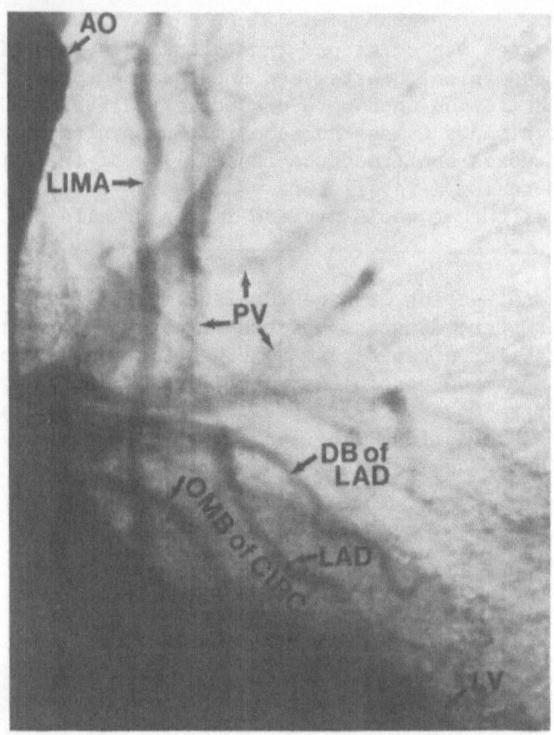

Figure 4 Transvenous synchrotron radiation
coronary angiogram (shallow right anterior
oblique) of a human subject following the
administration of Renograffin-76, 0.75 ml/kg,
at a rate of 12 ml/s. The angiogram was
recorded in April, 1987. The radiation dose
for this frame was 0.20 rad. The image shows
the aorta (AO), the left internal mammary
artery (LIMA), pulmonary veins (PV), the left
anterior descending coronary artery (LAD), a
diagonal branch of the left anterior coronary
artery (DB of LAD), an obtuse marginal branch
of the circumflex artery (OMB of CIRC), and
the left ventricle (LV). (SSRL)

The progress made in synchrotron radiation angiography in Germany and
in Japan, as well as in the United States, is reviewed in the Handbook on
Synchrotron Radiation, Volume 4 (13).

These studies have demonstrated that significant portions of the human
coronary artery circulation can be visualized by the transvenous
synchrotron radiation method, and confirmed that X-ray fluence should
increased (probably by a factor of three to four) in order to achieve a
signal-to-noise ratio that provides images comparable in quality to those
recorded in the canine model.

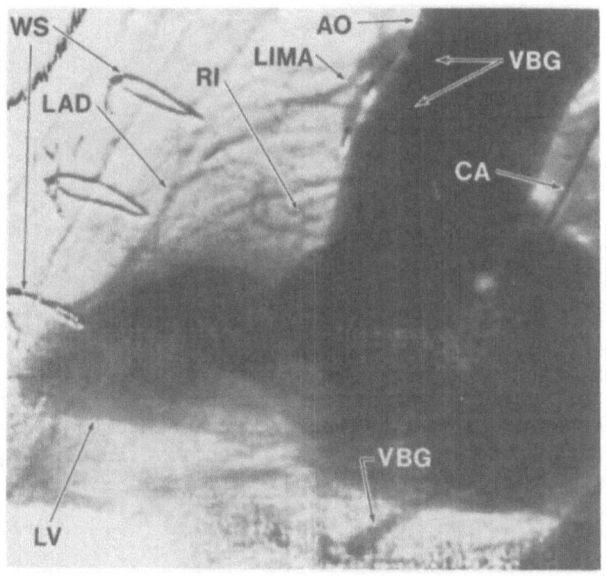

Figure 5 Lateral view of a transvenous synchrotron
radiation coronary angiogram recorded with the
dual-beam, dual detector optical system in March,
1989. The signal-to-noise ratio has been improved
by a factor of about 2.5 over that of previous
angiograms. The subject was a 62-year-old man with
severe angina pectoris who had undergone left
internal mammary artery and vein bypass graft
surgery four years earlier. Renografin-76 was
injected into the superior vena cava in a dose of
0.60 ml/kg at a rate of 12 ml/sec. The radiation
exposure was 0.49 rad. AO is the aorta; LIMA is
the left internal mammary artery; VBG is a vein
bypass graft; RI is the ramus intermedius artery;
LV is the left ventricle: CA is the catheter: CL
are surgical clips: WS are wire sutures. (SSRL)

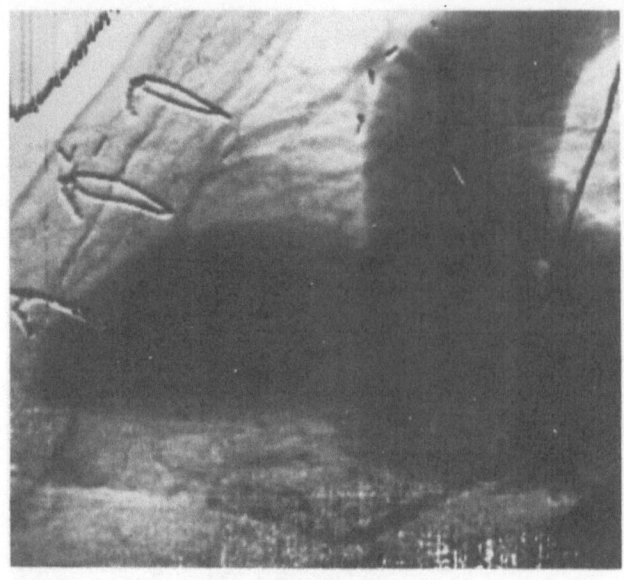

Figure 6   This image was recorded about 2 seconds
after the image shown in Figure 5. The passage of
most of the contrast agent out of the aorta allows
for the ready visualization of the overlapping vein
bypass grafts, which are not visible in Figure 5.
(SSRL)

DISCUSSION

The requisite attributes of imaging systems for the human coronary
circulation are: brief exposure times to freeze motion, probably on the
order of a few ms; spatial resolution fine enough to permit the
assessment of vascular narrowing, probably 0.25 to 0.5 mm; and an
adequate signal-to-noise ratio. The synchrotron radiation approach has
achieved the first two of these requirements. The third necessitates
increased X-ray fluence. The radiation available at the medical beamline
(X-17) at the National Synchrotron Light Source, Brookhaven National
Laboratory, will be evaluated in the near future in this regard.

Beyond the performance of the imaging system is the issue of how much
of the coronary artery circulation can be visualized directly by the use
of projection angles that throw the coronary artery segment into positions
that are not overlapped by contrast-agent containing structures. On the
basis of the limited number of experiments done to date on human subjects,
it seems reasonable to conclude that virtually the entire left anterior
descending coronary artery and most of the right coronary artery can be
readily imaged in this manner. Edge-enhancing techniques may be needed to
visualize the left main coronary artery and, in all likelihood, will be
required for the proximal portion of the circumflex artery; further
experimental data will clarify this matter. We believe that the results
obtained so far indicate that enough of the coronary circulation can be
imaged by the transvenous synchrotron approach to suggest that this method
is suitable for serial use in the evaluation of the natural history of
atherosclerosis and of its preventability, arrestability, and
reversibility.   The digitization of the data, which are acquired at time

intervals selected in relation to electrocardiographic signals, provides a convenient feature for comparative studies.

The size and cost of synchrotron radiation facilities are related to the electron beam energy and the X-ray fluence required. The narrowness of the bandwidth of the radiation diffracted by silicon crystals results in a severe loss of intensity. For this reason, our group is currently conducting experiments on the use of synthetic multilayers as diffracting elements. These transmit 40-90 times more radiation, at a bandwidth of 2.8 to 3.0%. The optimization of synthetic multilayers for angiography could have a significantly favorable impact on the application of the method for medical purposes. The use of vertically-focusing (bent Laue) crystals or germanium crystals also provide means of increasing the fluence of monochromatized beams.

This work was supported by National Institutes of Health Grant 1 R01 HL 39253-01 and Department of Energy Grant DE-FG03887 ER60527. Part of the work reported herein was done at the Stanford Synchrotron Radiation Laboratory, which is supported by the Department of Energy, Office of Basic Energy Sciences and the National Institutes of Health Biotechnology Resources Program, Division of Research Resources.

REFERENCES

1. See chapter by D. M. Kramsch, this publication.

2. B. Jacobson, Dichromatic absorption radiography. Dichromography, Acta. Radiol. 39:437 (1953).

3. E. Rubenstein, E.B. Hughes, L.E. Campbell, R. Hofstadter, R.L. Kirk, T.J. Krolocki, J.P. Stone, S. Wilson, H.D. Zeman, W.R. Brody, A. Macovski, A.C. Thompson, Synchrotron radiation and its application to digital subtraction, SPIE 314:42 (1981).

4. H. Winick, A. Bienenstock, Synchrotron radiation research, Ann. Rev. Nucl. Part. Sci. 28:33 (1978).

5. E.B. Hughes, H.E. Zeman, L.E. Campbell, R. Hofstadter, U. Meyer-Berkhout, J.N. Otis, J. Rolfe, J.P. Stone, S. Wilson, E. Rubenstein, D.C. Harrison, R. S. Kernoff, A.C. Thompson, and G.S. Brown, The application of synchrotron radiation to non-invasive angiography, Nuc. Instru. Methods Phys. Res. 208:665 (1983).

6. H.D. Zeman, E.B. Hughes, L. Finman Campbell, R. Hofstadter, A. Hudson, J.N. Otis, J. Rolfe, E. Rubenstein, D.C. Harrison, R.S. Kernoff, A.C. Thompson, and G.S. Brown, Evaluation of synchrotron x-rays for transvenous coronary angiography, Nuc. Instru. Methods Phys. Res. 222:308 (1984).

7. E.B. Hughes, E. Rubenstein, H.D. Zeman, G.S. Brown, M. Buchbinder, D.C. Harrison, R. Hofstadter, R.S.Kernoff, J.N. Otis, H.A. Sommer, A.C. Thompson, J.T. Walton, Prospects for non-invasive angiography with tunable x-rays, Nuc. Instru. Methods Phys. Res. B10/11:323 (1985).

8. E.B. Hughes, Rubenstein, E., Zeman, H.D., Brown, G.S., Buchbinder, M., Harrison, D.C., Hofstadter, R.S., Kernoff, Otis, J.N., A.C. Thompson, The angiography program at Stanford, Nuc. Instru. Methods Phys. Res. A246:719 (1986).

9. A.C. Thompson, H.D. Zeman, E. Rubenstein, J.N. Otis, R.H. Hofstadter, G.S. Brown, D.C. Harrison, R.S. Kernoff, J.C. Giacomini, H.J. Gordon, W. Thomlinson, Transvenous coronary angiography in dogs using synchrotron radiation, Internat. J. Cardiac Imag. 2:53 (1986).

10. E. Rubenstein, R. Hofstadter, H.D. Zeman, A.C. Thompson, J.N. Otis, G.S. Brown, J.C. Giacomini, H.J. Gordon, R.S. Kernoff, D.C. Harrison, W. Thomlinson, Transvenous coronary angiography in humans using synchrotron radiation, Proc. Nat. Acad. Sci. 83:9724 (1986).

11. A. Thompson, R. Hofstadter, J.N. Otis, H.D. Zeman, R.S. Kernoff, E. Rubenstein, J.C. Giacomini, H.J. Gordon, G.S. Brown, W. Thomlinson, Transvenous coronary angiography using synchrotron radiation, Nuc. Instru. Methods Phys. Res. A266, 252 (1988).

12. E. Rubenstein, J.C. Giacomini, H.J. Gordon, A.C. Thompson, G.S. Brown, R. Hofstadter, W. Thomlinson, H.D. Zeman, Synchrotron radiation coronary angiography with a dual beam, dual detector imaging system, Nuc. Instru. Methods Phys. Res. (in press).

13. E. Ebashi, E. Rubenstein, M. Koch, "Handbook on Synchrotron Radiation" Volume 4, North-Holland Physics Publishing, Amsterdam (in press, 1990).

B-MODE ULTRASOUND IMAGING CHARACTERIZATION OF ATHEROSCLEROSIS

M. Mercuri[1-3], M.G. Bond[1], H.L. Strickland[1], W.J. Bo[1],
C.P. Purvis[1], V. Challa[2]

Division of Vascular Ultrasound Research, Department of
Neurobiology and Anatomy[1], Department of Pathology[2], and Stroke
Research Center, Bowman Gray School of Medicine, 300 South
Hawthorne Road, Winston-Salem (NC) 27103, USA. II Department
of Internal Medicine[3], University of Perugia, 06100 Perugia,
Italy

INTRODUCTION

At present, prevention of atherosclerosis, or the effective
inhibition of the lesion progression, remains a primary medical research
objective (1). In the past 50 years efforts have been made to study and
understand the atherosclerotic process, and have resulted in several
achievements in basic sciences, epidemiology and medical management of the
disease. Using experimental and animal models, specific therapies have been
developed and tested and offer promising perspectives. However, it would
be of great help to detect the morphological characteristics of
atherosclerosis non-invasively and during plaque evolution in human
arteries.

The in vivo morphological evaluation of brain, lung, breast, bone and
other organs using radiography, Computer Tomography and Magnetic Resonance
Imaging (MRI) are diagnostic approaches widely used in clinical practice.
In part, these modalities provide an in vivo histopathologic interpretation
of specific tissue characteristics.

Methods used to study the morphological characteristics of
atherosclerosis in vivo include Radionuclide, Positron Emission Tomography,
MRI, angiography and ultrasound. They have been used to define
composition, physiologic state and viability of arterial tissues (2).

Imaging-based methods are widely used to evaluate atherosclerosis
including the vessel lumen and wall. Angiography is the "gold standard"
technique to study vessel lumen (3), but only high-resolution ultrasound
has the ability to characterize the vessel wall including thickness (4),
elasticity (5), and potentially the types of tissues that comprise plaques.
B-Mode ultrasound imaging provides two-dimensional images of arterial walls
by reflecting sound waves from tissue interfaces associated with the lumen-
intima, media-adventitia and adventitia-periadventitia boundaries (6).

In the past 20 years efforts have been made to apply ultrasound to
atherosclerosis research, and consistent results have been obtained in
measuring the extent and severity of atherosclerosis (7) and related
hemodynamic impairment (8). Future challenges in this field are to
demonstrate small changes in arterial wall thickness in large controlled
trials, and to confirm its utility in the early diagnosis and treatment of
atherosclerosis in high risk subjects.

Atherosclerotic Plaques, Edited by R.W. Wissler *et al.*
Plenum Press, New York, 1991

B-Mode ultrasound imaging is potentially useful for plaque tissue characterization. The ability to differentiate various components of lesions could be the most powerful predictor of plaque instability and active progression (9). However, the *in vivo* morphological interpretation of the atherosclerotic plaque components is still unsatisfactory.

Several attempts have been made to provide a morphological interpretation of ultrasound images of atherosclerotic plaques, however, these studies have led only to a qualitative interpretation of images (10-12). *In vitro* studies have shown that ultrasound provides useful information to differentiate several tissue components (12). Quantitative results were obtained by measuring attenuation and backsetter (13, 14), but unfortunately these methods require instrumentation not commercially available, and are difficult both to use and interpret.

The specific aim of this investigation is to determine, *in vitro*, the feasibility of applying conventional high-resolution B-Mode ultrasound imaging to quantitatively define arterial tissue components, and to differentiate normal from atherosclerotic arteries.

MATERIAL AND METHODS

In determining the capability of ultrasound to differentiate atherosclerotic plaques, it is required to compare one ultrasonic image to its precise histologic preparation. An *in vitro* experimental model has been designed to satisfy this requirement. Samples of fresh thoracic aorta were obtained at autopsy, washed in saline, freed of periadventitial tissues, opened longitudinally, and labelled. Rectangular strips 1.4 cm in length were prepared from these specimens, and a thin metallic pin was inserted longitudinally into the intima and used as a reference. The strips were suspended between two cork-plexiglass bands of a holder, and fixed in place with metallic pins in such a way that both intima and adventitia were freely exposed to the water bath. The specimens were then interrogated with a 90^0 incident ultrasonic beam.

The arterial strip was mounted in a water-tank and investigated with the ultrasound beam focus adjusted to a depth of 1 cm. Gain settings were chosen using data derived during a pilot investigation, and were maintained equally for all evaluations. A two dimensional X-Y translator platform allowed a precise positioning of the artery. Arterial strips were interrogated every 0.5 mm, and a consecutive series of motionless ultrasonic longitudinal images were obtained. The X-Y coordinates were recorded for each ultrasonic image, and were used to identify specific sites for the ultrasound-pathology comparison. Using this method it was possible to obtain bidimensional ultrasound images and histologic preparations with similar spatial configurations that demonstrated the intima, media and adventitia.

A Biosound 2000 II s.a. with a 8 MHz mechanical annular array transducer (dynamic range =70 dB, axial resolution =0.3 mm, lateral resolution =0.8 mm) was used. The instrument was interfaced with a Video-Densitometric Station which was equipped with an ultrasound scanner, a videorecorder, a high-resolution TV monitor, and a personal computer. A commercially available software which allowed digitation of the ultrasonic images and measures of gray scale characteristics of each artery was used.

After digitizing the ultrasonic image, an arterial window was selected and positioned to avoid inclusion of the reflection due to the media-adventitia interface. The actual intensity of each pixel was automatically calculated, labelled and stored to be analyzed for subsequent comparison with the histologic tissue characteristic.

The videodensitometric variables were the area and total, average, maximum and minimum gray scale intensities for each selected arterial window. Signal noise produced by artifactual reflections at primary interfaces was removed from the analyses using a digital filter, so that only the inner ectogenic area was included in the gray level analysis.

The B-Mode images were recorded on videotape for later analyses and image reproduction.

Arterial strips were fixed in 10% neutral buffered formalin for 24 hours, gross stained with Sudan IV, and processed in paraffin for hematoxylin-eosin and Verhoeff-Van Gieson stains. Tissues were characterized as normal (class 1), or as having diffuse intimal thickening (class 2), fatty streak (class 3), fibrous plaque (class 4), fibrous plaque with necrosis (class 5), plaque with mineral (class 6), plaque with cholesterol crystals (class 7), or as containing more than one of these complications (class 8). To take into account shrinkage artifact and magnification factors, microscopic slides were projected on a calibrated grid which allowed for dividing each microscopic image into areas resembling the size of the arterial window used for videodensitometric analyses.

Four hundred arterial segments were used to test the feasibility of application of high resolution B-Mode imaging ultrasound to characterize normal and atherosclerotic tissues.

A general descriptive statistical analysis was carried out for all videodensitometric variables. A simple linear model was used to correlate the variables. Depending on the characteristics and distribution of the data, appropriate parametric (ANOVA) or non-parametric (Kruskal-Wallis) tests were used (15). A value for $p<0.05$ after Bonferroni correction for multiple variables was considered statistically significant.

RESULTS

The numbers and distribution of the histologic arterial diagnosis were as follows: normal 100, diffuse intimal thickening 50, fatty streak 20, fibrous plaque 100, plaque with necrosis 15, mineralized plaque 50, plaque with cholesterol crystals 20, and other complicated plaques 45.

The internal consistency of videodensitometry was tested using the degree of concordance between the two main videodensitometric variables, i.e. maximum and average intensities. The coefficient of correlation in a simple linear model with 400 measures was $r=0.85$.

The precision was tested using the test-retest consistency approach. For this estimation 53 arterial segments, including normal and atherosclerotic tissue, were scanned twice in a blinded fashion and the average and maximum intensities were calculated for each of the samples. The mean difference (+/- SD) and the coefficient of variation were $0.15+/-0.94$ and 6.26% respectively. The correlation coefficient among two replicate and blinded readings was $r=0.90$. The predictive validity of the videodensitometric measurements of the ultrasound images was determined in 400 arterial normal and atherosclerotic segments using the qualitative histologic diagnosis as the discriminant factor. Parametric (ANOVA) and non-parametric (Kruskall-Wallis) tests showed significant differences for the average and maximum intensities according to the histopathologic diagnosis ($p<0.001$), and these were confirmed after Bonferroni correction for multiple rank variables (Table 1).

Table 1. B-Mode Imaging Ultrasound Average (A) and Maximum (M) Intensities according to Histologic Diagnosis. [Total N = 400].

	N	A*	M*
Normal	100	23.5+/-0.1	44.4+/-0.4
Diffuse Intimal Thickness	50	26.6+/-0.6	59.6+/-1.8
Fatty Streak	20	32.0+/-0.7	58.0+/-1.4
Fibrous Plaque	100	35.3+/-0.4	78.1+/-1.0
Necrosis	15	39.0+/-3.2	87.0+/-6.1
Mineral	50	46.0+/-1.5	99.4+/-3.2
Cholesterol Crystal	20	52.9+/-1.9	111.1+/-3.1
Other Complicated Plaque	45	58.5+/-1.6	113.7+/-1.7

(*) mean +/- S.E. ANOVA and Kruskal-Wallis Tests $p<0.001$

CONCLUSIONS

High-resolution B-Mode ultrasound imaging is a technique currently used for non-invasive quantification of the extent and severity of carotid artery atherosclerosis (16). However a primary advantage of this imaging technique, i.e. the ability to define the morphological characteristics of the vessel wall itself, has not been completely exploited.

Using digital technology it was possible to quantitatively determine echo reflectivity using commercially available instrumentation and software (17).

The in vitro model used in this study allowed for a precise comparison of bidimensional ultrasonic images with the histologic preparation. Using these methods we have shown that B-mode ultrasound imaging and its videodensitometric analyses provides a reliable and valid quantitative interpretation of tissue characteristics of the arterial wall.

Although these in vitro studies are quite encouraging several questions remain to be answered. It will be necessary to increase the sensitivity of the method using additional videodensitometric techniques (18). Additional experiments are necessary to compare the gray level intensities of B-Mode images with a quantitative histologic analysis. Perhaps most importantly we have to test these hypotheses on the near wall of arteries, and to extrapolate the method to the in vivo evaluation of arteries.

Considering the growing interest of epidemiologists and clinicians, the data obtained by various groups using different approaches, and the extensive application of the digital technology to improve ultrasound instrument performances, we may expect to see in the near future a consistent use of vascular ultrasound methods to study the morphologic characteristics of arterial tissues.

ACKNOWLEDGEMENTS

We gratefully acknowledge the following collaborators for their technical help: April Comer and Sarah Graham, Leonard Noble, David Clodfelder, Eddy Spencer and Mark Bell.

These studies were supported by National Institute of Neurologic and Communication Disorders and Stroke (NS-06655), the Division of Vascular Ultrasound Research, Center for Medical Ultrasound, and the Italian Ministry of Education.

REFERENCES

1. D. E. Strandness, Workshop overview, in: Clinical Diagnosis of Atherosclerosis, M. G. Bond, W. Insull, S. Glagov, A. B. Chandler and J.F. Cornhill, eds., p. 1, Springer-Verlag Inc., New York (1982).

2. J. F. Greenleaf, Tissue Characterization with Ultrasound, CRC Press Inc., Boca Raton (FL) (1986).

3. R. B. Rutherford, Evaluation and selection of patients for vascular surgery, in: Vascular Surgery, R. B. Rutherford, ed., p. 11, W.B. Saunders Co., Philadelphia (1989).

4. P. Pignoli, E. Tremoli, A. Poli, P. Oreste, and R. Paoletti, Intimal plus medial thickness of the arterial wall: A direct measurement with ultrasound imaging, Circulation 74:1399 (1986).

5. W. A. Riley, D. S. Freedman, N. A. Higgs, R. W. Barnes, S. A. Zinkgraf, and G. S. Berenson, Decreased arterial elasticity associated with cardiovascular disease risk factors in the young, Bogalusa Heart Study, Arteriosclerosis 6:378 (1986).

6.   M. G. Bond, K. S. Wilmoth, G. L. Enevold, and H. L. Strickland, Detection and monitoring of asymptomatic atherosclerosis in clinical trials, Am J Med 86(suppl. 4A):33 (1989).

7.   J. J. Ricotta, F. A. Bryan, M. G. Bond, A. Kurtz, D. H. O'Leary, J. K. Raines, A. S. Berson, M. E. Clouse, M. Calderon-Ortiz, J. F. Toole, J. A. DeWeese, S. N. Smullens, and N. F. Gustafson, Multicenter validation study of real-time (B-Mode) ultrasound, arteriography, and pathologic examination, J Vasc Surg 6:512 (1987).

8.   D. E. Strandness, Ultrasound in the study of atherosclerosis, Ultrasound in Med & Biol 12:453 (1986).

9.   C. K. Zarins and S. Glagov, Artery wall pathology in atherosclerosis, in: R.B. Rutherford, Vascular Surgery, p. 178, W.B. Saunders Co., Philadelphia (1989).

10. L. M. Reilly, R. J. Lusby, L. Hughes, L. D. Ferrel, R. J. Stoney, and W. R. Ehrenfeld, Carotid plaque histology using real-time ultrasonography, Am J Surg 146:188 (1983).

11. E. I. Bluth, D. Kay, C. R. B. Merrit, M. Sullivan, G. Farr, N. L. Mills, M. Foreman, K. Sloan, M. Schlater, and J. Stewart, Sonographic characterization of carotid plaque: Detection of hemorrhage, AJR 146:1061 (1986).

12. J. Weinberger, S. J. Marks, J. J. Gaul, B. Goldman, H. Schanzer, J. Jacobson, and S. Dikman, Atherosclerotic plaque at the carotid artery bifurcation. Correlation of ultrasonographic imaging with morphology, J Ultrasound Med 6:363 (1987).

13. B. Barzilai, J. E. Saffitz, J. G. Miller, and B. E. Sobel, Quantitative ultrasonic characterization of the nature of atherosclerotic plaques in human aorta, Circulation Research 60:459 (1987).

14. E. Picano, L. Landini, F. Lattanzi, C. Michelassi, M. Salvadori, F. Santarelli, A, Distante, A, L'Abbate, Ultrasonic tissue characterization of atherosclerosis: State of the art 1988, J Nucl Med & Allied Sciences 32:174 (1988).

15. Statgraphics: Statistical graphic system, Statistical Graphic Corporation, New York (1986).

16. M. W. Higgins and A. R. Sharrett, Ultrasound measurement of atherosclerosis: Directions for epidemiology, in: Pathobiology of the Human Atherosclerotic Plaque, p. 899, S. Glagov, W. P. Newmann, III and S. A. Shaffer, eds., Springer-Verlag, New York (1990).

17. D. J. Skorton, R. C. Chivers and S. M. Collins, Ultrasonic tissue characterization in cardiology, Am J Noninvas Cardiol 1:88 (1987).

18. S. M. Collins and D. J. Skorton, Computers in Cardiac Imaging. JACC 9:669 (1987).

NMR MICROSCOPY: A NEW TECHNIQUE IN ATHEROSCLEROSIS RESEARCH

Maurizio Soma[1], Tiziana Beringhelli[2], Rodolfo Paoletti[1], Maria Asdente[1], Winfried Kuhn[3]

[1]Inst. of Pharmacological Sciences, [2]Dept. of Inorganic and Metallorganic Chemistry, University of Milan, Milan, Italy, [3]Fraunhofer Institute, St. Ingbert, FRG

INTRODUCTION

Atherosclerosis is clinically silent until late in its course. Its diagnosis ordinarily depends on the detection of impaired blood flow or decreased blood pressure distal to an arterial narrowing. Angiographic visualization of deformity in the lumen of a vessel remains the best presumptive test of silent atherosclerosis (1). Recently, important advances have been made in developing non-invasive diagnostic instrumentation for visualizing blood vessels and atheroma. The new techniques, including B mode ultrasonography, computer-assisted tomography and radionuclear scanning, now allow for an earlier diagnosis of atherosclerosis (2,3). Even though these methods offer valuable morphological information about a diseased vessel, they give very little data on the physico-chemical structure of pathological alteration. The availability of a non-invasive method for the detection of morphological and physico-chemical features of atherosclerotic lesions and, possibly, the observation of their progression or regression, would represent a significant advance.

Proton Magnetic Resonance Imaging (MRI) and Nuclear Magnetic Resonance (NMR) spectroscopy is being extensively utilized in clinical and research fields in many areas. The application of NMR spectroscopy to biological systems has increased dramatically over the last decade along with an improvement in technical sophistication (4,5).

Atherosclerotic lesions affect the arterial wall, from non-protruding fatty streaks to more complex lesions, consisting of lipid, smooth muscle cells, fibroblasts, and occasional calcium deposits (6). The major objective of our work is to develop an NMR processing (imaging and spectroscopy) for the evaluation and the characterization of atherosclerotic lesions in vitro at various stages, which allows us to classify fatty streaks, atheroma, and calcified plaques. This work provides a basis for the methodology for evaluating atherosclerosis non-invasively at different pathological stages in vivo.

Atherosclerotic Plaques, Edited by R.W. Wissler *et al.*
Plenum Press, New York, 1991

Nuclear magnetic resonance imaging is somehow unique to non-invasive diagnostic methods for pathological tissues because it characterizes tissues giving both morphological and physico-chemical information according to changes in many different parameters, i.e. the spin-lattice and spin-spin relaxation times (T_1, T_2 respectively) and the chemical shift (CS).

NMR imaging

We first investigated how to recognize a normal and a pathological vessel using NMR, and what sequence was more suitable to reveal differences in the various atherosclerotic lesions, i.e. T_1, T_2, CS images and NMR spectra. All human autoptic specimens underwent the same sequential analysis i.e. multi-slice, CS, T_1, T_2 images, followed by NMR spectroscopy of the whole specimen and of its lipid extract. From the cross-section multislice images, particular slices were selected to perform the remaining measurements. Images were obtained with 36 /uM pixel resolution and 400 /uM slice thickness.

In general, water and the more mobile lipid components of the complex mixtures present in a lesion make the largest contribution to its proton image. The chemical shift (CS) of water protons, which is significantly different from that of lipid proton (- 3.3 ppm) (figure 1), allows their selective excitation in the presence of lipid protons (and vice versa). This has been utilized for producing vessel images in which signal strength (image brightness) is related only to water or to lipid distribution (chemical shift images).

Figure 2a shows the whole signal image of a selected aortic specimen and it can be compared to the images obtained from water signal (figure 2b) and from fat signal (fig. 2c). The lipid contrast in the entire signal (fig. 2a) is dependent on the time parameters used in the NMR sequence; while the lipid distribution in the vessel is isolated in fig. 2b, it is also distinguishable as the dark areas in Fig. 2c.

We observed previously (7,8) that when the vessels were normal, the internal profile and the wall thickness were regular. Furthermore, the lipid distribution along the normal wall, resulting from the CS images, was homogeneous. The aspect of a damaged vessel is quite different: figure 2 depicts the different features in the wall and the different distribution along the vessel wall.

Generally the whole signal of a lipid rich region is bright, while the one from necrotic and calcific areas is dark, as it is shown in the multislice images reported in figure 3.

These results show that MRI is capable of distinguishing the different types of structures occupying the lumen of an occluded vessel or within the arterial wall. A good agreement between NMR images, gross pathology, and histological analysis is generally found (7).

Other local information is based on the relaxation times T_1 and T_2,

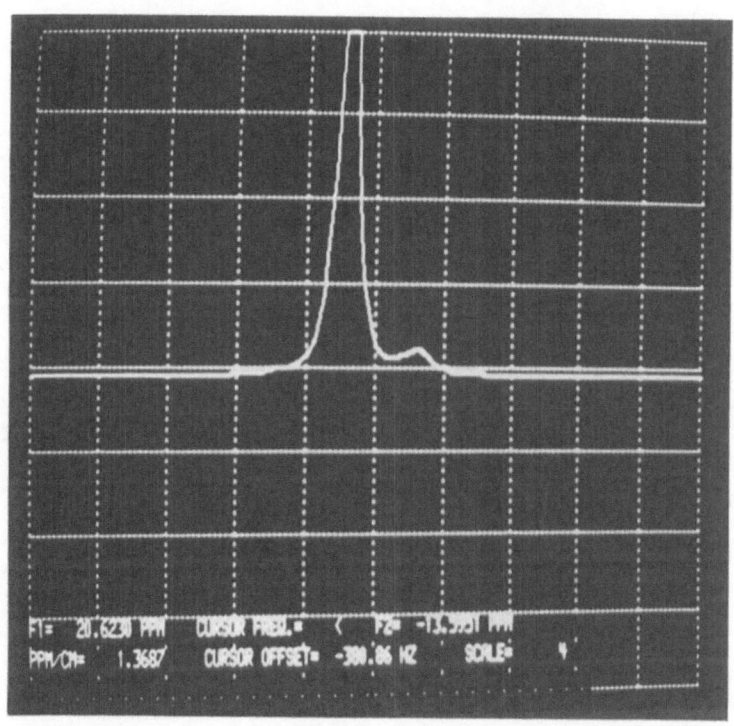

Fig. 1. High resolution ¹H spectrum of human atheroma plaque (see figure
2 for image), at 300 MHz on a Bruker AM300 spectrometer. The huge
peak belongs to protons from the water; the small peak is due to
lipid protons present in the lesion.

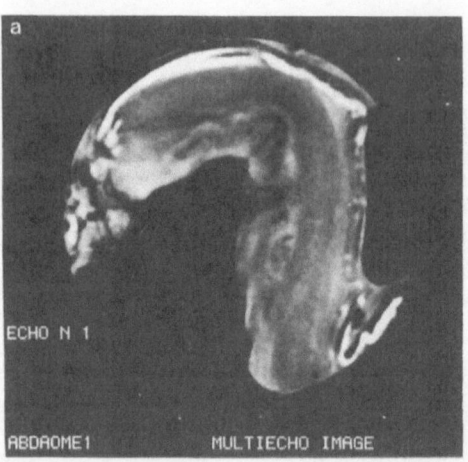

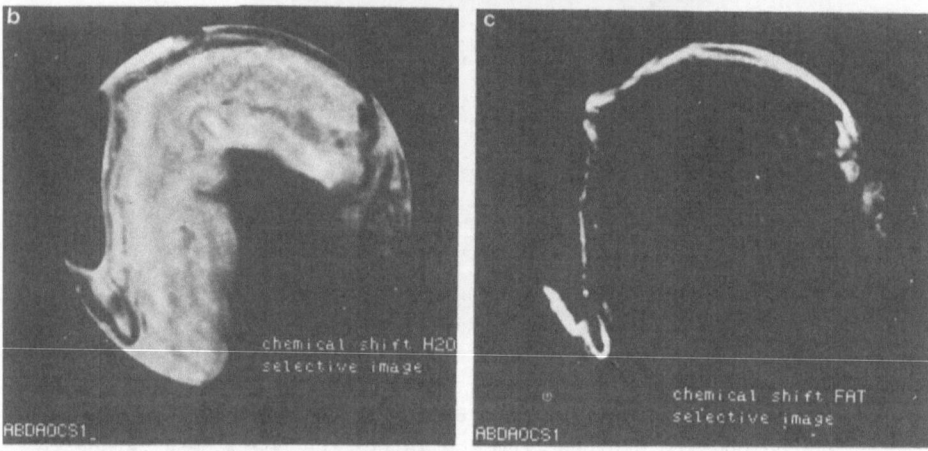

Fig. 2. Cross section NMR images of human atheroma. The autoptic sample was
isolated from the abdominal aorta of a 65 years old man. Figure
2a represents the image obtained from the whole proton signal (see
figure 1). Figure b and c, are the Chemical Shift (CS) selective
images obtained from the water and the lipid proton signals, respectively. Slice thickness 400 /uM; pixel resolution 36 /um.

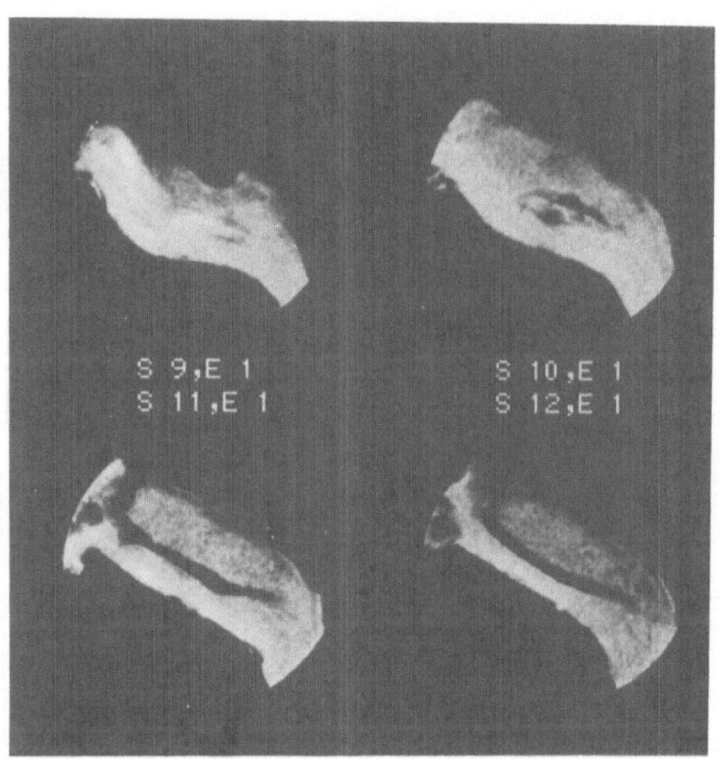

Fig. 3. Multi-slice cross section images of a human aortic calcific plaque. Slice thickness 400 / um; pixel resolution 36 / um. The cross sectional slices along the vessel reveal that a calcified region is present; it is not yet visible in slice 9, and begins to appear in slice N 10; the calcified region is clearly visible, as a dark region in slices N 11 and 12.

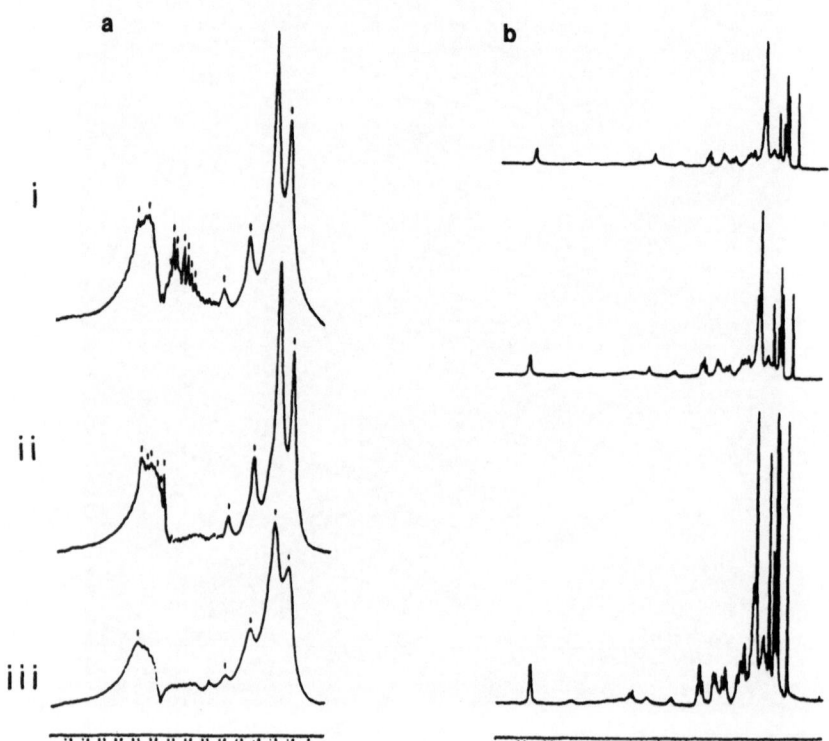

Fig. 4. ^{1}H spectra obtained from (a) whole samples and (b) related lipid
extracts of: (i) fatty streak; (ii) advanced plaque; (iii) compli-
cated-calcified plaque. In the left panel spectra, the huge water
signal was suppressed with particular sequences. All the spectra
are equally normalized.

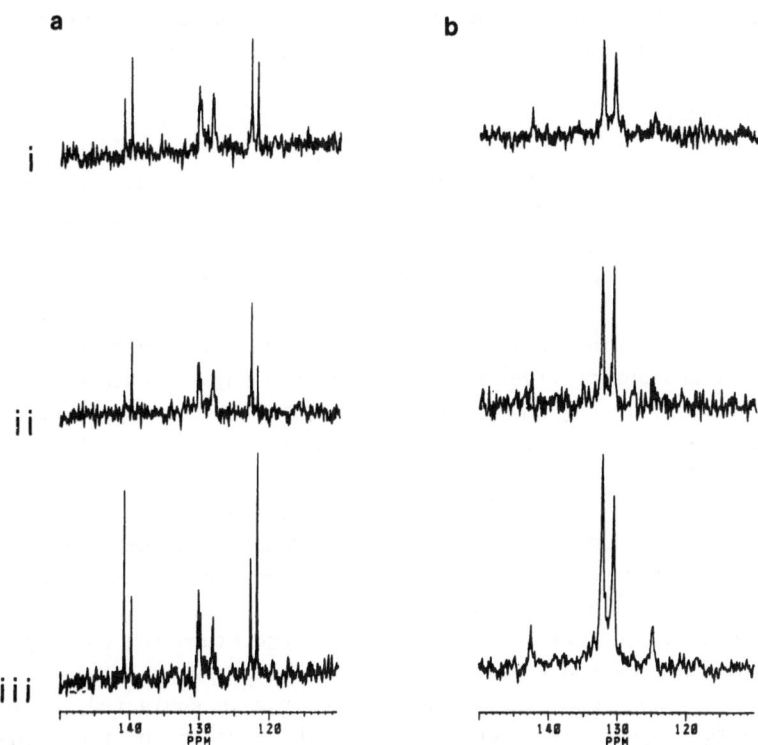

Fig. 5. ^{13}C spectra from the same sample (a) and extracts (b) as in figure 4.

which are related to the physical structure of the sample. (T_1-T_2) "measures" the solid degree of the molecular structure. In particular T_2 is very short in solids, as a consequence the peaks in the spectra from rigid samples are larger than the peaks from mobile structures, sometime so large that they merge in the baseline. In this case the corresponding molecules are not detectable with NMR and the information about the solid state phase is virtually lost. The lipid content in artery lesions is associated with the focal accumulation of three major classes of lipids: cholesterol, cholesteryl ester and phospholipid. At body temperature they can exist in distict, more or less rigid, physical states, from liquid to liquid crystal or crystal structure (6). Consequently, there is a problem of relating the intensity of the NMR lipid signal and the real lipid content. Furthermore, the phase of a particular compound in a mixture does not only depend on its own concentration but it is influenced by the concentration of the other lipid components of the mixture (6).

NMR Spectroscopy

In order to clarify this point a preliminary study has been undertaken aimed at verifying how and to what extent it is possible to characterize vessel lesions, both considering the "physical" and "chemical" aspect through localized T_1 and T_2 and chemical shift measurements.

While microimaging provides detailed information about the morphology of the wall, and qualitative information on the physico-chemical properties of tissues, magnetic resonance spectroscopy of the whole specimen provides more detailed information about the chemical composition of the wall.

We examined both ^1H and ^{13}C NMR spectra of the sample which had undergone NMR microscopy analysis as well as its total lipid extract. Figure 4 shows representative high resolution ^1H NMR spectra obtained from an aortic atheroma (a), at 37°C, along with the spectrum of their total lipid extracts (b). In the left panel, a selective presaturation was employed in order to suppress the huge signal of the water and to obtain a better description of the lipid region. The ^1H spectrum is dominated, beside the residual water signal, by tissue lipids which exist in the fluid phase at the measurement temperature. Based on analysis of chemical structure and observed shifts, the major spectral peaks were, allylic ($CH_2-CH=CH-$), methylene (CH_2-CH_2) and methyl protons (CH_3). The improvement in the resolution that allows the recognition of many other resonances such as the C-18 methyl protons (ppm = 0.68) and the protons bound to unsaturated carbons is clearly visible in the lipid extract (ppm = 5.33) (right panel). Thin layer chromatography studies showed that the largest constituent by weight of atheroma was cholesteryl ester (60%), followed by cholesterol (25%), phospholipid (10%) and triglyceride (5%).

Two observations can be pointed out:

1) The more advanced plaques (fig. 4iii) give the largest peaks to indicate more inhomogeneous and rigid structure (short T_2) of the chemical constituents under analysis. On the same sample a more rapidly decaying signal was also observed for each pixel signal directly in the time domain, in the T weighted images. The analysis of the T localized

values confirmed this trend, toward a more rigid structure for more advanced plaques: we obtained T_1 in range of 0.6-1 seconds (s) interval for normal vessels, 1-2 s for intermediate lesions, 2-3 s for advanced lesions (T_1 increases with the increasing of the sample rigidity). We found that both the chemical composition and the morphological structure of the lesion components are important.

2) While there is no noticeable difference in the areas of the same peaks in the spectra of the three tissue samples (i.e. there is almost the same quantity of "visible" lipids), there is a relevant difference in their corresponding lipid extracts (see fig. 4, sample iii). This indicates that in the more advanced plaques lipids are "lost" in the NMR image because of their more rigid structure. Indeed, cholesterol crystals were demonstrable in the histological analysis. The pattern observed in the ^{1}H spectroscopy analysis is confirmed by ^{13}C NMR spectroscopy (figure 5). The ^{13}C spectra obtained from the lipid extract (figure 5b, iii), revealed the presence of significant amounts of free cholesterol which were not detectable in the spectra obtained from the whole samples (figure 5a iii).

CONCLUSIONS

NMR imaging is able to characterize the qualitative composition and morphology of human plaques without having to open or manipulate the specimen as is done for typical pathological analysis. The more rigid and inhomogeneous structures of the advanced lesions are detectable but caution needs to be used to quantify the chemical structure of a vessel. A wider study of different kinds of plaques might improve the evaluation of the NMR imaging findings. These studies may be of clinical interest also, possibly allowing an assessment of the progression or the regression of the plaque following pharmacological treatments.

REFERENCES

1. B.G. Brown, E.L. Bolson and H.T. Dodge, Arteriographic assessment of coronary atherosclerosis, Arteriosclerosis, 2:2-15 (1982).
2. G.S. Tell, G. Howard and W.M. McKinney, Risk factors for site specific extracranial carotid artery plaque distribution as measured by B-mode ultrasound, J. Clin. Epidemiol. 42: 551-559 (1989).
3. R.S. Lees, A.M. Lees and H.W. Strauss, External imaging of human atherosclerosis, J. Nucl. Med. 24:154-156 (1983).
4. T.F. Budinger and P.C. Lauterbur, Nuclear magnetic resonance technology for medical studies, Science, 226:288-298 (1984).
5. B.M.W. Hitzig, J.W. Prichard, Kantor H.L., Ellington W.R., Ingwall J.S., C.T. Burt, S.I. Helman and J. Koutcher, NMR spectroscopy as an investigative technique in physiology, FASEB 1:22-31 (1987).
6. D.M. Small, Progression and regression of atherosclerotic lesions. Insights from lipid physical biochemistry, Arteriosclerosis 8:103-129 (1988).
7. M.Asdente, L. Pavesi, P.L. Oreste, A. Colombo, W.C. Kuhn and E. Tremoli, Evaluation of atherosclerotic lesions using NMR microimaging, Atherosclerosis 80:243-253 (1990).

8. M.Asdente, W.C. Kuhn, P.L. Oreste, L. Pavesi, M. Soma and E. Tremoli, 1H NMR microimages of carotid endarterectomy, AIFB V, in press (1990).

<u>Summary of Discussion following Session 4</u>

    <u>Paulin</u> called on <u>Wissler</u> to begin the discussion of his paper. <u>Wissler</u> pointed out that he wanted to ask <u>Paulin</u> one question about the prospects for future quantitation of plaque components by means of MRI and how close we are to the limits of resolution or speed that can be used in vivo to measure changes in plaques over time. <u>Paulin</u> responded by pointing out that, according to an old saying, it is increasingly difficult to say something about the future because "the future ain't anymore what it used to be." He then went on to say that MRI offers great opportunities for further development in technology. However, one has to make compromises between spatial and temporal resolution. He indicated that ultrafast MRI is developing very quickly and that one can now get a very reasonable picture within one heartbeat or within several heartbeats during one breath-holding interval, but at some sacrifice of resolution. <u>Kramsch</u> indicated that he would be interested to know whether with the proper improvement of the integrating algorithm one might be able to develop images that are comparable to contrast media angiography which would offer the advantages of being noninvasive and of eliminating the artifact of arterial dilatation due to contrast injection. He indicated that he hoped that, with time, the power would be good enough to see abnormalities in the carotid arteries that would help the surgeon make decisions. <u>Paulin</u> pointed out that MRI angiography already can provide images of the carotid arteries that fulfill such requirements. The coronary arteries pose a greater challenge because of the rapid motion of the heart and therefore cannot provide the same detail. He continued by saying that in the future MRI might enable one to observe laminar flow and to analyze the abnormalities of flow in the form of turbulence, which may indicate rough areas on the arterial surface associated with the first manifestions of atherosclerosis. <u>Bond</u> asked questions about the spatial resolution using the present magnetic resonance imaging, and <u>Paulin</u> replied that for human studies it is about 1 mm at present.

    <u>Bond</u> then went on to ask whether high sensitivity MRI might indicate qualitative changes in atherosclerosis which would be extremely important relative to our understanding of the arterial components of the disease and whether one might use a dual approach in which one injects certain types of media which could be taken up by the plaque or by macrophages or smooth muscle cells within the plaque which would then be even more meaningful when one looks at the plaques with MRI. <u>Paulin</u> pointed out that there are reports in the literature which indicate that there might be MRI contrast agents that could enter the pathologic areas, where they could be trapped. No conclusive date are available at present, but he agreed that this is a very important field for further investigation. <u>Siegel</u> asked <u>Paulin</u> whether the spectra that one can obtain with MRI might be of great value in understanding the pathophysiology of the plaque. <u>Paulin</u> was doubtful that MRI spectroscopy would permit the study of plaque metabolism in the near future, but he thought that it might be possible with existing spectroscopy equipment to elucidate regional myocardial abnormalities, which would be of considerable importance in patients who are about to develop clinical manifestations of ischemic heart

disease. <u>Paulin</u> said that a great deal of experimental work is now going on in the detection of possible shifts in spectra and what might happen when rather simple and straightforward changes occurred such as a shift in the pH of the diseased tissue. <u>Paulin</u> indicated that it is very difficult to gain conclusive results at present but that this is a very active and promising field of endeavor.

   The questions then turned to <u>Rubenstein's</u> and <u>Dix's</u> presentation. Questions were immediately raised regarding the cost of a dedicated system such as the one that these two investigators are using. <u>Rubenstein</u> pointed out that in his opinion the clinicians in the USA should rely on the two laboratories, one in Brookhaven, the other in Stanford, for long term serious studies of coronary disease. The facilities are already there, and further development and use in clinical research should cost relatively little beyond what we have already spent, which is several million dollars for each facility. <u>Rubenstein</u> pointed out that using a band width which is tolerable, that is in the range of 250 ev or up to 3x that amount, one can decrease both the cost and the size of these devices, but then one will image some bone. Under these circumstances, one might be able to decrease the cost and size of these devices by a huge amount. The essence of the system is the use of monochromatic radiation and there might be several other sources of monochromatic radiation without using electron storage rings. For example, one might be able to use the channeling of electrons through crystals. Perhaps in the next decade the research physicists will be able to develop a device about the size of a tape recorder, but one still has the problem of exposing the patient to ionizing radiation and that is something that most investigators and biomedical scientists would like to avoid.

   <u>Rubenstein</u> in response to a question from <u>Bond</u> about the time that is required to validate their approaches and their results, said that he thought that the first thing to do before further efforts at validation are undertaken would be to improve the system further. He then went on to indicate that after the components of the system are optimized it would take about a year to validate the system, but he did not believe that this would occur within the next two to three years. He also pointed out that a group at the Brookhaven National Laboratory in the USA have been involved in a TIMI trial and that there are a large number of patients at the Manhasset Hospital on Long Island who have had recent coronary arteriograms, and who might be benefited by comparing transvenous angiograms with coronary arteriograms, applying methods such as the ones <u>Kramsch</u>, <u>Blankenhorn,</u> and others have utilized and reported evidence of retardation or regression of plaques. They would like to initiate this study soon.

   <u>Bond</u> then went on to ask what the radiation dose is likely to be in the practical domain of a single coronary artery study. <u>Rubenstein</u> pointed out that <u>Dix</u> had indicated in his presentation that this is about 35 RADs. Part of this is expended in the exposure involving the positioning of the catheter and the localization of the tips of the catheter. The safety of the radiation is probably the same as the safety of the radiation when one utilizes an x-ray tube for ordinary diagnostic x-rays. The examination is done with a smaller dose of contrast media and the absence of arterial invasion is the main advantage. <u>Paulin</u> then asked whether the goal of the studies which <u>Rubenstein</u> is doing shouldn't be to develop a noninvasive screeening procedure so that one can apply it to the asymptomatic population to detect the early manifestation of atherosclerosis. Under these circumstances one would be looking for subtle changes that occur in the wall of the coronary arteries. In general, he stated his belief that contrast media angiography is not the right approach to use for this type of screening. <u>Rubenstein</u> responded that he and his group had no interest at all in screening populations at risk. He is much more interested in making these facilities available to coronary

arteriographers who already have some information on the extent of coronary disease and who are trying to follow progression, arrestability, or lack of arrestability of coronary disease. Rubenstein pointed out that at present they cannot see the left circumflex coronary artery adequately, but they think that with time they will be able to visualize it adequately by using enhancing techniques. His own point of view is that the ability to visualize the entire left anterior descending coronary artery and 80% of the right coronary artery should make it possible for the system to be used by coronary artery scientists to develop a large enough sample size to follow the natural history of coronary disease. Rubenstein went on to emphasize that at present they are really hoping to use this as a quantitative scientific research tool and not necessarily as a widely useful clinical tool. They hope that they can first of all make a valid comparison of what they can learn with the synchrotron by comparing it with known coronary arteriograms and then to decide what the correlations are between interpretation of results with the actual pathological study of the disease by using a serial longitudinal study of coronary disease in patients who may or may not be subjects of a number of intervention procedures. Paulin suggested using intravenous subtraction coronary arteriography, but Rubenstein stated he really needed to see the data that bore on this subject and that he was not sure that it was possible to take pictures of coronary tissues more than 4 milliseconds apart and get a useful image.

Following Mercuri's presentation, Berglund indicated that he thought that this presentation along with Landini's gave real hope for the possibility of tissue characterization during the development of the atherosclerotic process. Kramsch pointed out that this was a very timely and very useful validation of the ultrasound method and that he wondered why there was such an intensive brightness in the area of fibrous tissue. Could it be that some of the image was due to the presence of large quantities of elastin? To which Mercuri responded that they had not as yet validated many of these observations with specific quantitation of histopathological preparations. The next step is to increase the effectiveness of this type of study with quantitative micromorphometrically measured histopathological studies that will quantitate lipids, collagen, elastin, minerals, and necrosis in a really quantitative way which can include mapping of the lesion components. This is what their goal is at the present time. Kramsch pursued his questions about the areas of intense brightness which had many cholesterol crystals along the base and then the transition into a dark area, which might be caused by the crystals or by calcium. Mercuri pointed out that he thought at present the case was stronger that this indicated mineralization, although cholesterol crystals do give imaging at about the same intensity. Wissler complimented Mercuri on his study. He indicated that it would be particularly important to have not only micromorphometry of ordinary histology but also micromorphometry of high resolution fat stains and micromorphometry of the various fibrous elements. Wissler pointed out that his studies have indicated that there is a lot of lipid that is not appreciated in histological preparations which are not accompanied by a high resolution fat stain. In fact, in the study for which he is program director, the Pathobiological Determinants of Atherosclerosis in Youth (PDAY), lesions are being identified which help to eliminate the very large gap between a fatty streak and a fibrous plaque. These intermediate lesions, the identification of which is one of the main goals of definition by the PDAY study, are largely understood and in a sense classified by means of the fat stain, which also helps a great deal in interpreting the difference between diffuse fibrous thickening which is so common in coronary and carotid arteries, and lesions which may indicate the beginning and progression of the atherosclerotic process. Mercuri thanked Wissler and pointed out that the distribution of intensities in fibrous plaques is wide because of their morphological complexity. It is undoubtedly true that for the future one needs to study the specific composition of the arteries which are said to have raised lesions or fibrous plaques so that one can begin to delineate the various patterns of lesion components that accompany progression. Rubba pointed out that he thinks one of the important problems is to differentiate diffuse intimal thickening or focal intimal cushions from the early atherosclerotic process and that the mean intensity is almost the same for these two types of lesions. In his experience, the fatty streak or early fatty plaque shows a more diffuse enhancement of intensity. Mercuri pointed out that this is a very interesting point and that there are important differences between diffuse intimal thickening and the fatty streak. One of the limitations of the instruments is that the lateral resolution is only about 0.7 mm and this makes it difficult to identify specific characteristics of diffuse intimal thickening and the beginning of fatty depositions in the diffuse intimal thickening areas. Perhaps this can be overcome by future developments aimed at learning more about how to detect small amounts of lipid which are being deposited in areas of diffuse intimal thickening. In particular, the intravascular probe may give considerable additional information obtained from the inside of the artery. In fact, one may be able to use information gained from a combination of examinations from the inside and the outside of the artery in order to understand the interaction between ultrasound and the components of the diseased tissue.

Barbieri pointed out that he is interested in restenosis and he wondered if any of the individuals using ultrasound arteriography had studied enough examples of restenosis to know how this might vary from normal stenosis. No one appeared to have undertaken this kind of study, in all probability because of the limitations of using the ultrasound techniques for coronary arteriography. Bianciardi asked how many longitudinal planes one uses in Mercuri's studies and whether one is speaking of absolute intensity in relation to interpreting the tissue components. What does one use as an intensity reference? Mercuri pointed out that they have used only longitudinal scans and that these are basically 90° incident ultrasound beams that give a superficial strip view of the artery, and that the intensity studies thus far have utilized only relative intensity interpreted basically against background intensity.

The discussion following the presentations by Kuhn and Soma was initiated by Barbieri who found the MRI techniques fascinating because of the possibilities of studying insect embryos and other kinds of microscopic subjects from a functional point of view. Kuhn pointed out that these studies had only one limitiation, and that is that the subject being studied had to be smaller in size than 25 mm.

In the general discussion period, Bianciardi opened up the subjects that had been covered by asking Kuhn about the limits of the resolution of MRI. He pointed out that a few years ago it was much larger than it is at present and now it appears to be about 10 mm or less for NMR microscopy. He asked Kuhn whether it might soon be 100 microns or 10 microns or even a very small resolution dimension in vivo. Kuhn pointed out that there are a number of reasons for the limited resolution, one being the signal to noise ratio and the relationship of signal to noise to voxel size; when the signal to noise ratio goes down because the voxel size is limited, then the experimental times increase, and they increase to unusable time intervals for in vivo experiments or in vitro studies of living biological samples. Other limitiations include Brownian motion or diffusion from protons from one voxel to another during the measuring time. For in vitro samples the resolution is already 10 microns or less. There are other factors that limit resolution in solid fixed samples such as signal line width.

Siegel then asked a question about the spectra that Kuhn had demonstrated and used for the arteriosclerotic plaques, indicating that he was especially interested in changes of the correlation time. Kuhn indicated that these were two line spectra and that if Siegel is interested in correlation times, then it is difficult to estimate the correlation times of the molecules. It is possible with a very simple model, but he stated that they haven't done these calculations and that it is difficult to find the right model which describes the mobility of the molecules and the correlation between mobility and quantitative correlation between mobility and the capital T_1 or T_2 types. Siegel pointed out that he thought he had seen some line broadening as compared to results with sonication. However they had prepared the specimens with the lipids removed with solvents. He asked whether there is a line broadening under in vivo conditions. Soma answered this question and said that they had only used in vitro conditions, but since the sample was a piece of artery, there was rigidity and basically the spectrum was a summation of those series of spectra taken from the whole sample, which was 1x1 cm in size, so the signal was basically coming from the plaque suppressed in water and there was some broadening of the signals which were giving an idea of the rigidity of the sample. Kuhn added that they were working with solid state NMR on the plaque itself and that opens a whole new field. Solid state NMR is possible and it is not necessary to extract the plaque. We can do all the experiments that give us information about slow and fast motion of the molecules in the sample itself without any prior preparation. Siegel pointed out that this was very important information.

Kramsch asked Soma how they have been differentiating in their micro MRI between a solid crystal, a liquid crystal, and noncrystal. Soma responded that they were really trying to use the methodologies to see if they could characterize the state of the lipid in the plaque so they are trying to interpret the T_1 and T_2 measurements and their chemical shift. The reason for studying the spectra before and after extraction is to find out what is seen or not seen quantitatively by NMR, and possibly one can be even more precise and quantitative with the solid state NMR. Kramsch pointed out that for clinical quantitation, they will need to see what regresses or progresses and they will have to be able to measure the lipid in each different physical state. Soma agreed and said that that was their goal and that the one on the bottom was the broader line so that if they are able to repeat that kind of examination locally, then they can go back to the same spectrum and do the same spectra two months or two years later and interpret the composition because of the sharpness of the lines. Under these conditions they should be able to find out whether the sum of the lipids has moved and whether the sum of the lipids has changed. Soma pointed out that all of their studies so far were in vitro but he thought that in the fairly near future they should be able to make the same kind of observations in vivo, probably starting in an animal model. Wissler pointed out that Small and his group at Boston University have been measuring lipids in some of the developing plaques in the young people that are being studied in the PDAY research program. They have results which may help to indicate progression or nonprogression.

Wissler also noted that it would be helpful if one would show sections side by side viewed in the way the light microscopist ordinarily looks at fixed and stained tissue and the way these same sections look with the MRI micro-examination. It should be possible, he added, for one to make histopathologic sections in the same area which has been examined by MRI microscopy. Soma agreed that these types of examinations are just beginning and will be continued with Weber and his group.

Then Berglund asked for any thoughts that the presenters of the morning had that had not yet been expressed and Paulin indicated that his conclusion is that at present MRI does not have the power to show the histology of the artery wall during atherogenesis in vivo and that it appears to be more and more likely that ultrasonographic analysis, spectral analysis, etc. will be used for most quantitative analyses of plaque components in the near future. On the other hand, Paulin pointed out, MRI is a powerful tool and it should be of great value in analyzing the functional parameters of the target organ, especially the myocardium. Rubenstein indicated that he and Dix agree that we will be able to see significant proportions of the proximal coronary circulation adequate for making long term evaluations of the prevention, arrestability, or reversibility of coronary atherosclerosis. Mercuri indicated that we should welcome the efforts that are being made using a number of methodologies and that we should concentrate on studying the natural history of atherosclerosis using contrast media angiography, the MRI, the synchrotron angiography, spectrum analysis, and ultrasound. This multiple methodology approach is the only way in his opinion to overcome the big problems related to atherogenesis. Soma said that he agreed that we need the multiple approaches and that he hoped that NMR imaging and spectroscopy will soon be feasible and probably be able to be used along with ultrasound to detect much more of what is going on in the artery wall and that ultrasound may really be coming quickly to the point where it can be used intravascularly with profitable results. He indicated that selective studies on highly selected patients who have the most puzzling problems should be rewarding.

HOW AN UNDERSTANDING OF HDL'S METABOLISM MAY HELP US DISCOVER NEW WAYS TO

EVALUATE ATHEROSCLEROSIS AND ITS RISK OF PROGRESSION IN THE LIVING PATIENT

Gerd Assmann

Institut für Klinische Chemie und Laboratoriumsmedizin
und Institut for Arterioskleroseforschung
Münster, Germany

Prospective studies of recent years have demonstrated the existence of a reverse relation between plasma HDL (high density lipoproteins) concentration and the incidence of coronary artery disease (1-3) (Table 1). Also, in cohort studies patients with verified coronary artery disease present with lower mean HDL concentrations than healthy controls (Figure 1). A study group of the European Atherosclerosis Society (EAS) has, in a recent policy statement (4), agreed on 35 mg/dl HDL cholesterol as a provisional cutoff value for risk assessment. This cutoff corresponds to the 16th percentile of the HDL cholesterol distribution in adult males in West Germany (Figure 2). Plasma concentrations below this cutoff may be associated with increased risk for premature onset of atherosclerosis.

Whereas epidemiologic and clinical data suggest a major role of low HDL cholesterol in the formation of atherosclerosis, comparatively little is known on the metabolic origin of HDL deficiency. Similarly, the precise metabolic events by which drugs affect the plasma concentration of HDL cholesterol are only understood to a limited degree.

Table 1.   Cohort studies (men): CHD risk change (%)
per 1 mg/dl increment in HDL cholesterol level

Study	None	Cholesterol Covariates LDL	Non-HDL	Total
FHS	– 1.9 %	– 1.9 %	– 1.6 %	– 2.0 %
LRCF*	– 2.7 %	– 3.6 %	– 2.7 %	– 3.3 %
CPPT	– 3.0 %	– 2.3 %	– 1.8 %	– 2.8 %
MRFIT	– 1.7 %	– 2.0 %	– 1.1 %	– 2.0 %
BRHS	———	———	– 1.0 %	– 2.0 %
PROCAM	– 3.6 %	– 4.0 %	– 3.4 %	– 3.6 %
All except those in the "None" column have been adjusted for age, cigarette smoking, systolic blood pressure and BMI. * CHD mortality				

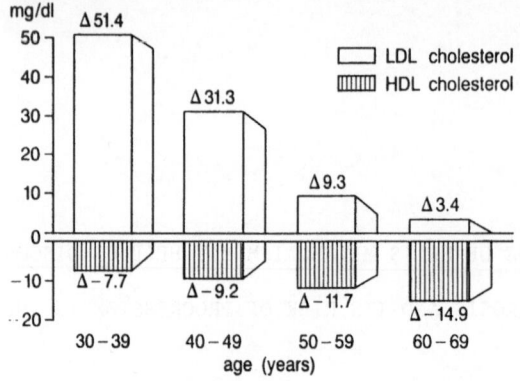

Fig. 1. HDL cholesterol and LDL cholesterol. Differences of mean serum concentrations between male MI survivors (four age decades) with angiographically verified coronary artery disease and an age and sex matched control group. Results are given in absolute values.

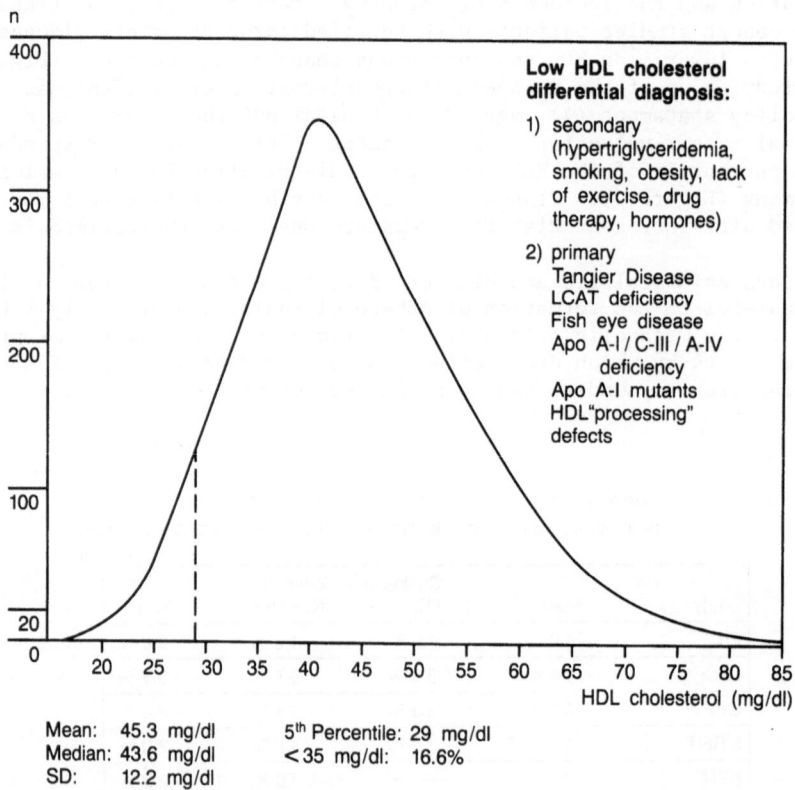

Fig. 2. Frequency distribution of HDL cholesterol serum concentrations in a German male population (n = 11402).

HDL are a heterogeneous population of lipid/protein complexes. Their common feature is a relatively high protein content that is responsible for the high density of these lipoproteins. There is a choice from about 10 different proteins, called apolipoproteins, which can associate with lipids to form plasma lipoproteins. The existence of a variety of HDL subpopulations is caused by differences in the types and numbers of apolipoproteins per particle and by their proportion and types of lipids.

HDL particles derive from discoidal precursors that are synthesised in the liver and the small intestine. The predominant structural components of these discs are phospholipids and apolipoprotein A-I. Similarly composed and shaped are surface remnants of chylomicrons which are synthesised by the small intestine in response to dietary fat intake (5). Acquisition of cholesterol, mainly in the form of cholesteryl esters, the product of the LCAT (lecithin: cholesteryl acyltransferase) reaction, leads to the formation of spherical HDL particles.

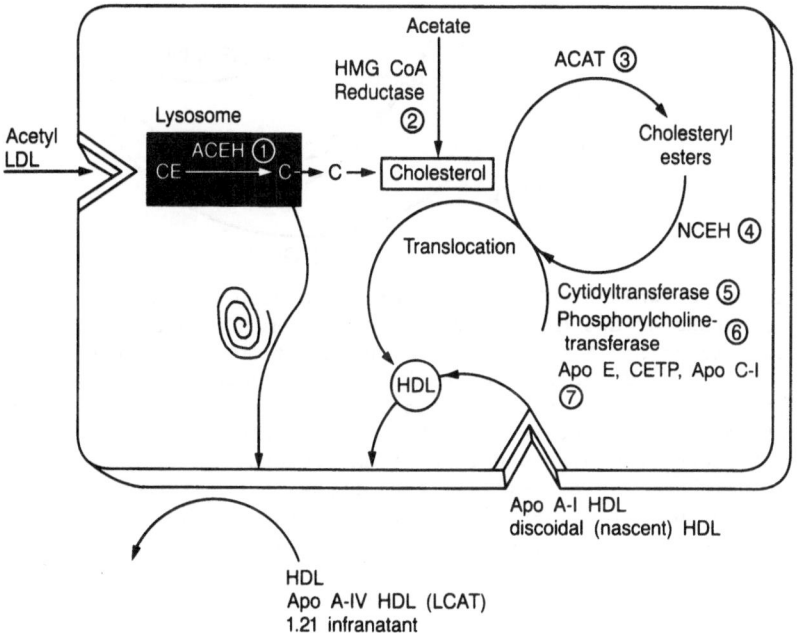

Fig. 3. Schematic drawing of cellular interactions of HDL. 1. ACEH (acid cholesteryl ester hydrolase) is a lysosomal enzyme that hydrolyses cholesteryl esters. 2. HMGCoA-reductase is the key enzyme in cellular de novo synthesis of cholesterol. 3. ACAT (acylcoenzyme A: cholesteryl acyl transferase) is a microsomal enzyme that reesterifies cholesterol. 4. NCEH (neutral cholesteryl ester hydrolase) is a cytoplasmic cholesteryl ester hydrolysing enzyme. Together with ACAT it controls the cellular cholesterol pool size. 5 and 6. Enzymes of phopholipid metabolism important in lipoprotein particle assembly. 7. Apolipoprotein E, CETP (cholesteryl ester transfer protein) and apolipoprotein C-I are thought to be important for lipid translocation.

While it is a major function of other lipoproteins to deliver lipids to cells, the main metabolic role of HDL appears to be the acceptance of excess cholesterol from peripheral cells and its delivery to the liver for final deposition (6). Although peripheral cells have the capability of synthesising cholesterol in addition to its acquisition by endocytosis of

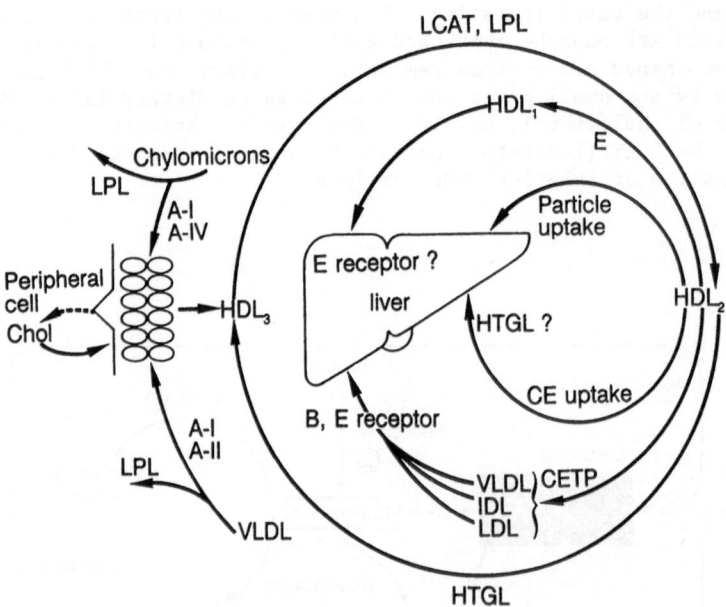

Fig. 4. Major pathways by which HDL mediate reverse cholesterol transport. 1. Uptake of apo E-rich HDL_1, formed from HDL_3 and HDL_2 by a postulated apo E receptor. 2. Uptake of apo A-1 containing HDL particles. 3. Selective uptake of HDL_2 cholesteryl esters involving hepatic triglyceride lipases. 4. CETP mediated transfer of cholesteryl esters from HDL_2 to LDL, IDL, or VLDL leading to a LDL-receptor mediated uptake of cholesterol. Abbreviations: LCAT = lecithin: cholesteryl acyltransferase, LPL = lipoprotein lipase, CETP = cholesteryl ester transfer protein, HTGL = hepatic triglyceride lipase, CE = cholesteryl esters.

lipoproteins they are unable to catabolise cholesterol. Instead they have at their disposal a very effective system for elimination of cholesterol. A pathway termed "reverse cholesterol transport" uses HDL to carry excess cholesterol to the liver (7-9). Whether this process requires the presence of a cholesteryl ester transfer complex (10) or a direct interaction of HDL with the cells is currently not known. Likewise unclarified is the role of the recently cloned and sequenced cholesteryl ester transfer protein.

Table 2. Influence of lipid lowering drugs on HDL-
cholesterol concentration

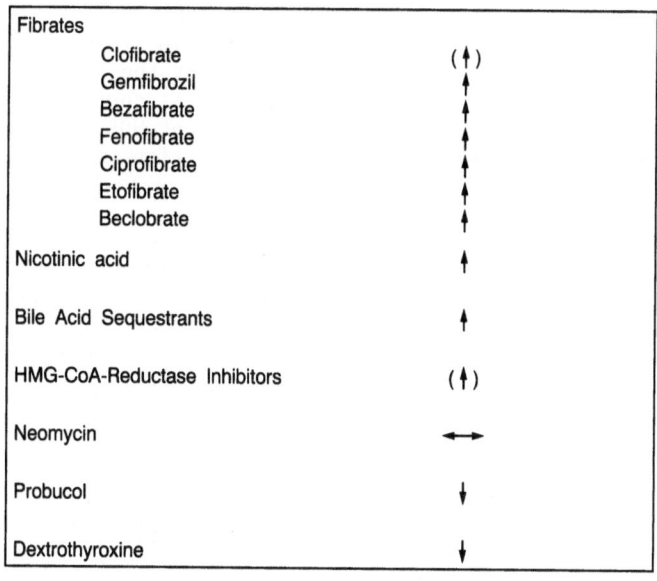

Fibrates	
Clofibrate	(↑)
Gemfibrozil	↑
Bezafibrate	↑
Fenofibrate	↑
Ciprofibrate	↑
Etofibrate	↑
Beclobrate	↑
Nicotinic acid	↑
Bile Acid Sequestrants	↑
HMG-CoA-Reductase Inhibitors	(↑)
Neomycin	↔
Probucol	↓
Dextrothyroxine	↓

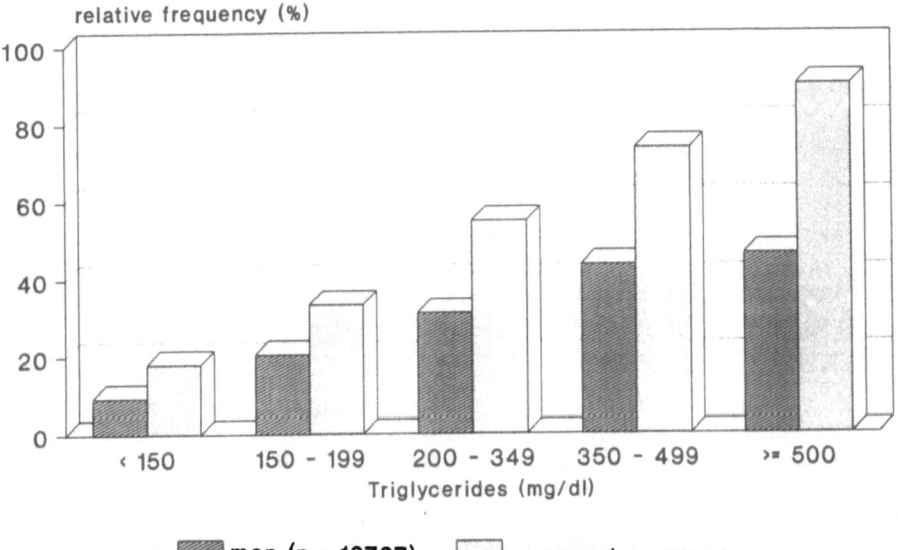

Fig. 5. Procam study: relation between low HDL-cholesterol (men < 35
mg/dl, women < 45 mg/dl) and serum triglycerides.

In this context the recent discovery of a retroendocytosis pathway for HDL (11, 12) may be of crucial importance. This pathway, which so far has only been demonstrated in vitro, consists of a receptor mediated endocytosis of HDL precursors by macrophages and the subsequent export of these particles after cholesterol and apolipoprotein E have been added (11, 13). In Tangier disease, which is characterised by the nearly complete absence of HDL from plasma, an impairment of the retroendocytosis pathway may be of physiological importance. In this concept HDL are acceptors for excess intracellular cholesterol which by the addition of apolipoprotein E are marked for liver uptake.

Complementary to this system of cholesterol return a second pathway has been postulated in which HDL particles are docking to a cell surface receptor. The docking process in this concept is thought to trigger signals that lead to the delivery of cholesterol to HDL without a necessity for particle uptake (14). Both the retroendocytosis pathway and the docking pathway are shown in a schematic drawing in Fig. 3.

In vitro studies on the lipoprotein metabolism of the plasma compartment have shown that there can be a fast and effective exchange of apoproteins and lipids among different lipoprotein classes (15). In this process, the cholesterol ester transfer protein can probably facilitate the transfer of cholesterol esters from HDL to lipoproteins of a lower density. In case this reaction is of quantitative importance, this adds another dimension to the role of HDL in reversed cholesterol transport via an integration of this pathway into the cholesterol homeostasis system of the low-density lipoprotein (LDL) receptor. Figure 4 shows a summary of possible pathways for reversed cholesterol transport (16).

HDL CHOLESTEROL AND SERUM TRIGLYCERIDES

Elevation of serum triglycerides is frequently associated with low HDL cholesterol (Fig. 5) Based upon the findings of the PROCAM study a subgroup of individuals can be defined, where the combined anomaly of high cholesterol/HDL cholesterol ratios (>5) and hypertriglyceridemia (>200 mg/dl) is associated with high risk of atherosclerosis (Fig. 6).

HYPOLIPIDEMIC DRUGS AND HDL CHOLESTEROL

There has not yet been a randomized trial to test the hypothesis that raising low HDL cholesterol will reduce CHD risk. However, post hoc analysis of primary prevention trials (Lipid Research Clinics - Coronary Primary Prevention Trial, Helsinki Heart Study) using cholesterol-lowering agents (cholestyramine or gemfibrozil) with concomitant HDL-raising effect have yielded promising preliminary results.

For other hypolipidemic drugs (Table 2) results from primary prevention trials are not available. Their modes of action differ substantially (Table 3) (17, 18). Theoretically, increased activity of lipoprotein lipase observed with nicotinic acid and various fibrates should account for the observed triglyceride lowering and HDL cholesterol raising effects of these drugs, a mechanism which should be considered anti-atherogenic. Further results from clinical trials are urgently needed to document that these drugs not only beneficially affect plasma lipoproteins but also retard the progression of atherosclerosis. Basic clinical meta-bolic studies are required to ascertain the most promising avenues of HDL metabolism which may be used to investigate and perhaps develop clinical tests which will correlate with active progression of atherosclerosis.

Table 3. Possible mechanism of drugs affecting HDL-cholesterol

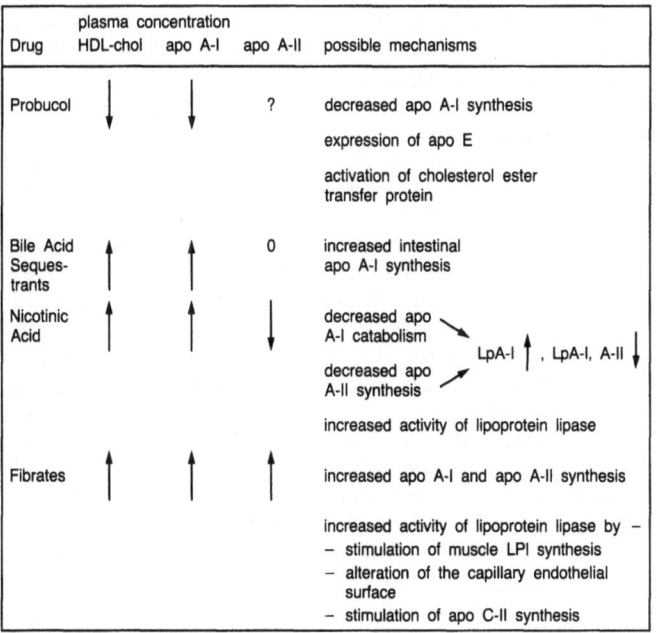

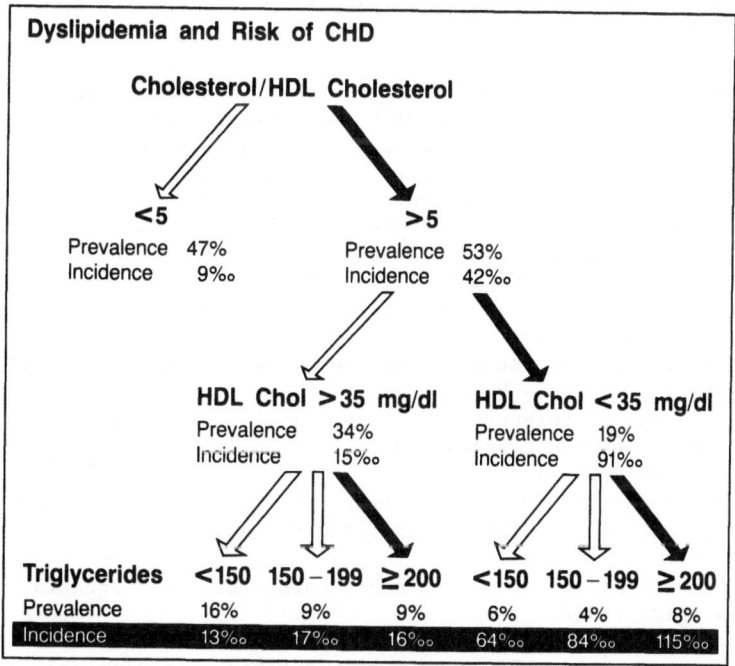

Fig. 6. Procam study: data refer to male participants, age 40-65, of this study.

REFERENCES

1. T. Gordon, W. B. Kannel, W. P. Castelli, and T. R. Dawber, Lipoproteins, cardiovascular disease, and death. The Framingham Study, <u>Arch. Intern. Med.</u> 141:1128-1132 (1981).

2. G. Assmann and H. Schulte, "PROCAM-Trial," Panscientia Verlag, Hedingen, Zurich (1986).

3. H. M. Frick. Helsinki Heart Study - primary prevention trial with gemfibrozil in middle aged men with dyslipidaemia, <u>New Engl. J. Med.</u> 317:1237-1245 (1987).

4. Study Group, European Atherosclerosis Society, Strategies for the prevention of coronary heart disease: A policy statement of the European Atherosclerosis Society, <u>Europ. Heart J.</u> 8:77-88 (1987).

5. T. G. Redgrave and D. M. Small, Quantitation of the transfer of surface phospholipid of chylomicrons to the high density fraction during catabolism of chylomicrons in the rat, <u>J. Clin. Invest.</u> 64:162-171 (1979).

6. C. Koo, T. L. Innerarity, and R. W. Mahley, Obligatory role of cholesterol and apolipoprotein E in the formation of large cholesterol-enriched and receptor active high density lipoproteins. <u>J. Biol. Chem.</u> 260:11934-11943 (1985).

7. R. Ross and J. A. Glomset, The pathogenesis of atherosclerosis, <u>New Engl. J. Med.</u> 295:364-377 & 420-425 (1976).

8. R. J. Havel, Role of the liver in atherosclerosis, <u>Arteriosclerosis</u> 5:569-580 (1985).

9. J. M. Hong, S. J. Demosky Jr., S. B. Edge, R. E. Gregg, J. C. Osborne, and H. B. Brewer Jr., Characterization of a human hepatic receptor for high density lipoproteins, <u>Arteriosclerosis</u> 5:228-237 (1985).

10. P. E. Fielding and C. J. Fielding. A cholesteryl ester transfer complex in human plasma, <u>Proc. Natl. Acad. Sci. (USA)</u> 77:3327-3330 (1980).

11. G. Schmitz, R. Niemann, B. Brennhausen, R. Krause, and G. Assmann. Regulation of high density lipoprotein receptors in cultured macrophages: role of acyl-CoA: cholesterolacyltransferase, <u>EMBOJ</u> 4:2773-2779 (1985).

12. G. Schmitz, H. Robenek, U. Lohmann, and G. Assmann, Interaction of high density lipoproteins with cholesteryl ester-laden macrophages: biochemical and morphological characterization of cell surface receptor binding, endocytosis, and resecretion of high density lipoproteins by macrophages. <u>EMBOJ</u> 4:613-622 (1985).

13. G. Schmitz, G. Assmann, H. Robenek, and B. Brennhausen, Tangier disease: a disorder of intracellular membrane traffic. <u>Proc. Natl. Acad. Sci. (USA)</u> 82:6305-6309 (1985).

14. J. P. Slotte, J. F. Oram, and E. L. Bierman, Binding of high density lipoproteins to cell receptors promotes translocation of cholesterol from intracellular membranes to the cell surface, <u>J. Lipid Res.</u> 26:487-494 (1985).

15. S. Eisenberg, Preferential enrichment of large-sized very low density populations with transferred cholesteryl esters, <u>J. Lipid Res.</u> 26:487-494 (1985).

16. G. Assmann and G. Schmitz, Familial HDL deficiency: Tangier disease, <u>in</u>: "Metabolic Basis of Inherited Disease," McGraw-Hill, New York (1989).

17. G. Assmann, "Lipid Metabolism and Atherosclerosis," Schattauer Verlag, Stuttgart (1982).

18. G. Assmann, ed., Fettstoffwechselstörungen und koronare Herzkrankheit. Primärprävention, Diagnostik und Therapie - Leitlinien für die Praxis, MMV Medizin Verlag, München (1988).

THE USE OF RADIOLABELED LOW DENSITY LIPOPROTEIN FOR EVALUATING

ATHEROSCLEROSIS: PRESENT STATUS AND FUTURE PROMISE

Rick Hay

Department of Pathology
The University of Chicago
Chicago, Illinois (USA)

INTRODUCTION

Emerging noninvasive techniques such as magnetic resonance imaging, vascular ultrasound, and synchrotron angiography promise in vivo detection and analysis of atherosclerosis in ways that could only be imagined a decade ago. Conventional invasive arteriography, verified whenever possible by dissection and lesion component morphometry, remains the gold standard for revealing atheroma location and lesion-associated stenosis. Yet the newer modalities are acquiring the power and the resolution that may permit accurate assessment of plaque size and shape; of spatial disposition of lipid, mineral, and tissue components within a plaque; and of structural distortions and adaptations in the artery wall adjacent to an atherosclerotic lesion.

Nonetheless, all these are inherently anatomic modalities. They suggest little about the actual or potential behavior of a plaque at any given time. Only from repeated studies can one infer whether a lesion of interest has been growing or shrinking, remodelling or quiescent during a selected time interval. A different kind of noninvasive strategy, specifically one that reveals the metabolic and physiologic status of individual plaques at the time of analysis, can provide a powerful adjunct to the structural approaches.

Growing atheromata characteristically acquire lipid, specifically cholesteryl ester, through uptake of particles including low density lipoproteins (LDL) as depicted in Figure 1. Even though the relationships between plaque growth, LDL uptake, and LDL turnover within the plaque are not kinetically simple, it is reasonable to propose that growing or otherwise metabolically active plaques should acquire LDL and/or retain LDL-derived components at greater rates than do shrinking or quiescent plaques. Guided by this hypothesis, over the last few years our group and a few others have been developing nuclear imaging methods suitable for experimental and clinical evaluation of LDL biodistribution in vivo, including noninvasive detection of atheromata by virtue of their ability to acquire radiolabeled LDL.

Atherosclerotic Plaques, Edited by R.W. Wissler *et al.*
Plenum Press, New York, 1991

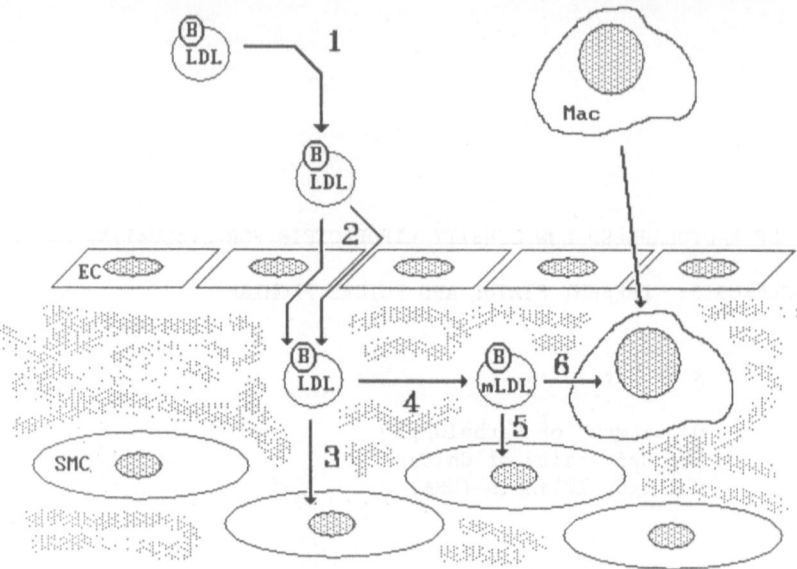

Fig. 1. Probable pathway for in vivo acquisition of LDL particles
by the artery wall. Step 1, Native LDL is moved by
hemodynamic forces from regions of laminar flow to the
intima-plasma interface, where interactions with
endothelial cells (EC) can occur. Step 2, Native LDL
particles traverse or pass between EC and bind to
components of the subintimal extracellular matrix. Step
3, Some native LDL particles are taken up by subintimal
cells, including smooth muscle cells (SMC). Step 4,
Oxidation and other phenomena generate structurally
modified LDL particles (mLDL), which may undergo
preferential uptake by SMC (step 5) and by activated
monocyte-macrophages (Mac; step 6).

THE ISSUES

    Two central issues have so far dominated research in this field:
identifying the most suitable derivative to serve as a radiotracer for LDL
biodistribution, and establishing whether sufficient LDL-associated
radioactivity can be incorporated into individual atheromata to permit
their detection and evaluation by nuclear imaging techniques. Progress in
each area is summarized below.

What is the most suitable LDL derivative?

    The ideal species of radiolabeled LDL for biodistribution studies
would be prepared quickly and easily, in radiochemically stable form, at
high specific and total activity. The radionuclide employed would be safe
for use in the population at risk for developing atherosclerosis, and it
would be readily monitored by external gamma camera imaging. The resultant
radiolabeled derivative should accurately mimic native LDL in its
biological behavior prior to uptake of the particle by individual cells,
yet it should resist intracellular degradation so that cumulative
acquisition of LDL by even low-uptake tissues might be measured.

LDL particles radioiodinated by classical methods--commonly used for in vitro experiments and for assessing the turnover of intravascular lipoproteins--fail to meet most of these biodistribution criteria. However, LDL labeled with I-125 or I-131 via the tyramine cellobiose (TyC) method developed by Pittman et al.[1] has previously been shown to be satisfactory on all counts except for imageability. Therefore, both we and Moerlein et al.[2] have successfully adapted Pittman's method to label LDL with I-123, a radionuclide with suitable nuclear imaging properties and a physical half-life of 13 hours. As another alternative to classically radioiodinated LDL, in 1985 Lees and his colleagues described a method for labeling LDL with Tc-99m,[3] a readily imaged radionuclide with a physical half-life of six hours.

We have compared the biodistribution of human I-123-TyC-LDL with that of Tc-99m-LDL in rabbits, rhesus monkeys, and human subjects.[4-7] In normolipemic rabbits, we determined that the distribution of tissue-associated I-123 activity was similar to that observed by Pittman for I-125 injected as I-125-TyC-LDL (personal communication). In all three species, however, we documented significant metabolic differences between I-123-TyC-LDL and Tc-99m-LDL. Renal uptake and urinary excretion (in humans) or total excretion (in rabbits and monkeys) of radionuclide were dramatically lower with I-123-TyC-LDL, and the fractional catabolic rates (FCR) calculated for I-123-TyC-LDL were only about one-third those obtained for Tc-99m-LDL. Adrenals and gonads, steroidogenic tissues rich in LDL receptor content, showed higher uptake of I-123 than of Tc-99m. We also found that I-123 remained stably associated with circulating LDL even 48 hours after injection of I-123-TyC-LDL, whereas about half of Tc-99m injected as Tc-99m-LDL was lost to higher density fractions of plasma. Finally, the FCR values we have observed for intravascular I-123-TyC-LDL (0.015 $\pm$ 0.003/h) in human subjects are comparable to those reported by Kesaniemi and Grundy for conventionally prepared I-125-LDL.[8] From these results we conclude that I-123-TyC-LDL is a more representative tracer of native LDL metabolism in vivo than is Tc-99m-LDL.

Despite this encouraging finding, practical considerations make I-123-TyC-LDL far from ideal as a routine clinical radiopharmaceutical agent. Its preparation is technically demanding and expensive. Because the physical half-life of I-123 is much shorter than the biological half-life of circulating I-123-TyC-LDL, high blood pool activity interferes with lesion detection throughout the potential imaging period. In addition, the short physical half-life of I-123 would render important tissue validation studies--such as microscopic autoradiography of atherosclerotic lesions surgically excised after imaging--virtually impossible. Because of these shortcomings, in 1988 we began searching for other ways to radiolabel LDL without compromising its biological properties.

Drawing on recent advances in radiolabeling monoclonal antibodies for experimental and clinical tumor radioimmunotherapy, we have synthesized and evaluated a derivative of human LDL labeled with indium-111, a radionuclide with relatively advantageous imaging properties and a physical half-life of 67 hours.[9] We chose to use the bifunctional chelate SCN-Bz-DTPA, or 1-(p-isothiocyanatobenzyl)-diethylenetriaminepentaacetic acid,[10] since both physical[11] and biological data[10,12] predict the octadentate structure of [SCN-Bz-DTPA]-LDL to be a more stable chelator for In-111 than the heptadentate structure created by covalently binding the cyclic anhydride of DTPA (cDTPA) to LDL as other investigators have done.[12-15]

We have found that In-111 routinely binds with high efficiency ($\geq$ 90%) to [SCN-Bz-DTPA]-LDL, at less than one-third the cost of preparing I-123-TyC-LDL; and that In-111-[SCN-Bz-DTPA]-LDL is stable in the circulation for at least 48 hours postinjection. We detected no significant differences at necropsy 24 hours postinjection with respect to tissue biodistribution of activity between normolipemic rabbits injected with In-111-[SCN-Bz-DTPA]-LDL and those receiving I-123-TyC-LDL. In a rabbit injected simultaneously with In-111-[SCN-Bz-DTPA]-LDL and I-131-TyC-LDL, the values for FCR and the percent of injected activity corrected for physical decay (%IA) recovered in each organ at 48 hours postinjection were identical for both radionuclides, with two exceptions. For In-111, about 10% IA was recovered in the liver and about 20% IA in the upper large intestine, whereas the corresponding values for I-131 were 20% and 10%, respectively. (We believe these offsetting differences reflect more rapid lysosomal turnover, and consequently enhanced biliary excretion, of apolipoprotein B degradation products containing In-111-[SCN-Bz-DTPA] compared to those containing radioiodine-TyC. This phenomenon of accelerated hepatic clearance may permit injection of higher doses of In-111-[SCN-Bz-DTPA]-LDL than we originally estimated.)

When tested in vitro, In-111-[SCN-Bz-DTPA]-LDL showed behavior comparable to that of conventional I-125-LDL in a competitive binding assay using McA-RH7777 rat hepatoma cells. And in the first human subjects to receive autologous In-111-[SCN-Bz-DTPA]-LDL, the calculated values for fractional catabolic rate, hepatic uptake, and renal uptake of In-111 were very close to those for I-123 injected as I-123-TyC-LDL.

Two additional advantages of In-111-[SCN-Bz-DTPA]-LDL became apparent during our studies. First, because of its comparatively long physical half-life, we were able to monitor human blood samples and excreta for In-111 activity for longer than three weeks, compared to only about one week for I-123-TyC-LDL. This feature allowed us to collect a more complete set of biodistribution data, and to demonstrate that more than 90% of the In-111 activity injected as LDL is eventually excreted in urine and stool. Secondly, also due to its physical half-life, we were able to image tissue-associated In-111 activity for several days postinjection in rabbits and in human subjects, with considerably reduced blood background compared to that following injection of I-123-TyC-LDL.

In summary, we have found that both In-111-[SCN-Bz-DTPA]-LDL and I-123-TyC-LDL are reliable tracers for the biodistribution of native LDL, but that Tc-99m-LDL, at least in our experience, is not. Because In-111-[SCN-Bz-DTPA]-LDL offers practical advantages over I-123-TyC-LDL, including ease and cost of preparation and the opportunity to conduct extended imaging and biodistribution analyses, as well as improved radiochemical stability compared to In-111-LDL synthesized via cDTPA, we feel it is the most suitable LDL derivative presently available for experimental and clinical use.

Can lesion-associated LDL be detected by nuclear imaging?

Tc-99m-LDL, directly radioiodinated LDL, radioiodine-TyC-LDL, and In-111-LDL can all be incorporated into experimental arterial lesions in vivo.[9,16,17] In some instances direct scintigraphic and/or autoradiographic confirmation of focal radionuclide accumulation by the lesions has been obtained. For example, two days following injection of 0.5 mCi of In-111-[SCN-Bz-DTPA]-LDL into a cholesterol-fed rabbit we were able, with short film exposure times, to generate satisfactory en face autoradiograms of In-111 activity in the aorta. These clearly demonstrated that the distribution of In-111 activity matched the distribution of fatty lesions, and that even the smallest lesions grossly visible were active in LDL uptake (Figure 2).

However promising the pictures, extrapolating from these results to the clinical setting raises some points of caution. First, the relative

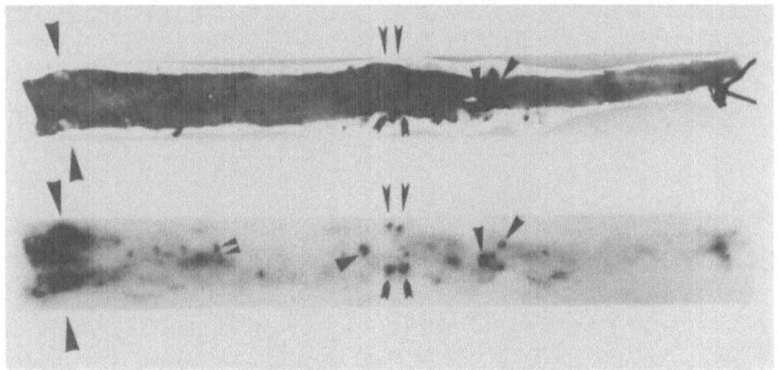

Fig. 2. In-111 accumulation in rabbit atheromata. A rabbit
fed an atherogenic diet for six weeks was injected
intravenously with In-111-[SCN-Bz-DTPA]-LDL (0.5
mCi) and was necropsied two days later. Arrows
indicate early atheromata (white lesions on gross
photograph of opened and fixed aorta, upper panel)
and corresponding regions of focal In-111 activity
(lower panel, 24-hour autoradiogram).

amount of injected radionuclide that accumulates in experimental lesions is
low--on the order of 0.02 %IA per gram of tissue by two to six days
postinjection (R. Hay et al., unpublished).[15] Assuming that the same
relationship holds for human atheromata, and permitting some assumptions
about lesion geometry and radionuclide detection, one can estimate that
active lesions in the range of 0.1-0.5 gram will be near the limits of
gamma camera visualization two days following a 1 mCi injection of
In-111-[SCN-Bz-DTPA]-LDL. On the other hand, if human atheromata are an
order of magnitude less active in LDL uptake, as the findings of Lees et
al. suggest,[18] only correspondingly larger plaques will be visualized by
external scintigraphy. Second, included in this level of radionuclide
accumulation as "tissue background" is the mosaic pattern of radiolabeled
LDL uptake seen in normal vessels. Even in the absence of a lesion,
atherosclerosis-prone regions may accumulate between one-third and one-half
as much activity per gram tissue as do grossly visible fatty lesions (R.
Hay et al., unpublished).[15,19] Third, as discussed below, focal
accumulation of radionuclide by lesions tends to be obscured by the
activity associated with circulating LDL. And fourth, since enhanced LDL
uptake is to be expected of virtually any healing or inflammatory process
of the artery wall, not all focal uptake of radiolabeled LDL seen in the
arteries of human subjects can be assumed to represent atherosclerosis.

Despite these concerns, promising external scintigrams of known and
likely atherosclerotic lesions in situ have been obtained from human
subjects injected with autologous radiolabeled LDL. In 1983 Lees, Lees,
and Strauss demonstrated focal uptake of I-125-LDL at symptomatic and
asymptomatic carotid stenoses.[20] In a subsequent series of 17 patients
with known atherosclerosis, Lees et al. reported focal accumulation of
radionuclide in the carotid region of one subject and in the iliofemoral
regions of three subjects within one day following injection of autologous
Tc-99m-LDL.[18] When the single imageable carotid lesion was surgically
excised and retrieved for histopathological examination, the region of
highest radionuclide accumulation was found to be rich in foam cells and
macrophages with evidence of recent hemorrhage, features suggesting plaque
destabilization.

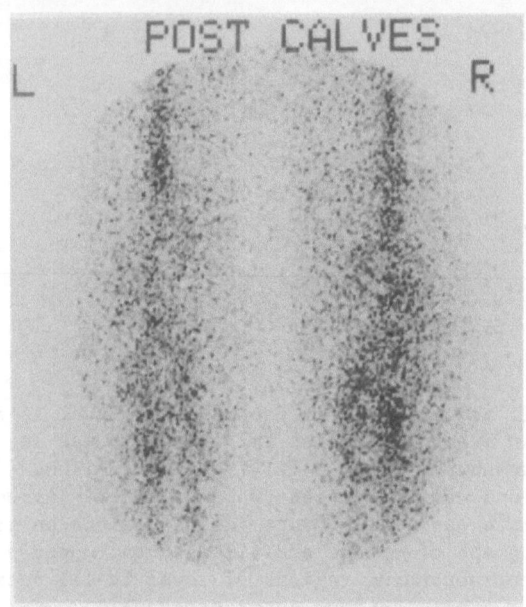

Fig. 3. Accumulation of I-123 in calf
vessels of a human subject. A
human subject with known coronary
and peripheral atherosclerosis
developed claudication in the
right leg. Two days after
injection of autologous I-123-
TyC-LDL, posterior gamma camera
images of the legs were obtained.
Note the inhomogeneous uptake in
a vascular pattern, with
prominent accumulation of
activity just distal to the right
arterial trifurcation.

In our series of eight subjects receiving autologous I-123-TyC-LDL,
including five with previously known or clinically suspected
atherosclerosis, we have observed focal accumulation of I-123 by two days
postinjection in the legs of two subjects (e.g. Figure 3) and in the
cardiac regions of three. Upon repeat study of one subject with
In-111-[SCN-Bz-DTPA]-LDL, focal cardiac accumulation of In-111 persisted
between the third and seventh days postinjection. Unlike Lees et al.,[18]
however, we have not been able to detect focal vascular uptake of
Tc-99m-LDL.

Thus, even with unprocessed or minimally processed images, it does
appear that some vascular lesions in some individuals can be visualized by
external scintigraphy of radionuclides injected in the form of LDL.

THE FUTURE

There are currently three major obstacles to elevating the status of
atherosclerotic lesion detection with radiolabeled LDL to that of a useful
clinical tool. The first is confirming at the tissue level that positive

external images actually represent localization of native LDL in metabolically active plaques. This task will require careful correlation of nuclear images with the better-established modalities for plaque detection, as well as detailed histopathologic and autoradiographic analysis of radiolabeled lesions retrieved at atherectomy or at necropsy. Such studies are impractical if LDL labeled with short-lived radionuclides such as Tc-99m or I-123 is used. However, with the development of longer-lived, radiochemically stable, and metabolically faithful imaging agents such as In-111-[SCN-Bz-DTPA]-LDL, they should prove feasible.

The second hurdle is to improve upon existing methods for preparing radiolabeled LDL. Current labeling procedures--albeit successful at providing imageable derivatives of LDL--are cumbersome, personnel- and time-intensive, and involve a level of radiation exposure for the subject that cannot be overlooked. Were we to rely upon an available agent such as In-111-[SCN-Bz-DTPA]-LDL for all future clinical imaging studies, these shortcomings could seriously impede widespread clinical application and patient care benefits resulting from this approach. Both Shih et al.[21] and our group (unpublished data) have been exploring the use of synthetic and semisynthetic analogues of LDL, the labeling of which involves considerably less preparation time and effort. Despite their attractive features, it remains to be established to what extent these analogues mimic the biological behavior of LDL, or even how well they are taken up by true atherosclerotic lesions.

Another promising approach is to design radiolabeled derivatives of LDL that are slowly cleaved in the circulation, so that atheroma uptake of LDL might be preserved even while the total body clearance of radionuclide is accelerated. Yet another approach, now just in its infancy, is to apply the biochemistry lessons we have learned from generating radiolabeled LDL to the development of LDL-based contrast agents for magnetic resonance imaging, a modality with no radiation hazard and with superior image resolution.

The third challenge, one that is shared with all the other imaging modalities, is to improve the signal-to-noise ratio of the images generated, and in turn, to maximize the information retrieved about a plaque. As mentioned earlier, the major background problem with radiolabeled LDL is its long biological half-life (two to three days) in the circulation, which results in high blood pool activity surrounding the lesions of interest. Synthesis of slowly cleavable derivatives of LDL might reduce the blood background; however, we are convinced that implementing appropriate computer-based image processing strategies will be required to eliminate it. One simple strategy is to align sequential postinjection images normalized for activity in the region of interest, and then to subtract an early image (representing blood pool only) from the later images (representing the sum of blood pool and tissue accumulation of radionuclide). The resulting "difference" images should therefore display net tissue accumulation. An example of the results possible with this strategy is shown in Figure 4. A more sophisticated but otherwise similar strategy is to inject the subject with a blood pool agent, such as Tc-99m-labeled erythrocytes, shortly before the time of imaging; and to use dual isotope acquisition programs to generate simultaneous, perfectly aligned images of blood pool and radiolabeled LDL distribution.

These are not trivial obstacles, nor are the proposed solutions free of controversy or potential artefact. Nevertheless, if we continue to improve the production and the detectability of radiolabeled LDL or its analogues at the same rate as we have during the last five years, imaging atherosclerotic lesions by virtue of their lipoprotein uptake should prove a viable clinical modality for the next century.

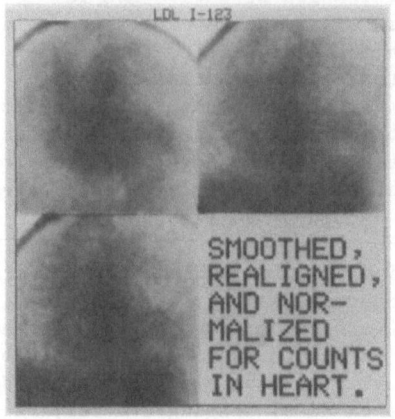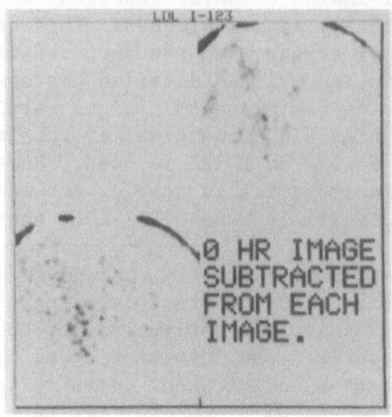

Fig. 4. Processed cardiac images of hypercholesterolemic subject.
Gamma camera images of the cardiac region were obtained
at 0 hours (upper left field of each panel), 24 hours
(upper right fields), and 48 hours (lower left fields)
after injection of autologous I-123-TyC-LDL. The images
were realigned and normalized for counts in the heart
(left panel), and the zero time image representing blood
pool was subtracted by computer from the 24-hour and 48-
hour images to generate difference images (right panel).
A persistent, arborizing pattern of activity suggestive
of the course of the right coronary artery is seen in the
lower left quadrants of both difference images.

REFERENCES

1. R. C. Pittman, T. E. Carew, C. K. Glass, S. R. Green, C. A. Taylor,
   Jr., and A. D. Attie, A radioiodinated, intracellularly trapped
   ligand for determining the sites of plasma protein degradation in
   vivo, Biochem. J. 212:791 (1983).
2. S. M. Moerlein, K. B. Dalal, S. N. Ebbe, Y. Yano, and T. F. Budinger,
   Residualizing and non-residualizing analogues of low-density
   lipoprotein as iodine-123 radiopharmaceuticals for imaging LDL
   catabolism, Nucl. Med. Biol. 15:141 (1988).
3. R. S. Lees, H. D. Garabedian, A. M. Lees, D. J. Schumacher, A. Miller,
   J. L. Isaacsohn, A. Derksen, and H. W. Strauss, Technetium-99m low
   density lipoprotein: Preparation and biodistribution, J. Nucl.
   Med. 26:1056 (1985).
4. R. Hay, R. Fleming, V. Stark, K. Lathrop, and P. Harper,
   Biodistribution of low density lipoprotein in normal and
   hyperlipemic animals, Cor Notes 3:5 (1988).
5. J. W. Ryan, P. V. Harper, R. V. Hay, K. A. Williams, K. A. Lathrop,
   V. J. Stark, and R. M. Fleming, Human biodistribution of I-123 and
   Tc-99m labeled LDL, J. Nucl. Med. 29:803 (1988).
6. J. W. Ryan, P. V. Harper, R. V. Hay, K. A. Williams, K. A. Lathrop,
   V. J. Stark, and R. M. Fleming, Comparison of radiolabeled LDLs
   for detection of atherosclerotic plaques in humans, Eur. Heart J.
   9 (Suppl.1):158 (1988).
7. R. V. Hay, R. M. Fleming, J. W. Ryan, K. A. Williams, V. J. Stark,
   K. A. Lathrop, and P. V. Harper, Nuclear imaging analysis of human
   low density lipoprotein biodistribution in rabbits and monkeys, J.
   Nucl. Med. in press (1991).

8. Y. A. Kesaniemi, and S. M. Grundy, Significance of low density lipoprotein production in the regulation of plasma cholesterol level in man, J. Clin. Invest. 70:13 (1982).

9. R. V. Hay, J. W. Ryan, K. A. Williams, R. W. Atcher, M. W. Brechbiel, O. A. Gansow, V. J. Stark, R. M. Fleming, R. J. Donati, K. A. Lathrop, and P. V. Harper, Indium-111-[SCN-Bz-DTPA]-low density lipoprotein: A new agent for extended nuclear imaging and detection of atheromata, in: "Cardiovascular Science & Technology: Basic and Applied, I," J. Norman, ed., Oxymoron Press, Louisville (1989).

10. J. M. Esteban, J. Schlom, O. A. Gansow, R. W. Atcher, M. W. Brechbiel, D. E. Simpson, and D. Colcher, New method for the chelation of Indium-111 to monoclonal antibodies: biodistribution and imaging of athymic mice bearing human colon carcinoma xenografts, J. Nucl. Med. 28:861 (1987).

11. H. R. Maecke, A. Riesen, and W. Ritter, The molecular structure of indium-DTPA, J. Nucl. Med. 30:1235 (1989).

12. M. D. Gross, R. W. S. Skinner, S. W. Schwendner, L. E. DeForge, R. E. Counsell, and R. S. Newton, Indium-111-DTPA-low density lipoprotein (LDL) imaging of LDL-receptor activity, J. Nucl. Med. 30:768 (1989).

13. J. M. Nicolas, B. Leclef, H. Jardez, A. Keyeux, J. A. Melin, and A. Trouet, Imaging atherosclerotic lesions with In-111-labelled low density lipoproteins, J. Nucl. Med. 30:788 (1989).

14. J. M. Rosen, S. P. Butler, H. N. Ginsberg, G. E. Meinken, T. S. T. Wang, S. C. Srivastava, and P. O. Alderson, Development of In-111 labeled LDL for imaging atherosclerotic lesions, J. Nucl. Med. 30:787 (1989).

15. J. M. Rosen, S. P. Butler, G. E. Meinken, T. S. T. Wang, R. Ramakrishnan, S. C. Srivastava, P. O. Alderson, and H. N. Ginsberg, Indium-111-labeled LDL: A potential agent for imaging atherosclerotic disease and lipoprotein biodistribution, J. Nucl. Med. 31:343 (1990).

16. R. S. Lees, A. M. Lees, A. J. Fischman, and H. W. Strauss, External imaging of active atherosclerosis with 99mTc-LDL, in: "Pathobiology of the Human Atherosclerotic Plaque," S. Glagov, W. P. Newman III, and S. A. Schaffer, eds., Springer-Verlag, New York (1990).

17. D. C. Schwenke, and T. E. Carew, Initiation of atherosclerotic lesions in cholesterol-fed rabbits. I. Focal increases in arterial LDL concentration precede development of fatty streak lesions, Arteriosclerosis 9:895 (1989).

18. A. M. Lees, R. S. Lees, F. J. Schoen, J. L. Isaacsohn, A. J. Fischman, K. A. McKusick, and H. W. Strauss, Imaging human atherosclerosis with 99mTc-labeled low density lipoproteins, Arteriosclerosis 8:461 (1988).

19. D. C. Schwenke, and T. E. Carew, Initiation of atherosclerotic lesions in cholesterol-fed rabbits. II. Selective retention of LDL vs. selective increases in LDL permeability in susceptible sites of arteries, Arteriosclerosis 9:908 (1989).

20. R. S. Lees, A. M. Lees, and H. W. Strauss, External imaging of human atherosclerosis, J. Nucl. Med. 24:154 (1983).

21. I.-L. Shih, R. S. Lees, M. Y. Chang, and A. M. Lees, Focal accumulation of an apolipoprotein B-based synthetic oligopeptide in the healing rabbit arterial wall, Proc. Natl. Acad. Sci. USA 87:1436 (1990).

PLATELET LABELLING IN ATHEROSCLEROSIS

Helmut Sinzinger, Irene Virgolini, and Peter Fitscha

Atherosclerosis Research Group (ASF) Vienna, Atherosclerosis Research Group of the Austrian Academy of Sciences,
Vienna, and 2nd Department of Internal Medicine, Poli-
clinic Vienna, Austria

INTRODUCTION

Three mechanisms are centrally involved in human atherogenesis, i.e.,
the role of the coagulation system: encrustation theory (C. von Rokitansky
1), cellular reaction to injury (Virchow 2), and lipid entry (Anitschkow 3)
are well defined. Bizzozero (4) more than one century ago stressed the
role of platelets. In recent years the early diagnosis of atherosclerosis
using radioisotopic techniques has been frequently attempted. The most
extensive information available concerns the involvement of the coagulation
system using radiolabelling of either fibrinogen or platelets. In this
brief overview all three of these processes of atherogenesis will be
considered with special attention to use of labelled platelets. At present
atherosclerosis can be functionally monitored at least partially to permit
further insights into the development of the disease, but there are still
limitations to be overcome.

COAGULATION SYSTEM

Plasmatic Coagulation

Only few labelling data are available using imaging approaches to
identify, diagnose, and follow the course of plasmatic coagulation in
arterial thromboembolic events (5). After the introduction of radiolabelled fibrinogen into diagnosis of arterial thrombi (6), the use of
123I-fibrinogen has been claimed as a useful imaging agent to detect human
atherosclerosis in vivo non-invasively. These promising preliminary
findings, however, were not supported by later reports in the literature.
In 24 patients with active disease we were not able to discover any true
positive lesion site. Similarly, the promise of fibronectin (7) labelled
either with 111In or 131I has thus far not been sustained.

Platelets

Mathew Thakur in 1976 (8) discovered 111Indium-oxine as a new
platelet labelling agent. It offered the advantage of external imaging as
well as parallel kinetic monitoring. Other major advantages are a low
elution and reutilisation rate. Using experimental abrasion of the

endothelial coverage of the abdominal aortic segment, he was able to prove the usefulness of this new tracer. A variety of indium tracers, such as acetylacetone, tropolone, merc (MPO), oxine, oxine-sulfate, and choloro-tetraphenyl-porphyrine as well as 99mTc-oxine and -HMPAO have been examined without establishing significant advantages over 111In-oxine. Due to its short half-life and the possible radiation damage 99mTc-oxine was only occasionally used.

Labelling Techniques

Almost every investigator has a preferred labelling technique. Almost all of them represent a slight modification of the one originally proposed by Thakur (8). We feel that an incubation temperature of 37°C, a cell concentration of at least 10^9 cells per ml, and a pH of 6.2 are the key requirements to achieve optimal results (9). An optimal radiolabelling of platelets is not so much reflected by the labelling efficiency as it is by a good recovery indicating the in vivo metabolic activity of the cells. An injection of a non-viable platelet population does not permit one to monitor normal kinetics. We found that the addition of prostacyclin (PGI2) and nitric oxide (NO, one of the active compounds of the endothelial derived relaxing factor (EDRF), 10) both result in an improvement in platelet metabolic activity, especially if the processing of the cells was not very skillfully carried out. Thus, the addition of these substances may be especially helpful for the beginner. Interestingly enough, elevated cholesterol and LDL-cholesterol significantly impair the labelling efficiency (11).

EXPERIMENTAL DATA

Thakur in his pioneering work (8) was the first to show platelet deposition in dog carotid arteries. Morphological control experiments in rabbits demonstrated that endothelial abrasion of a large abdominal segment with subsequent platelet deposition results in positive imaging. In contrast, however, segmental desquamation of endothelium followed by platelet accumulation did not cause positive images. Local lesions may result in a local disturbance of haemostasis associated with an enhanced platelet uptake. Even in the absence of any visible lesion, a number of lesions not being imaged under the gamma-camera may well result in a severely shortened platelet survival, reflecting systemic haemostatic imbalance. In experimental lesions labelling is regularly performed before the lesioning. They thus appear much more frequently positive as compared to human lesions, which are labeled at a later stage and appear to be less extensive.

HUMAN DATA

Autologous platelet labelling in humans has been performed in quite a wide range of clinical conditions (Table 1). Labelling with 111In-oxine has the advantage of parallel monitoring of platelet survival; it is a quite useful clinical measure for systemic haemostasis and its alteration either due to pathological platelet consumption (shortening) or therapeutic improvement (prolongation).

Morphological Control

Morphological study of human atherosclerotic lesions indicates that part of the radioactivity seen is due to platelets deposited on the surface (parie-tal thrombus, ulcerated lesion), while the majority can be found as

Table 1. Platelet imaging in patients

1. Atherosclerosis
carotid artery	Davis et al. 1980
femoral artery	Fitscha et al. 1985
coronary artery	Ezekowitz et al. 1982
aneurysms	Heyns et al. 1982
thrombogenicity	Sinzinger et al. 1982
therapeutic monitoring	Sinzinger et al. 1985

2. Surgical interventions
endarterectomy	Price et al. 1982
angioplasty	Pope et al. 1985

3. Synthetic material
graft patency	Goldman et al. 1983
bypass grafts	Dewanjee et al. 1985
thrombogenicity	Price et al. 1982

4. Thrombosis
left ventricular	Ezekowitz et al. 1982
venous thrombosis	Moser et al. 1985

5. Transplantation
kidney	Leithner et al. 1981
pancreas	Sinzinger et al. 1984

6. Kinetics
haematology	Peters et al. 1982
survival	Harker et al. 1977

(for references see (5))

cellular debris incorporated into vascular wall cells mostly taken up by macrophages.

Incidence of Positive Lesions

The incidence of so-called "active" visible lesions in patients suffering from preclinical atherosclerosis ranges below 10%, in clinically manifest disease up to 50% (12), while in certain cases, such as juvenile stroke patients (13) this incidence increases up to 100%. Platelet uptake is generally used to quantify the severity of the atherosclerotic ulceration or the tendency toward thrombosis.

Vascular Regions

Carotid Arteries: The carotid arteries were originally investigated by Davis et al. in 1980 (14). The incidence of visible lesions in the carotid arteries in general appears to be higher as compared to femoral arteries or other arterial segments which can be visualized.

Femoral Arteries: Femoral artery lesions occasionally can be imaged. However, no correlation with the severity and extent of the disease has been demonstrated. Like the carotid arteries these lesions are very well suited to test the efficacy of drugs in rendering vascular surfaces less thrombogenic. This has been shown for a variety of compounds like aspirin, prostaglandins, and others.

Coronary Arteries: While in experimental conditions a platelet deposition can be imaged in the coronary arteries after severe intimal injury, the positive findings in humans are anecdotal and thus far can apparently be of use only in selected cases. For example, in only 25% of patients suffering from myocardial infarction who were studied within 24 hours of the onset of chest pain could an area of increased 111In-oxine uptake corresponding to an obstructed coronary vessel be detected by angiography. Reliable imaging is prevented by problems of high background movement, small vessels, and a relatively small lesion to background ratio.

LIPIDS

Low-Density Lipoproteins; Tracers: A variety of different tracers (123-Iodine [I], 125-I (15), 131-I, 99mTc, and 111-In) has been tested using various radiolabelling and separation (ultracentrifugation, immunoffinity chromatography) techniques. Others, such as cholesteryl ester analogues, HDL, and VLDL have been applied in experimental studies. Clinical studies have also been reported indicating localization of labelled LDL in atherosclerotic plaques in human subjects.

Receptor Behavior: LDL binding to the liver in normal humans results in an immediate trapping of radiolabelled LDL (figure 1). The corresponding kinetic curve shows a continuous increase over the first 16 minutes (figure 2) after reinjection. In contrast, in familial hypercholesterolmia the total uptake (figure 3) is much less (as assessed by whole-body quantification), the kinetic curve showing perfusion, i.e., a decrease after an initial peak (figure 4) within the first two minutes.

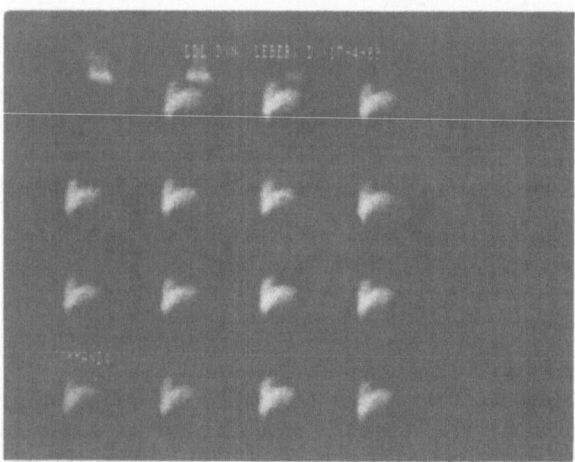

Fig. 1.   Accumulation of 123I-labelled LDL in the liver of a healthy normocholesterolemic adult. Sequence of initial 16 frames each lasting for 1 minute.

184

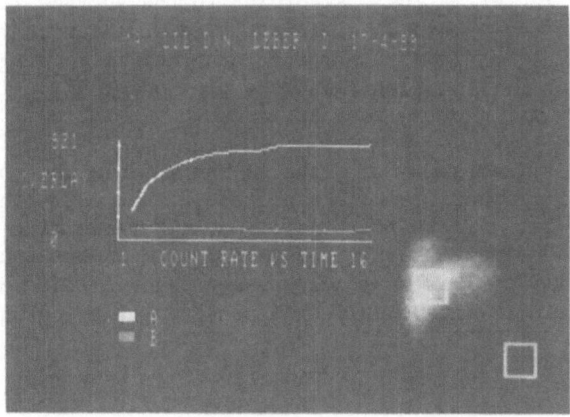

Fig. 2.   The kinetic curve summarizing the 16 frames shows a continu-
usly increasing activity over the liver; the lower curve
represents the blood background.

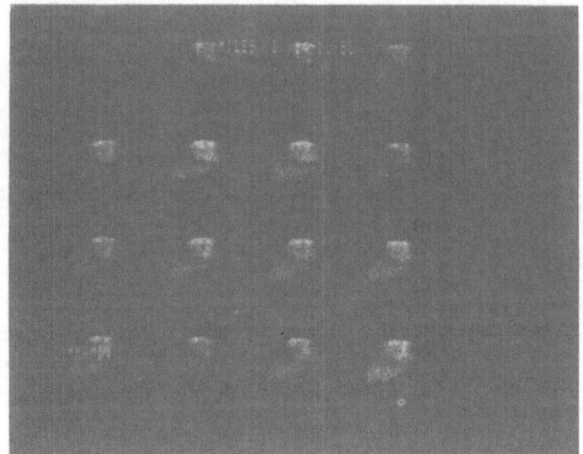

Fig. 3.   Severely decreased LDL-uptake in the liver of a hypercholes-
erolemic patient. The liver activity remains low, the back-
round and the heart activity are rather high.

Lesion Imaging: Lipid lesions are characterized by an enhanced LDL-
entry (15, 16). Normocholesterolemics almost completely lack areas of
visible enhanced LDL-entry while computerized kinetic analysis may very
well identify a pathological behaviour. In contrast, in hypercholesterolmia the incidence and number both increase dramatically while more advanced
plaques and complicated lesions have only a moderately increased to normal
LDL entry depending on their lipid content. The highest LDL-uptake is
found at the edge of the lesion as compared to the center. The total
uptake correlates well to the number of foam cells found as well as to the
lipid content per foam cell. Extra- and intracellular lipid deposition
cannot be differentiated.

Surface Characterization: According to the surface lining, three different kinetic curves can be differentiated in experimental animals and in humans as well. In areas with intact endothelial coverage (type I) the total LDL-entry is very low, an immediate peak after injection with a decrease of the kinetic curve thereafter can be monitored.

Deendothelialized segments (type II) show a maximum uptake at 2-6 hours with a drop thereafter. The amplitude of the curve, however, is significantly higher. The third type (type III) reflecting reendothelialized segments shows a continuously increasing tracer uptake up to 48 hours monitoring time (17). This approach has been proven to be useful in monitoring therapeutic intervention (physical activity, drug treatment).

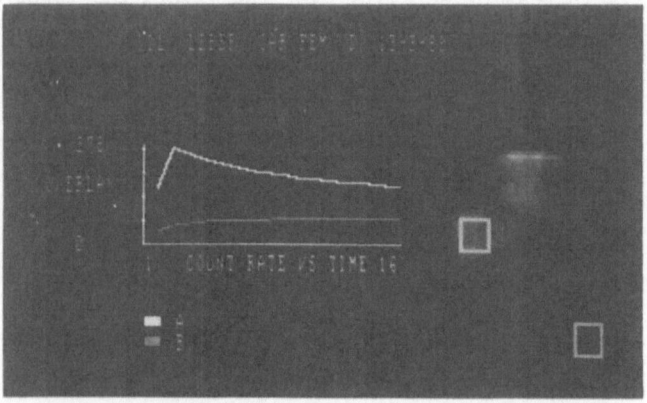

Fig. 4.   The kinetics over the liver of the familial hypercholesterolmic patient demonstrates that after an initial peak there is a decrease of liver activity while the background steadily increases.

CELLS

Monocytes: The major problem for monocyte labelling is to isolate a sufficient cell number (apheresis), to achieve a clean preparation of viable cells and to titrate radioactivity (<20 uCi 111In-oxine/10^8 cells).

Kinetics: The kinetics of mononuclear cells after reinjection are quite complicated and not yet completely understood. Possible differences in the decay between healthy controls and patients with manifested disease seem to occur.

Lesion Imaging: In experimental animals (baboons (18)) and in humans (19) preliminiary evidence of positive monocyte imaging exists.

OTHER MARKERS FOR LESIONS

Besides the briefly mentioned techniques, the use of monoclonal antibodies, porphyrins, fibronectin, non-specific polyclonal immunoglobulin G, and other precursors has been attempted with varying success (for review, see (5)).

Acknowledgements

We thank Drs J. Kaliman, Graziana Lupattelli (Perugia, Italy), B. Pramsohler, and F. Rauscha for their sustained cooperation. The valuable laboratory assistance of Judith Bednar, Gabriele Cafourek, Susanne Granegger, Ulli Horvath, and Brigitte Jankovic, as well as the secretarial services of Eva Unger in preparing and typing the manuscript, are gratefully acknowledged.

REFERENCES

1. C. von Rokitansky, "Über einige der wichtigsten Krankheiten der Arterien," K.K. Hof-und Staatsdruckerei, Wien (1852).

2. R. Virchow, "Phlogose und Thrombose im Gefässystem. Gesammelte Abhandlungen zur wissenschaftlichen Medizin," Hirsch, Berlin (1856).

3. N. N. Anitschkow, Experimental arteriosclerosis in animals, in: "Arteriosclerosis. A Survey of the Problem," E. C. Cowdry, ed., MacMillan, New York (1933).

4. J. Bizzozero, Über einen neuen Formbestandteil des Blutes und dessen Rolle bei der Thrombose und der Blutgerinnung, Virchows Archiv Pathol. Anat. 90:261 (1882).

5. H. Sinzinger and I. Virgolini, Nuclear medicine and atherosclerosis: A review, Eur. J. Nucl. Med. 31:in press (1990).

6. L. R. Erhardt, T. Lundman, and H. Mellstadt, Incorporation of 125I-labelled fibrinogen into coronary arterial thrombi in acute myocardial infarction in man, Lancet I:387 (1973).

7. A. Uehara, Y. Isaka, K. Hashikawa, K. Kimura, T. Kozuka, T. Kamada, H. Etani, S. Yoneda, and M. Imaizumi, 131-Iodine-labeled fibronectin: potential agent for imaging atherosclerotic lesion and thrombus, J. Nucl. Med. 29:1264 (1988).

8. M. L. Thakur, M. J. Welch, J. H. Joist, and R. E. Coleman, Indium-111-labelled platelets: studies on preparation and evaluation of in vitro and in vivo functions, Thromb. Res. 9:345 (1976).

9. H. Sinzinger, H. Kolbe, E. Strobl-Jäger, and R. Höfer, A simple and safe technique for sterile autologous platelet labelling using "Monovette" vials, Eur. J. Nucl. Med. 9:320 (1984).

10. X. Wagner, S. Granegger, A. Dembinska-Kiec, and H. Sinzinger, Nitric oxide (NO) for radiolabelling of human platelets, in: "Radiolabelled Cellular Blood Elements," H. Sinzinger and M. Thakur, eds., Facultas, Vienna (1989).

11. H. Sinzinger, K. Widhalm, J. Flores, and S. Granegger, Low density lipoproteins decrease labelling efficiency of human platelets, Nucl. Med. Commun. (submitted) (1990).

12. C. Kessler, R. Reuther, J. Berentelg, and B. Kimmig, The clinical use of platelet scintigraphy with 111-In-oxine, J. Neurol. 229:255 (1983).

13. B. Pramsohler, G. Lupattelli, H. Scholz, and H. Sinzinger, Platelet scintigraphy and survival in juvenile stroke patients, in: "Radiolabelled Cellular Blood Elements," H. Sinzinger and M. Thakur, eds., Alan R. Liss, Inc., New York, 71-80, (1990).

14. H. H. Davis , B. A. Siegel, L. A. Sherman, W. A. Heaton, T. P. Naidich, J. H. Joist, and M. J. Welch, Scintigraphic detection of carotid atherosclerosis with indium-111-labeled autologous platelets, J. Nucl. Med. 21:548 (1980).

15. R. S. Lees, A. M. Lees, and H. W. Strauss, External imaging of human atherosclerosis, J. Nucl. Med. 24:154 (1983).

16. J. Kaliman, H. Sinzinger, H. Bergmann, and C. Kolbe, Value of 123-I- low density lipoproteins (LDL) in the diagnosis of human atherosclerotic lesions, Circulation 72:300 (1985).

17. I. Virgolini, P. Angelberger, G. Lupattelli, J. Pidlich, and H. Sinzinger, In-vivo-Einstrom autologer radioaktiv markierter Low-density-Lipoproteine (LDL) in menschliche Gefässe, Wr. klin. Wschr. 101:798 (1989).

18. A. duP. Heyns, H. Pieters, and A. C. Steyn, Isolation and labelling with In-111 of a viable population of blood monocytes, in: "Radiolabelled Cellular Blood Elements," H. Sinzinger and M. Thakur, eds., Alan R. Liss, Inc., New York, 261-270, (1990).

19. I. Virgolini, C. Müller, P. Fitscha, P. Chiba, and H. Sinzinger, Radiolabelling autologous monocytes with 111-Indium-oxine for reinjection in patients with atherosclerosis, in: "Radio- labelled Cellular Blood Elements," H. Sinzinger and M. Thakur, eds., Alan R. Liss, Inc., New York, 271-280 (1990).

USE OF MONOCLONAL ANTIBODIES TO FIBRINOGEN, FIBRIN AND

FIBRIN(OGEN) DEGRADATION PRODUCTS IN ATHEROSCLEROSIS

Alessandra Bini[1], Bohdan J. Kudryk[2]

[1]Istituto di Ricerche Farmacologiche Mario Negri,
Consorzio Mario Negri Sud, S. Maria Imbaro,Italy and
Department of Pathology, College of Physicians and
Surgeons of Columbia University, New York, USA;
[2]Lindsley F. Kimball Research Institute, The New York
Blood Center, New York, USA

I. INTRODUCTION

Fibrinogen is a soluble protein which is converted into an
insoluble gel, fibrin, by thrombin. Fibrin formation is involved
in the physiology of hemostasis and wound repair and in a number
of pathological processes such as thrombosis, atherosclerosis,
tumors, renal disease and inflammation.

Fibrinogen is a large symmetrical blood glycoprotein (M_r
340,000), composed of three pairs of non-identical polypeptide
chains, $A\alpha$, $B\beta$, and γ, held together by 29 disulfide bonds. The
central domain, N-DSK, the aminoterminal disulfide knot of
fibrinogen [$(A\alpha1-51, B\beta1-118, \gamma1-78)_2$], can be chemically separated
from the rest of the molecule by cleavage with cyanogen bromide.

Proteolysis of fibrinogen by thrombin releases fibrinopeptide
A (FPA, Aα1-16) and fibrinopeptide B (FPB, Bβ 1-14), two moles
each per mole of fibrinogen, leading to desFPA, desFPB fibrin
(fibrin II) formation. This fibrin is further stabilized by Factor
XIII-mediated crosslinking of both the α- and γ-chains in their
terminal domains. Cleavage of fibrinogen by plasmin converts
fibrinogen to Fragment X that retains the trinodular structure.
Further cleavage leads to Fragment Y and Fragment D. Fragment Y is
further degraded to Fragment D and Fragment E. In crosslinked
fibrin, Fragment D-Dimer is obtained by proteolysis of two
adjacent fibrin molecules. Results from clinical and experimental
studies led to the formulation of the hypothesis of the relative
proteolysis of fibrinogen by thrombin and plasmin. [1] According to
this scheme, if thrombin action prevails over plasmin, fibrin is
formed, possibly leading to occlusive thrombosis. If plasmin
action predominates, formation of Fragment X would act as a
regulatory mechanism depleting substrate for fibrin II formation.
To verify this hypothesis the basic question to be answered was on
the similarity between a clot formed in vitro and a thrombus
formed in vivo. The biochemical changes occurring in the

fibrinogen-to-fibrin transition from purified components have previously been analyzed in detail. [2]

II. IMMUNOCHEMICAL AND IMMUNOHISTOCHEMICAL CHARACTERIZATION OF FIBRINOGEN AND FIBRIN IN ATHEROSCLEROTIC PLAQUES

Surgically removed human thrombi, normal and atherosclerotic vessels obtained at surgery or autopsy were studied to characterize their molecular composition of fibrinogen-derived protein. [3]

The samples were analyzed immunochemically and immunohistochemically. In the first part of the study, normal aortas, atherosclerotic lesions and acute and organized thrombi were degraded with cyanogen bromide and tested with radioimmunoassays for FPA, FPB, as well as fragments $B\beta 1-42$, $B\beta 15-42$ and N-DSK. Arterial specimens were classified according to histological criteria as normal aortas, fatty plaques, fibrous plaques and complicated plaques. In both acute and organized thrombi, 50-70% of the total protein was fibrinogen-derived and of this, approximately 80% represented fibrin II and 20% represented Fragments X, Y or E, with trace amounts of fibrinogen and fibrin I (desFPA fibrin). There was no significant difference between acute and organized thrombi. The content of fibrinogen-derived protein in arterial samples was only about 5%. In normal aortas, most of the fibrinogen-derived protein was intact fibrinogen (80%), with the remainder being desFPA fibrin and Fragments X, Y or E. Fatty plaques had less fibrinogen (about 55%), increased desFPA fibrin (fibrin I about 30%), desFPA desFPB fibrin (fibrin II about 10%) and Fragments X,Y or E (about 10%) than normal aortas. In fibrous plaques, fibrinogen and fibrin I decreased with an increase of fibrin II to 20 %, and 25% of Fragments X,Y or E. In complicated plaques, the amount of the different molecular forms of fibrinogen was comparable to both acute and organized thrombi with mostly fibrin II, less than 5% fibrinogen and fibrin I and about 20% of Fragments X, Y or E. These data showed intact fibrinogen as the main molecular form present in normal aortas with a progression to mostly fibrin II in complicated plaques. Increasing amounts of fibrin(ogen) degradation products were also present with increasing severity of the lesion.

In a further study, a number of acute and organized thrombi, previously degraded with CNBr, were gel-filtered on Sephacryl-200 and fractions assayed for immunoreactivity. [4] Gel-filtration of a CNBr-digest of a thrombus (abdominal aortic aneurism) showed that about 50% of the $B\beta$ 15-42 immunoreactivity was associated with N-DSK, and that less than 2% was present as free peptide. These results suggest that the N-DSK immunoreactivity was due to approximately equal amounts of fibrin II and Fragments X, Y, and E. Similar results were obtained for two other thrombi and an embolus.

Immunohistochemical identification of the distribution of different molecular forms of fibrinogen-derived protein in normal and atherosclerotic arteries and thrombi was accomplished by using previously characterized monoclonal antibodies (MAbs) with the avidin-biotin complex immunoperoxidase technique. The antibodies used were: MAb1-8C6, anti $B\beta 1-42$, identifies both fibrinogen and fibrin I, MAb T2G1, anti-$B\beta 15-42$, reacts fully with fibrin II, and MAb GC4, anti-Fragment D which also cross-reacts with Fragment D-Dimer.[5] Acute and organized thrombi reacted with all the antibodies although in organized thrombi the detection of fibrinogen/fibrin I was much weaker. Fragment D/D-Dimer was more concentrated in the central area of thrombi. In normal aortas, fibrinogen/fibrin I was detected in only 2 out of 12 samples and traces of fibrin II in only 1 of these. Fragment D-Dimer was not seen in normal vessels. In early lesions, fibrinogen/fibrin I was present in the intima and subintima in short threads in areas of loose connective tissues, around foam cells, macrophages and smooth muscle cells. Fibrin II was present on the endothelium only in one coronary artery and in small flecks around vessel wall cells. In fibrous plaques, fibrinogen/fibrin I were detected in the vessel wall as short threads or bundles, or around smooth muscle cells and macrophages with a patchy, stellate appearance. Fibrinogen/fibrin I were also detected on luminal thrombi together with fibrin II. Fibrin II was distributed in long threads and bundles in the intima and media or around cells. Fragment D/D-Dimer was detected in large areas of fibrin deposition but was rarely seen around cells. In advanced lesions, fibrinogen/fibrin I were distributed in large areas in loose connective tissue, around macrophages and smooth muscle cells, and in areas of cholesterol crystals and calcium deposits. In these lesions, long threads of fibrin II were observed parallel to the luminal surface, suggestive of incorporation of mural thrombus. Fibrin II and Fragment D/D-Dimer were distributed around cholesterol crystals and calcium deposits.

In summary, the results of these studies suggest that increased fibrin formation and degradation in atherosclerotic vessels is associated with increasing severity of the lesions. The observed distribution of the different molecular forms of fibrinogen in the vessel wall indicates that biochemical changes of fibrinogen-derived protein during the progression of atherosclerosis is not related solely to thrombus formation or to increased permeability of the endothelium. The detection of the different molecular forms of fibrin(ogen) around macrophages suggests active participation of these cells in the process of fibrin formation and/or degradation in the vessel wall. [6]

The functional effects which fibrinogen-derived protein might have on the endothelium in atherosclerosis is being investigated in parallel studies where preliminary results have shown that LMW FDPs [Low Molecular Weight Fibrin(ogen) Degradation Products] have a time-dependent and dose-dependent effect on the release of mitogenic activities from endothelial cells in culture. [7]

III. PLASMA FIBRINOGEN LEVELS AND HERITABILITY ASSOCIATED WITH THROMBOSIS AND ATHEROSCLEROSIS

A number of recent studies (reviewed by Di Minno and Mancini 1990) [8], including The Framingham Study, [9] The Northwick Park Heart Study (NHPS), [10,11], the Goteborg Study, [12] and a few others, [13,14,15] have correlated the incidence of ischemic heart disease (IHD) with elevated fibrinogen level, comparable to or higher than that with cholesterol levels. The studies, which investigated both myocardial infarction (MI) and stroke, considered fibrinogen levels ranging from 310 to 700 mg% [9,10,11,12] as increased, while in the studies on myocardial infarction alone, high levels of fibrinogen were those above 350-400 mg%. [13,14,15]

Other factors that affect fibrinogen values were advancing

age [9],[16],diabetes and its complications, [15] oral contraceptive use [12] smoking and obesity. [9],[10]

A study on plasma fibrinogen level in 85 families of probands with early myocardial infarction compared with 85 families randomly selected from the general population, showed that the genetic heritability for plasma concentration of fibrinogen is 51%, which has been shown to be higher only for serum cholesterol and LDL cholesterol among the generally accepted risk factors for coronary heart disease (CHD).[17] The mode of inheritance remains to be established. Studies on the genetic variation at the fibrinogen locus defined by RFLPs (restriction fragment length polymorphism) have detected the presence of two different alleles for the alpha and two pairs for the beta chain of the fibrinogen genes with the probes used. [18] The individuals with genotype B2B2 have shown higher mean values of plasma fibrinogen (370 mg%), compared to the other genotypes. The authors point out that if the findings of the NHPS study apply to these values, they would represent an increase in risk of 75% for developing IHD in the next five years. However, the genetic variation defined by RFLPs described accounts only for 15% of the total variation. It is possible that these values are underestimated as other studies in progress show other RFLPs at the beta and gamma fibrinogen chain loci. [19]

IV. THROMBOSIS AND ATHEROSCLEROSIS

The presence of thrombi at sites of narrowing or occlusion of injured vessels has been demonstrated in a large number of detailed pathological studies. [20], [21] This work has been reviewed by Saffitz et al.[22], and Davies.[23] Clinical angiography has shown early thrombotic occlusion of a stenotic artery at the time of infarction. [24] Angiographic data in patients with acute myocardial infarction and in unstable angina showed predominant obstructive morphology infrequently found in patients with stable angina. [25]

Postmortem examination of epicardial arteries and myocardium has shown presence of thrombi associated with myocardial infarction, sudden death and unstable angina [26],[27],[28] (reviewed by Davies[23]). Reconstruction of these coronary thrombi from serial sectioning has shown a common morphologic feature of plaque rupture and fissuring with recent thrombi in the intima and/or in the lumen with total occlusion of the vessel, or with a lesser degree of luminal thrombus in the case of sudden death.[21],[28],[27] Fissuring of a plaque on a severely damaged arterial wall releases a pool of extracellular lipid within the intima that can stimulate thrombus formation.[28],[29] Microemboli were mostly found distal to thrombi in arteries that contained an acute thrombus, showing that thrombus formation and fragmentation is a dynamic process. [26],[27]

A very recent study has analyzed morphometrically the composition of atherosclerotic plaques in coronary arteries of patients after acute myocardial infarction (AMI) and sudden cardiac death. In the coronary arteries of the AMI group, the atherosclerotic plaques with more than 75% narrowing consisted of significantly more amorphous debris (containing cholesterol clefts and presumably rich in extracellular lipids), less calcium and less cellular fibrous tissue than in the sudden death group, which might predispose to the formation of intramural thrombi. [30] Earlier studies detected both LDL and fibrin(ogen)-related antigens in atherosclerotic lesions suggesting that a common mechanism exists for entry of fibrinogen and lipoprotein in the vessel wall.[31,32,33]

A more recent study has found a correlation between total fibrin related antigens and LDL in each group of atherosclerotic lesions.[34] Deposits of both fibrin(ogen) and LDL were localized by immunofluorescence in human cerebral arteries with increased associated deposits found in more severe lesions. Fibrin(ogen) deposition was found only in the intima of early lesions, suggesting fibrinogen deposits might precede the deposition of LDL in the development of cerebral atherosclerosis.[35]

V. USE OF MONOCLONAL ANTIBODIES AS DIAGNOSTICS IN THROMBOSIS: CURRENT STUDIES AND FURTHER DEVELOPMENTS

Monoclonal antibodies T2G1 and GC4 have been used successfully in imaging fresh and aged experimentally induced thrombi in dogs.[36,37] Both In-111 F(ab')2 T2G1 and Tc-99m Fab' T2G1 are currently being used in clinical trials as clot imaging agents in patients with deep vein thrombosis.[38] Monoclonal antibody 59D8[39], was recently shown to be indistinguishable from T2G1. The Fab fragment of 59D8 has been labelled with In-111 via DTPA chelate and preliminary data from the clinical trials in deep vein thrombosis have been recently reported.[40,41,42] It should be feasible to use these antibodies in patients with myocardial infarction. Imaging their coronaries after thrombolytic therapy should provide information on the state of recanalization and possible reocclusion.

Fibrinogen levels cannot be modified by diet. The effect of dietary lipids on thrombosis and atherosclerosis has been recently reviewed.[43] The results of a randomized controlled trial to examine the effect of dietary intervention in the secondary prevention of myocardial infarction have been published recently.[44] A large number of subjects (2033 men) who recovered from myocardial infarction were given advice to reduce their fat intake, and to increase their ratio of polyunsaturated to saturated fat as well as their intake of fatty fish and cereal fibre. Total mortality after 2 years was 29% lower in the fish advice group, which the authors attribute entirely to a reduction in IHD. The subjects who could not tolerate fish were given EPA (eicosapentaenoic acid).

Clinical and experimental data from these studies might stimulate a multidisciplinary study to analyze the different aspects described, and thus elucidate the role of fibrinogen in the development of atherosclerosis. Patients undergoing vascular surgery could be the better subjects for a long-term study. Their preoperative fibrinogen levels and fibrinogen polymorphism would be measured in blood samples. Imaging of the endarterectomy patients with B-mode ultrasonography and with labelled monoclonal antibodies T2G1 and GC4 before surgery, and with a follow-up of one to five years should be possible and would provide information on the degree of atherosclerosis in their vessels and possibly on their fibrin and degraded fibrin deposits. Tissue samples from these patients will be studied for the distribution of the different molecular forms of fibrinogen in the excised atherosclerotic plaques. Patients after MI would also be good candidates for a multidisciplinary study of this kind since they might undergo bypass surgery, but these tissues are obtainable only in a very limited number of cases, as the affected coronaries are seldom removed. Furthermore, these patients after surgery will probably modify their exercise, smoking and diet habits according to recently formulated recommendations[45,46] and this could provide further grouping criteria. In fact, although fibrinogen levels are not altered by dietary intervention, a change in the levels of total serum cholesterol, LDL cholesterol, serum triglycerides, and VLDL cholesterol might lead to reduction and partial regression of preexisting atherosclerosis that could result in decreased accumulation and deposition or increased degradation of fibrinogen-derived protein in the vessel wall.

ACKNOWLEDGMENTS

Supported by Grants HL-15486, HL-21006, HL-24230 from the National Heart, Lung and Blood Institutes, National Institutes of Health, Bethesda, MD, NATO Collaborative Research Grant (CRG-890569), Agenzia per la Promozione dello Sviluppo del Mezzogiorno, deliberazione n.6166, PR1 and Progetto Finalizzato CNR 3603-3605/3608.

REFERENCES

1. H. L. Nossel, Relative proteolysis of the fibrinogen Bß thrombosis, Nature 291:165 (1981).
2. B. Blombäck, B. Hessel, D. Hogg, and L. Therkildsen, A two-step fibrinogen-fibrin transition in blood coagulation, Nature 257:501 (1978).
3. A. Bini, J.J.Jr.Fenoglio, J. Sobel, J. Owen, M. Fejgl, and K.L.Kaplan, Immunochemical characterization of fibrinogen, fibrin I, and fibrin II in human thrombi and atherosclerotic lesions. Blood 69:1038 (1987).
4. A. Bini,J.Sobel and K.L. Kaplan, Separation and characterization of fibrinogen-derived fragments in human arterial thrombi, in: "Fibrinogen and its Derivatives",Muller-Berghaus G., U. Scheefers-Borchel, E. Selmayr and A. Henschen ed., Elsevier Science Publishers, Amsterdam (1986).
5. A. Bini, J.J. Jr Fenoglio., R. Mesa-Tejada, B.J. Kudryk, and K.L. Kaplan, Identification and distribution of fibrinogen, fibrin, and fibrin(ogen) degradation products in atherosclerosis. Arteriosclerosis 9:109 (1989).
6. K. L. Kaplan, A. Bini, Thrombosis in atherogenesis. Crit. Rev. Oncol. Hematol. 9:305 (1989).
7. R. Lorenzet, J.H. Sobel, A. Bini, and L.D. Witte, The release of mitogenic activity from endothelial cells is enhanced by low molecular weight fibrinogen-degradation products. Circulation 78:394 (1988).
8. G. Di Minno, and M. Mancini, Measuring plasma fibrinogen to predict stroke and myocardial infarction. Arteriosclerosis 10:1 (1990).
9. W. B. Kannel, P.A. Wolf, W.P. Castelli, and R.B. D'Agostino, Fibrinogen and risk of cardiovascular disease, The Framingham study. J.A.M.A. 258:1183 (1987).
10. T. W. Meade, R. Chakrabarti, A. Haines, W.R.S. North, Y. Sitirling, and S.G. Thompson, Haemostatic function and cardiovascular death: Early results of a prospective study, Lancet I:1050 (1980).

11. T. W. Meade, M.C. Brozovic, R.R. Chakrabarti, J.D. Imeson, S. Mellows, G.J. Miller, W.R.S. North, Y. Stirling,and S.G.Thompson, Haemostatic function and ischaemic heart disease: principal results of the Northwick Park Heart Study. Lancet II:533 (1986).

12. L. Wilhelmsen, K. Svardsudd, K. Korsan-Bengtsen, B. Larsson, L. Welin, and G. Tibblin, Fibrinogen as a risk factor for stroke and myocardial infarction, N. Engl.J. Med. 13. N. Cristal, A. Slonim, I. Bar-Ilan, and A. Hart, Plasma fibrinogen levels and the clinical course of acute myocardial infarction, Angiology 34:693 (1983).

14. N. T.J. O'Connor, S. Cederholm-Williams, S. Copper, and L. Cotter, Hypercoagulability and coronary artery disease, Br. Heart J. 52:614 (1984).

15. A. Hamsten, M. Blomback, B. Wiman, J. Svensson, A.Szamosi, U. de Faire, and L. Mettinger, Haemostatic function in myocardial infarction. Br. Heart J. 55:58 (1986).

16. T. W. Meade, R.Chakrabarti, A.P. Haines, W.R.S. North, and Y. Stirling, Characteristics affecting fibrinolytic activity and plasma fibrinogen concentrations. Br.Med.J. 1:153 (1979).

17. A. Hamsten, U. De Faire, L. Iselius, and M. Blomback, Genetic and cultural inheritance of plasma fibrinogen concentration, Lancet II:988 (1987).

18. S. E. Humphries, M.Cook, M. Dubowtiz, Y. Stirling, and Meade TW, Role of genetic variation at the fibrinogen locus in determination of plasma fibrinogen concentration. Lancet I:1452 (1987).

19. I. K. Murray, K. Buetow, D. Chung, and A. Aschbacher, Linkage disequilibrium of RFLP's at the beta fibrinogen (FGB) and gamma fibrinogen (FGG) loci on chromosome 4. Cytogenet, Cell Genet. 40:707 (1985).

20. R. L. Ridolfi, and B.M.Hutchins, The relationship between coronary artery lesions and myocardial infarcts: ulceration of atherosclerotic plaques precipitating coronary thrombosis. Am. Heart J. 93:468 (1977).

21. M. J. Davies, and A. Thomas, Thrombosis and acute coronary-artery lesions in sudden cardiac ischemic death. N. Engl. J. Med. 310:1137 (1984).

22. J. E. Saffitz, R.C. Fredrickson, and W.C. Roberts, Relation of size of transmural acute myocardial infarction impact to mode of death, interval between infarction and death and frequency of coronary arterial thrombus, Am. J. Cardiol. 57:1249 (1986).

23. M. J. Davies, Thrombosis in acute myocardial infarction and sudden death, Cardiovasc. Clin. 18:151 (1987).

24. M. A. De Wood, J. Spores, R. Notske, L.T. Mouser,R. Burroughs, M.S. Golden, and H.T. Lang, Prevalence of total coronary occlusion during the early hours of transmural myocardial infarction, N. Engl. J. Med.303:897 (1980).

25. J. A. Ambrose, S.L. Winters, R.R. Arora, J.I. Haft, J.Goldstein, K.P. Rentrop, R. Gorlin, and V. Fuster, Coronary angiographic morphology in myocardial infarction: a link between the pathogenesis of unstable angina and myocardial infarction, J. Am. Coll. Cardiol. 6:1233 (1985).

26. R. J. Frink, P.A. Rooney, J.O. Trowbridge, and J.P. Rose, Coronary thrombosis and platelet:fibrin microemboli in death associated with acute myocardial infarction, Br. Heart J. 59:196 (1988).

27. E. Falk, Unstable angina pectoris with fatal outcome: dynamic coronary thrombosis leading to infarction and/or sudden death. Autopsy evidence of recurrent mural thrombosis with peripheral embolization culminating in total vascular occlusion, Circulation.71:699 (1985).

28. M. J. Davies, and A.C. Thomas: Plaque fissuring-the cause of acute myocardial infarction, sudden ischaemic death, and crescendo angina, Br.Heart J. 53:363 (1985).

29. V. Fuster, and J.H. Chesebro, Mechanisms of unstable angina, N. Engl. J. Med. 315:1023 (1986).

30. A. H. Kragel, S.G. Reddy, J.T. Wittes, and W.C. Roberts, Morphometric analysis of the composition of atherosclerotic plaques in the four major epicardial coronary arteries in acute myocardial infarcation and in sudden coronary death, Circulation 80:1747 (1989).

31. E. B. Smith, K.M. Alexander, and I.B. Massie, Insoluble "fibrin", soluble fibrinogen and low density lipoprotein. Atherosclerosis 23:19 (1976).

32. E. B. Smith, E.M. Staples, H.S. Dietz, and R.H. Smith, Role of endothelium in sequestration of lipoprotein and fibrinogen in aortic lesions, thrombi, and graft pseudo-intimas. Lancet I:8812 (1979).

33. E. B. Smith, and E.M. Staples, Intimal and medial plasma protein concentrations and endothelial function, Atherosclerosis 41:295 (1982).

34. E. B. Smith, G.A. Keen, A. Grant, and C. Stirk, Fate of fibrinogen in human arterial intima. Arteriosclerosis 10:263 (1990).

35. S. Sadoshima, and E. Tanaka, Fibrinogen and low density lipoprotein in the development of cerebral atherosclerosis, Atherosclerosis 34:93 (1979).

36. Z. D. Grossman, S.F. Rosebrough, J.G. McAfee, G. Subramanian, C.A.Ritter-Hrncirik, L.S. Witanowski, and G. Tillapaugh-Fay, Imaging fresh venous thrombi in the dog with I-131 and In-111 labeled fibrin-specific monoclonal antibody and its F(ab')2 and Fab fragments, Radiographics 7:913 (1987).

37. S. F. Rosebrough, Z.D. Grossman, J.G. McAfee, B.J. Kudryk, G. Subramanian, C.A. Ritter-Hrncirik, L.S. Witanowski, G. Tillapaugh-Fay, Urrutia, and C. Zapf-Longo, Thrombus imaging with indium-111 and iodine-131-labeled fibrin-specific monoclonal antibody and its F(ab')2 and Fab fragments, J. Nucl. Med. 29:1212 (1988).

38. B. J. Kudryk, A. Bini, S.F. Rosebrough, and T.F. Schaible, Fibrinogen-fibrin: preparation and use of monoclonal antibodies as diagnostics, in: Biotechnology of Blood, Stoneham, MA, (ed): Butterworths (1990, in press).

39. K. Y. Hui, E. Haber, and G.R. Matsueda, Monoclonal antibodies to a synthetic fibrin-like peptide bind to human fibrin but not fibrinogen, Science 222:1129 (1983).

40. M. Jung, K. Kletter, R. Dudczak, R. Koppensteiner, E. Minar, and P .Kahls, A. Stumpflen, P. Pokieser, and H. Ehringer, Deep vein thrombosis: Scintigraphic diagnosis with In-111-labeled monoclonal antifibrin antibodies, Radiology 173:469 (1989).

41. L. Lusiani, P. Zanco, A. Visonà, G. Breggion, A. Pagnan, and G. Ferlin, Immunoscintigraphic detection of venous thrombosis of the lower extremities by means of human antifibrin monoclonal antibodies labeled with ^{111}In, Angiology 40:671 (1989).

42. A. Alavi, H. Palevsky, N. Gupta, M.A. Kelley, A.D. Jatlow, J.F.
      Schaible, J. Brown, and H.J. Berger, Radiolabelled
      antifibrin antibody in the detection of venous thrombosis:
      preliminary results, Radiology 175:79 (1990).
43. A. Nordoy, and S.H. Goodnight, Dietary lipids and thrombosis.
      Relationships to atherosclerosis, Arteriosclerosis 10:149
      (1990).
44. M. L. Burr, J.F. Gilbert, R.M. Holloday, P.C. Elwood, A.M.
      Fehily, S. Rogers, P.M. Sweetnam, and N.M. Deadman, Effects
      of changes in fat, fish, and fibre intakes in death and
      myocardial infarction/diet and reinfarction trial (DART),
      Lancet II:757 (1989).
45. J. C. La Rosa, D. Hunninghake, D. Bush, M.H. Criqui, G.S. Getz,
      A.M. Gotto, S.M. Grundy, L. Rakita, R.M. Robertson, M.L.
      Weisfeldt, and J.I. Cleeman, Task Force on Cholesterol
      Issues, American Heart Association: The cholesterol facts. A
      summary of the evidence relating dietary fats, serum
      cholesterol, and coronary heart disease. Circulation 81:1721
      (1990).
46. E. Ernst,T. Weihmayr, V. Schmid, M. Baumann, and A. Matrai,
      Cardiovascular risk factors and hemorheology. Physical
      fitness, stress and obesity, Atherosclerosis 59:263 (1986).

Summary of Discussion following Session 5

Following Assmann's presentation, Bond asked whether the apparent decrease in LDL cholesterol in the patients who had myocardial infarcts wasn't due to the well known phenomenon, i.e., those with the most elevated LDL died at a younger age. Assmann agreed with this interpretation. Then the discussion turned to whether the HDL cholesterol concentrations were definitive in relation to the decreasing LDL concentrations which were being affected by diet or drugs. Assmann preferred the interpretation that the young individuals are not particularly affected by low HDL concentrations whereas the older individuals may show the effects of HDL cholesterol as a much more potent risk factor. Kramsch indicated that he admired the results Assmann had presented. He pointed out that in the CLAS study where the HDL cholesterol values increased by 37% they could not find an independent beneficial effect of raising HDL cholesterol. Assmann responded that the HDL cholesterol determinations in the laboratory are not very sophisticated in that they measure the conglomerate of numerous lipoproteins of very different importance in reverse cholesterol transport. For instance, the HDL particles containing both A-I and A-II do not interact with HDL receptors, yet these contribute a major part of the analysis in the blood of HDL cholesterol. The next step in coronary angiography studies is to ask questions about the Al particle concentrations because this is a much more direct way to measure the effects of the HDL cholesterol family of lipids as affected by the lipase mediated particle availablity. He predicted that the drugs in the future should be monitored for Al particles versus Al-A2 particle concentrations as well as lipoprotein lipase function. Kramsch indicated that in the CLAS study Alupovich of the Oaklahoma Research Foundation did measure the Al particles and could not find any evidence that these reflected protection. However, he did discover that the C3 apolipoprotein had a remarkable deleterious effect on the protection rendered by maximal lowering of the low density lipoproteins. Those patients who showed progression of their lesions in spite of very effective lowering of their low density lipoproteins were those who had definitely elevated apoprotein C3 levels. Assmann responded by indicating that there is some evidence that C3 modulates the uptake of chylomicron remnants and that in certain individuals postprandial plasma contains high concentrations of highly atherogenic particles which are absent from the fasting plasma. Kramsch noted that individuals showing the most high progression were also the ones who in general had higher levels of triglyceride rich lipoproteins. Assmann concluded that the sophisticated regression studies which will be done during the next decade should include many more lipoprotein measurements in addition to LDL cholesterol and HDL cholesterol.

Assmann responded to a question from J. Campbell about reverse cholesterol transport by smooth muscle cells. He noted that these cells also have receptors for HDL but that cells such as the smooth muscle cells which regulate cholesterol primarily via LDL receptors do not depend so much on reverse cholesterol transport as the monocyte-derived macrophages do. He believes that these cells are dependent only to a minor degree upon effective reverse cholesterol transport mechanisms. In fact he believes that macrophages depend upon effective HDL cholesterol removal mechanisms.

Volpe then entered the discussion and asked whether the varied risk conditions indicated by E2/E3 polymorphism as compared to E3/E4 and in relation to the LDL/HDL ratio and the apo B/A_1 ratio were altered by nutritional factors. Assmann responded that the genes and the environmental factors interact with each other so that individuals affected by E3/E4 heterozygosity or E4 homozygosity are at higher risk due to absorbing more cholesterol from their diet. The key therapeutic consideration in these individuals is to limit cholesterol intake. Despite this genetic condition, they are not at increased risk and should not be treated a priori with a reductase inhibitor because cholesterol in the diet is the key problem. Wissler then entered the discussion and pointed out that in the PDAY study, Komatsu and he are finding many more macrophages in the thoracic aorta, where lesions generally do not progress, than in the lower abdominal aortic lesions where we know that in general progression is most likely to occur. Assmann found that observation to be very interesting because in his study of the literature it was quite clear that in homozygous familial hypercholesterolemia the results of the LDL cholesterol receptor deficiency leads to extremely severe lesions in the thoracic aorta and not in the lower abdominal aorta, so that the observations about macrophage reverse cholesterol transport might help to explain this reversal of the usual pattern that is seen when the LDL (apo B) receptors are present and functioning. Wissler pointed out that in his experience the lesions are more prevalent in the thoracic aorta in early adolescence and that it is only with time, usually in the middle or late third decade (i.e., in the middle or late 20s) that the lesions become more severe in the abdominal and in particular in the lower abdominal aorta.

Soma asked how Assmann measured Lp(a) and if Assmann knew of modulation by HDL of lipoprotein lipase. Assmann pointed out that his group measured Lp(a) by immunoelectrophoresis and that there are also very good ELISA techniques available. He went on to point out that the fibrates and nicotinic acid are very useful when the HDL cholesterol is depleted because they affect lipoprotein lipase. Assmann went on to explain that when HDL is lowered the depletion is frequently due to lipoprotein lipase deficiency. What we don't know is the cause of the lipoprotein lipase depletion.

Following Hay's presentation, Paulin opened the discussion by saying that the nuclear medicine scans which Hay had shown may be difficult to interpret and that MRI might be more promising because it will give much better spatial resolution and that even now MRI can be rather simply gated to the cardiac cycle. Liu complimented Hay on his presentation and pointed out that the fact that he sees a lot of kidney activity with technetium suggests that technetium actually is coming off the LDL and being excreted. He suggested that the compound is not stable enough for the label to be maximally effective. He asked Hay whether he had any idea as to how much of the LDL activity can be concentrated in the plaques and how firmly it is anchored there. Hay agreed that the technetium labeled LDL is not as stable as it needs to be and indicated that in the studies he is doing with Harper as much as 50% of the label does come off. He is not convinced that since the activity in the kidney appears to last for a long time, it is merely the result of the technetium being excreted there. Hay went on to point out that a few nanocuries into the plaque are necessary in order to visualize it, and that he believes that the immediate goal in his studies is to compare plaques that have a high uptake with those that have a low uptake and to then be able to figure out how they are different in terms of their cellular composition, metabolism, and so forth.

Heistad asked whether Hay and his coworkers had enough data to talk about LDL uptake in the edges versus the center of the rabbit plaque. Hay indicated that lesions following balloon catheter stripping of endothelium are quite different from the generation of a plaque following cholesterol feeding in the rabbit in the absence of extensive endothelial damage. Hay indicated that in the plaque resulting from sustained hyperlipidemia without mechanical endothelial injury there is uptake throughout the plaque and not just at the edge of the lesion. He suggested that the rabbit plaque is not ideal for these purposes, and that one really needs to study the plaques produced in monkeys where one can simulate the human plaque much more closely. Kramsch asked about the indium-111 and whether one might be able to do high resolution autoradiography at the microscopic level with this isotope, to which Hay replied in the affirmative. Sinzinger then entered the discussion and also complimented Hay on his results. He asked whether the images changed in either the experimental animal or in the individuals that had been studied if one looked at them at one day versus two days versus three days. Hay responded that they did change, but at present they need more cases in order to know exactly what the variations mean. Bonnet indicated that they have been labeling plaques with smooth muscle cell monoclonal antibodies but that they have a large interference by nonspecific uptake by the liver. Hay pointed out that earlier studies indicated that LDL is largely disposed of in the liver and they really expected it to be there in high concentrations.

Following Sinzinger's presentation, Bassenge asked how much of the label is generally taken up by the average lymphocyte. Sinzinger responded that one has to be sure that the lymphocytes are not interfering and generally speaking they only make up about 20% of the cell population being tested. Bassenge pursued his questioning about the methods employed to eliminate lymphocytes from the cells being studied. Sinzinger replied that elutriation was very effective in eliminating the lymphocytes but the main problem in the studies he has been doing are the platelets rather than the lymphocytes.

Gerrity then asked how long it took for the monocyte labeling of the lesions and Sinzinger said that when they did the imaging they always did it after twenty-four hours, although the images he presented of the liver and spleen were done almost immediately after injection; in general, they did not change very much during the period of observation. He went on to indicate that they had studied some intervals before twenty-four hours but that these did not work very well because the noise to background ratio with indium presented problems. At present, his group believes that they will probably have to work with more than one tracer and possibly as many as three, although they do not really know what the third one may be at this point. Gerrity then pointed out that the reason he was interested in the time sequence is that there is very little information concerning how long it takes monocytes to enter the vessel wall and what the residence time is after a cell sticks to endothelium and enters a lesion. He wondered whether this form of technology might help answer these important questions. Sinzinger said that at least in animals one ought to be able to find out how long monocytes take to migrate into experimental lesions and how long their residence times are.

Weber then asked how the low and high shear stresses affected the endothelial cells relative to the sticking of platelets or monocytes or other important elements that might indicate that lesions are likely to develop. Sinzinger said that with platelets it is well known in animal experiments and under in vitro conditions such as perfusion chambers that dynamics play a key role. On the other hand in humans, he has seen little evidence that hemodynamics have very much effect, and that may be principally due to the lack of sensitivity of the methodology being used for in vivo studies in humans.

Bassenge then asked whether he had understood correctly and that there was a steep increase of labeled LDL going to the myocardial area of the patients who had a hypercholesterolemia. He asked whether Sinzinger had any explanation for that phenomenon. <u>Sinzinger</u> said that it is a transient phenomeon and that there is little evidence that it has localized in the myocardiaum for any lengthy period.

<u>Wissler</u> also requested more information from <u>Sinzinger</u> about the localization in animals, and particularly in hypercholesterolemic animals, of labeled LDL, platelets, or labeled monocytes. <u>Sinzinger</u> said that as far as he knew this had not been done with low density lipoproteins, but with platelets it had been done and the main localization appeared to be in the areas where lesions are likely to develop and not in the shear stress areas.

<u>Siegel</u> then asked <u>Sinzinger</u> why there is still localization of platelets in the lesions following treatment with PGI$_2$. <u>Sinzinger</u> responded that he did not mean "adherence," what he really meant was "residence" because it is much more difficult using the current technology to tell very much about "adherence." If you give any antiplatelet agent, then there is not much effect on platelet residence.

<u>Bond</u> indicated that he was impressed with the images which showed the accumulation of LDL within the ventricles and the atria of the heart. He was curious as to why there was not also localization in the lung fields since the label would have to go through the pulmonary circulation as it traveled from the right heart to the left heart. <u>Sinzinger</u> indicated that this phenomenon also occurs if one just injects technetium with no attachment to any pathogenetic agent such as platelets or LDL. He believes that this phenomenon of myocardial localization is a matter of spatial and volume distribution and that similar phenomena have also been observed in the kidney.

The discussion of <u>Bini's</u> presentation then took place and the first questioner was <u>Weber</u>, who asked whether there were more fibrin breakdown products or evidence of fibrinogen localization in the cerebral arteries as compared to other parts of the arterial system. He also asked what criteria <u>Bini</u> was using to define complicated lesions. <u>Bini</u> pointed out that calcification was not the best indicator, although when one sees calcium in the lesions, that almost always means that there will be fibrin localization in the necrotic center. In regard to the cerebral circulation, she pointed out that so far she had not been able to study any of the intracranial arteries inside the calvarium.

<u>Bond</u> asked <u>Bini</u> what she thought of the several reports showing that fibrinogen levels are indeed a risk factor, strongly statistically significant, but that they are very low in relation to asymptomatic carotid artery atherosclerosis diagnosed with high resolution B-mode ultrasound. He noted that these observations fit very well with <u>Bini's</u> findings. He also noted that hemorrhage into the plaque appears to be independent of mural thrombosis and that he believes that rupture of the neovascularization of the plaque by vasa vasorum was probably the major cause of hemorrhage into the atherosclerotic plaque, in contrast to the many studies which indicate that there is almost always a fracture of the fibrous plaque which leads to the appearance of hemorrhage in the plaque if one studies it at some distance from the point of the fracture. <u>Bini</u> indicated that one of the things that the low molecular weight fibrinogen degradation products do is to stimulate release of growth factors from endothelial cells and therefore to stimulate angiogenesis.

<u>Siegel</u> then called on <u>Wissler</u> who asked whether <u>Bini</u> had done any postangioplasty studies. He thought that such studies might be very revealing since somehow restenosis, which occurs so frequently after angioplasty, might to some extent be related to thrombosis following angioplasty. He suggested that it might be worthwhile to study the genetic variations in people undergoing angioplasty which would or would not favor thrombosis. <u>Bini</u> agreed that this area deserved a great deal more study so that we will better understand the role of thrombosis as a complication of ballon angioplasty used for treatment of ischemic heart disease.

Liu opened the general discussion. He described studies which had just been completed in which one long term changes are observed following angioplasty of atherosclerosis in the rabbit. Even after three months there is still evidence of endothelial dysfunction both by staining and by the inability of acetylcholine stimulation to release EF causing vasodilatation. He thinks that perhaps acetylcholine injection and its effect on coronary tone may be helpful in assessing endothelial dysfunction since normal endothelium should support dilatation of the artery while abnormal endothelium would support paradoxical coronary constriction. Gerrity said that one of the messages that he hoped to get across in his presentation is that we don't really have any good methods right now for assessing endothelial function and that these suggestions that are being made during the discussion may be of very great value.

G. Campbell then commented on the production of EDRF by newly proliferated endothelial cells described by Van Houtte et al. He indicated that the Campbells had performed a number of studies in which they had endothelial denuded arteries of experimental animals and then looked at the activity of the resulting neointima. He pointed out that in many cases these vessels were lined by modified smooth muscle cells and not by regenerated endothelium. These smooth muscle cells do not produce EDRF. It is difficult to distinguish areas lined by endothelium from areas lined by smooth muscle cells without the use of Evan's Blue and it is therefore easy to misinterpret results. G. Campbell asked whether Gerrity had observed post-stenotic dilatation in his studies. Gerrity responded that in his experience there was more pre-stenotic dilatation than post-stenotic dilatation but that downstream from the coarctation there is the generation of areas which stain avidly with Evan's blue. G. Campbell mentioned a number of studies in which it appeared that the media within the dilatation showed considerable degeneration and alteration of function of the smooth muscle cells. He wondered, therefore, if the vessel in the areas of dilatation was lined by smooth muscle cells, as well as endothelial cells. He asked Gerrity whether he had stained his preparation with Factor VIII and Gerrity responded that so far he had not tried to definitely identify the endothelial cells using this marker but that in general he believes he would have been able to recognize the difference between endothelial cells and smooth muscle cells in his preparation.

J. Campbell then entered the general discussion and asked Hay if he would like to comment on what Gerrity had just shown in relation to the uptake of labeled LDL in the same place where he has seen Evan's blue staining and whether he, Hay, feels that the labeled uptake he sees in the region of the developing lesions is extracellular or intracellular. She was particularly interested in whether the labeled lipoproteins are being recognized by receptors on smooth muscle cells or macrophages or whether the label that he uses actually interferes with receptor mediated uptake. Hay indicated that he thought his data and Gerrity's data were very much in agreement and that the evidence that they have developed so far indicates that indium-labeled LDL localizes and reacts with receptors just as classically iodinated LDL iodine-tyramine cellobiose labeled LDL does. In fact there is some evidence that indium labeling might represent a modest improvement over iodination methods. They are planning some high resolution radioautography that will give more evidence of where precisely LDL is in the artery wall relative to the cells. G. Campbell then indicated that there may be difficulties in using labelled low density lipoprotein to mark areas of regression or progression of lesions. It may be a good indicator when localized within smooth muscle cells, and could mark areas where modified smooth muscle cells were proliferating. However, if the labelled LDL is sequestered by the extracellular matrix, then staining would not necessarily indicate lesion progression. Therefore, he did not believe that the localization of LDL would give valuable information as to where lesions were developing into more advanced plaques.

Hay indicated that it is his belief that as one looks at morphologic changes in a particular part of the artery wall, differences in residence time of LDL in these areas are going to be very important. As the labeled LDL level in the plasma falls, there should be a remarkable decrease in image activity, but in the lesion-prone areas it would probably decrease much more slowly than in the lesion-resistant areas. He thinks that after several hours the lesion vs. non-lesion discrimination may increase, and that one should be able to identify active lesions between 48 and 96 hours post-injection. These quantitative parameters should emerge as one does more studies correlating the lesion components with retention of the label in various parts of the artery wall.

QUANTITATIVE MICROSCOPIC MORPHOMETRY OF THE

MAJOR COMPONENTS OF THE ATHEROSCLEROTIC PLAQUE

Robert W. Wissler

The University of Chicago
Chicago, IL USA

INTRODUCTION AND OBJECTIVES

This report has three main goals. The first is to summarize the
major components of the advanced atherosclerotic plaque as seen
microscopically and to document some of the relatively simple and
inexpensive quantitative approaches to micromorphometry of these
components. The second is to present a summary of the evidence indicating
that the microarchitecture of the plaque is very important in understanding
the potential clinical effects of a lesion. The third is to summarize a
few of the preliminary quantitative microscopic observations which have
been reported from the study of the pathobiological determinants of
atherosclerosis in youth and to indicate their possible importance in
predicting the potential for progression to clinically important disease.

Atherosclerotic plaques vary widely in their microscopic and chemical
components. Even in their early phases of development the relative
quantities of lipid and the types, location, and number of cells, the
quantities of extra- and intracellular lipid, and the relative quantities
of the connective tissue elements can be very different from one part of
the arterial tree to another, and from one individual to another.
Furthermore, in general, plaques do not constitute any real threat of
clinical complications until they narrow the lumen of the artery
substantially and/or contain a large, soft, grumous, necrotic, cholesterol-
rich core relative to the fibrous cap which overlies this atheroma.
Therefore, it would be highly desirable to be able to measure the major
components of the atherosclerotic plaque during its development in the
living person in order to predict the potential pathological effects which
the plaque might be expected to produce.

THE MICROARCHITECTURE AND MAJOR CLINICAL EFFECTS

As recently summarized (1) there is now substantial agreement about
the major mechanism by which thrombotic occlusion of medium sized muscular
arteries such as the coronary, carotid, or femoral arteries develops.
Fracture of the fibrous cap and the resulting exposure of the underlying
thromboplastic components of the artery wall to the circulating blood
appears to be consistently present when looked for diligently. The major
components of the clinically significant atherosclerotic plaque which are

Atherosclerotic Plaques, Edited by R.W. Wissler *et al.*
Plenum Press, New York, 1991

likely to give the most important information relative to these major effects of atherosclerosis, namely stenosis and thrombosis, are listed in order of priority:

o   The amount of lipid deposited in the artery wall and particularly the amount of extracellular cholesterol and other fatty components,

o   The numbers and kinds of cells in the plaque's cap and shoulders,

o   The quantity, density, and location of the major synthetic products of the smooth muscle cells in the atherosclerotic plaque with special emphasis on collagen,

o   The size and location of the plaque relative to the artery wall including the microarchitecture of the lesion and the extent of involvement of the media of the artery, and

o   The degree of calcification of the plaque components.

Table 1.   The approaches used to quantitate the gross and microscopic effects of regression regimens on the atherosclerotic lesions in nonhuman primates for the nine studies which have been completed and reported.

Exp#	Date of Study	Method of Lesion Quantitation
Rh-18	1968 - 1971	Extent and severity of coronary and aortic disease subjectively graded and tabulated by two observers and then averaged for the aorta and for the coronary arteries (6).
Rh-27	1973 - 1975	Three studies with very similar protocol in which the extent and
Rh-31	1974 - 1976	severity of gross and microscopic aortic atherosclerosis was quantitatively determined by point
Rh-32	1975 - 1979	counting on both coronary and aortic samples by computer assisted micromorphometry of plaque components (8).
Cy-35	1977 - 1979	Four studies in which progression and regression of atherosclerosis
Rh-37	1978 - 1980	were quantitatively evaluated by computer assisted micromorphometry
Rh-38	1979 - 1981	of plaque components at four month intervals using cynomolgus monkeys and
Cy-39	1980 - 1982	rhesus monkeys in which lesion induction was accomplished with peanut oil and cholesterol or with coconut oil and butter plus cholesterol (22).
Rh-39	1980 - 1982	Probucol and cholestyramine were given combined and separately to treat advanced atherosclerosis while atherogenic diet was continued and the results measured by computer assisted micromorphometry and other methods (9).

METHODOLOGY

In the following passage a brief overview of some of the methods
which have been used to measure lesion components in young people will be
described and evaluated. These methods have been successfully used in
experimental animals, especially to evaluate lesions in the nonhuman
primate models of atherosclerosis by measuring the components of developing
or regressing plaques.

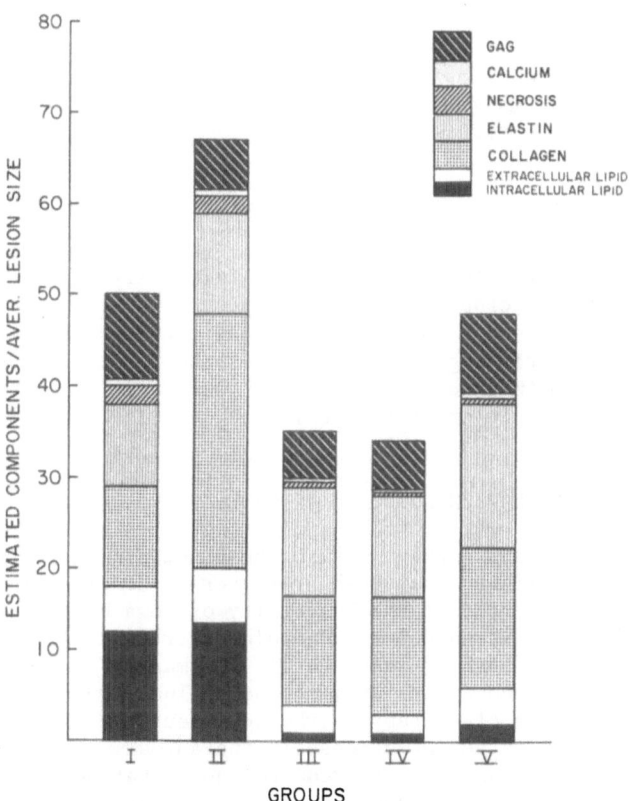

Fig. 1. Bar graph of "point-counting" results of aortic lesion components
from various experimental groups, adjusted to unit area of lesion
size. Data for intra- and extracellular lipid, collagen, elastin,
necrosis, calcification, and glycosaminoglycans are shown. The
total height of each bar represents the average lesion size for
each group. The experimental groups for this particular experiment
are as follows: I and II: Autopsied after one year and two years
of receiving a high fat high cholesterol diet. III:
Arteriosclerotic components of group treated with a low fat,
cholesterol free diet for the second year, IV same as II except
that cholestyramine was added to the diet throughout the second
year and group V was continued on the atherogenic ration with
cholestyramine added for the second year.

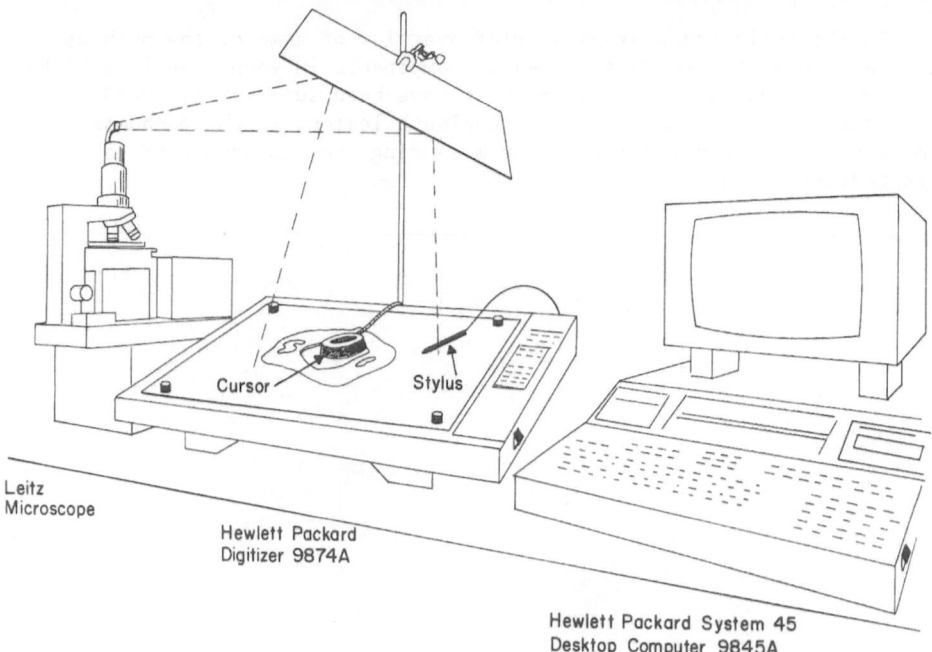

Leitz
Microscope

Hewlett Packard
Digitizer 9874A

Cursor   Stylus

Hewlett Packard System 45
Desktop Computer 9845A

Fig. 2.   Apparatus for performing morphometric analysis: Computer
            linked to microprojection and digitizer system.   The computer
            is programmed so that the basic calculations are performed
            prior to printing the hard copy of the results which are
            presented in a form which can be readily utilized for basic
            tables, graphs or statistical analyses (12).

EXAMPLES FROM EXPERIENCE WITH NONHUMAN PRIMATE ATHEROSCLEROSIS

        Utilizing the rhesus monkey model of human atherosclerosis developed
by Bruce Taylor and colleagues at Rush Presbyterian Hospital in Chicago (2)
and profiting from work done at the University of Iowa by Armstrong,
Connor, and Warner (3), we have performed over thirty studies with this
animal model during the past 25 years (4-5).   In many of these studies
animals with advanced plaque were utilized to evaluate quantitatively the
effects of various types of therapy on the components of the plaques as
well as on the overall extent of disease in the animal.   As is indicated in
Table 1, a number of the experiments required quantitative comparisons of
the plaques and their components before and after therapy both grossly and
microscopically (6-10).
        In the first of these studies we used relatively crude but time-
honored, well defined subjective methods of measuring plaque extent and
severity microscopically by means of a zero to four plus scale and by an
estimated percent of lumen stenosis similar to those used by others.   We
have been able to develop and utilize progressively more sophisticated
methods of lesion and plaque component evaluations as the studies have
continued (11).   Throughout the nine regression studies on which we have
reported results we have consistently utilized a method of standard
sampling so that small standard segments of arteries from the same
anatomical part of the same artery can be compared in different animals
and/or different experimental groups.   As shown in Figure 1, the second
system utilized to measure plaque components microscopically consisted of a
rather slow and tedious point-counting approach which nevertheless yielded
very rewarding and reproducible results (11).

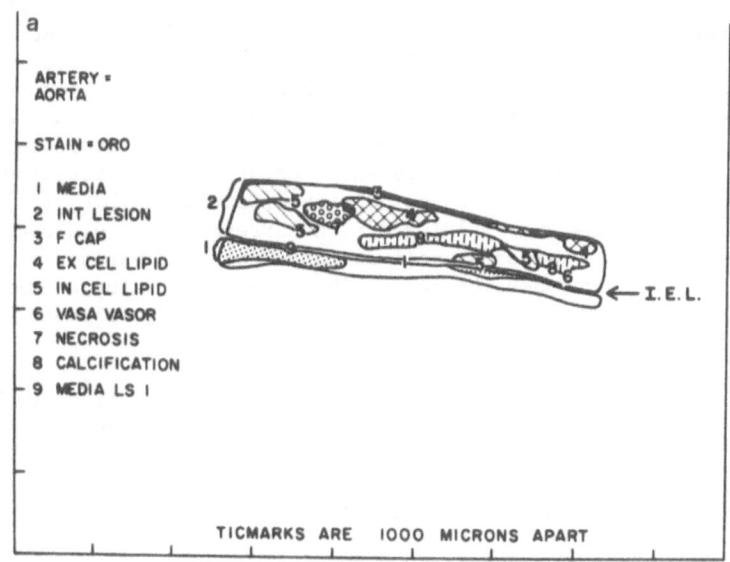

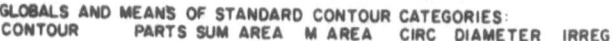

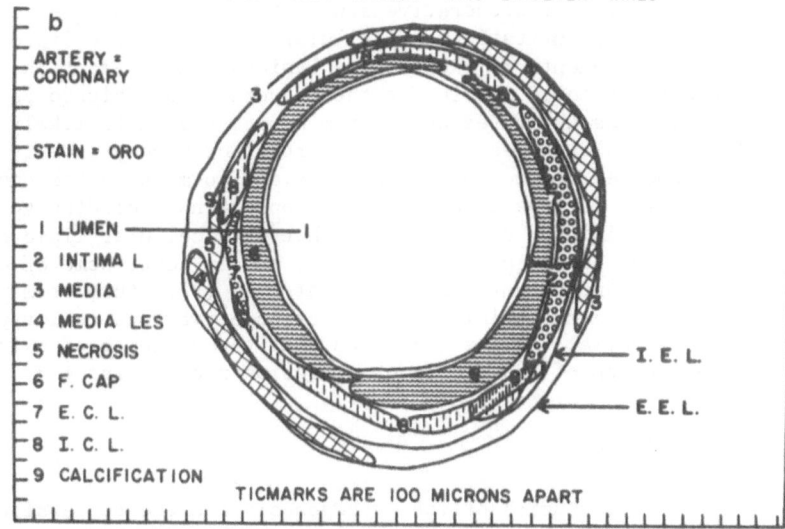

Figure 3a. Advanced rhesus aortic lesion from abdominal sample.
Figure 3b. Advanced coronary artery lesion from cynomolgus monkey showing extensive medial involvement.

Each computer printout shows contour of lesions. The lumen is shown for intact muscular arteries. The whole artery and the media, as well as lesion components, are digitized in order to evaluate lesion size, shape and the area occupied by intra- and extracellular lipid, fibrous caps, necrotic areas, calcification, fibrosis, medial involvement, etc. Special programs have been developed to allow recording and analysis of lines, points, and contours resulting in a hard copy of the total tracing with accompanying calculations. This method is highly reproducible, accurate and time conserving. It convincingly documents the qualitative and quantitative changes which occur during induction and regression of atherosclerosis (12).

This in turn has been replaced by a computer assisted digitizing micromorphometric approach (Figure 2) developed with the help and support of Dr. Gene Bond (12). More recently we are exploring even more sophisticated scanning techniques as applied to histopathology to measure both cell populations and the distribution and extent of various lesion components including intra- and extracellular lipids, apolipoproteins, and the population of cells which have recently undergone proliferation (13) as well as the epitopes of oxidized low density lipoprotein (LDL) (14). These quantitative approaches are yielding a rich harvest of new discoveries about atherosclerotic plaques as well as the effects of various etiologic factors in the development of the plaque utilizing a number of different food fats (15, 16), the regression of the plaques under the influence of various types of therapeutic intervention (8), and the effects of circulating immune complexes on the microarchitecture of the plaque and its potential for effective regression (17). Examples of micromorphometry of cynomologus and rhesus advanced lesions are shown in Figure 3.

STUDIES OF DEVELOPING ATHEROSCLEROSIS IN YOUNG PEOPLE

Many of these methods utilized for quantitative studies of the pathogenesis and the regression of atherosclerosis in the rhesus monkey model are now being applied to the study of the pathobiological determinants of atherosclerosis in youth (PDAY) (18). Even in the early stages of this multi-center cooperative study it is clear that there is much to be learned by quantitating the cellular as well as the lipid and the fiber protein components of these human lesions. At present the preliminary results of these studies at the University of Chicago PDAY Center indicate that as the research program progresses it is likely to be very valuable to be able to measure the proportion of monocyte-derived macrophages as compared to smooth muscle cells and to measure the amount and identify location of several of the apolipoproteins including Lp(a) (18, 19). Other preliminary data indicate that extracellular lipid may be a strong predictor of lesion progression (20), and in fact, some of our preliminary observations strongly support that view (21), that it may be possible to monitor recent cellular proliferation of various cell types in these postmortem arterial samples (13), and that the epitopes of oxidized LDL may be a reflection of factors favoring lesion progression (14).

SUMMARY AND CONCLUSIONS

It is clear from studies of the pathogenesis and the regression of atherosclerosis in rhesus monkeys that there is much to be learned by being able to measure the components of the atherosclerotic lesions during progression and regression. In fact, we have recently reported a number of studies of this disease process at various intervals during progression and regression which definitively document the importance of various nutritional and immunological variables on the lesion components affecting both the histogenesis and the response of lesions to therapy (22). It is now becoming increasingly clear that micromorphometric studies of lesion components in the developing atheromatous disease in young people will also be extremely valuable in evaluating the potential of plaques for progression and ultimately for clinical effects or for regression. These studies, in turn, emphasize how valuable it will be to be able to measure in the living individual the variations in plaque components that occur during the development of atherosclerosis using non-invasive sequential observations of the artery wall with emphasis on what is happening in the lesion in conjunction with what is happening in the lumen of the artery. This conference and this monograph provide evidence that that is an attainable goal and one for which it is highly justifiable to strive.

REFERENCES

1. P. Constantinides. Plaque hemorrhages, their genesis and their role in supra-plaque thrombosis and atherogenesis, in: "Pathobiology of the Human Atherosclerotic Plaque," pp. 393-411. S. Glagov, W.P. Newman III, and S.A. Schaffer, eds., Springer Verlag, New York (1990)
2. C. B. Taylor. Experimentally induced arteriosclerosis in nonhuman primates, in: "Comparative Atherosclerosis," pp. 215-243. J.C. Roberts, Jr. and R. Straus, eds., Harper & Row, New York (1965)
3. M. L. Armstrong, W.E. Connor, and E.D. Warner. Tissue cholesterol in the hypercholesterolemic rhesus monkey, Arch. Pathol. 87:87-92 (1969)
4. R. W. Wissler. Recent progress in studies of experimental primate atherosclerosis, in: "Progress in Biochemical Pharmacology," vol. 4, pp. 378-392. C.J. Miras, A.N. Howard and R. Paoletti, eds., S. Karger, Basel (1968)
5. R. W. Wissler, and D. Vesselinovitch. Atherosclerosis in nonhuman primates, in: "Advances in Veterinary Science and Comparative Medicine," vol. 21, pp. 351-420. C.A. Brandly, C.E. Cornelius, and C.F. Simpson, eds., Academic Press, New York (1977)
6. D. Vesselinovitch, R.W. Wissler, K. Fischer-Dzoga, R. Hughes, and L. DuBien. Regression of atherosclerosis in rabbits. I. Treatment with low fat diet, hyperoxia and hypolipidemic agents. Atherosclerosis 19:259-275 (1974)
7. D. Vesselinovitch, and R.W. Wissler. Requirement for regression studies in animal models, in: "Atherosclerosis IV (Proc. 4th Int. Symp.), pp. 259-263. G. Schettler, Y. Goto, Y. Hata, and G. Klose, eds., Springer-Verlag, Berlin (1977)
8. R. W. Wissler and D. Vesselinovitch. Interaction of therapeutic diets and cholesterol-lowering drugs in regression studies in animals, in: "Regression of Atherosclerotic Lesions," pp. 21-41. M.R. Malinow and V.H. Blaton, eds., Plenum, New York (1984)
9. R. W. Wissler and D. Vesselinovitch. Combined effects of cholestyramine and probucol on regression of atherosclerosis in rhesus monkey aortas. Appl. Pathol. 1:89-96 (1983)
10. R. W. Wissler and D. Vesselinovitch. Can atherosclerotic plaques regress? Anatomic and biochemical evidence from nonhuman animal models. Am. J. Cardiol. 65:33F-40F (1990)
11. D. Vesselinovitch and K. Fischer-Dzoga. Techniques in pathology in atherosclerosis research. Adv. Lipid Res. 18:1-63 (1981)
12. R. W. Wissler, D. Vesselinovitch, T.J. Schaffner, and S. Glagov. Quantitating rhesus monkey atherosclerosis progression and regression with time, in: "Atherosclerosis V (Proc. Vth Int. Symp.)," pp. 757-761. A.M. Gotto, Jr., L.C. Smith, and B. Allen, eds., Springer-Verlag, New York (1980)
13. D. Gordon, M.A. Reidy, E.P. Benditt, and S.M. Schwartz. Cell proliferation in human coronary arteries. Proc. Natl. Acad. Sci. USA 87:4600-4604 (1990)
14. W. Palinski, M. E. Rosenfeld, S. Yla-Herttuala, G. C. Gurtner, S. S. Socher, S. W. Butler, S. Parthasarathy, T. E. Carew, D. Steinberg, and J. L. Witztum. Low density lipoprotein undergoes oxidative modification in vivo. Proc. Natl. Acad. Sci. USA 86:1372-1376 (1989)
15. D. Vesselinovitch, G.S. Getz, R.H. Hughes, and R.W. Wissler. Atherosclerosis in the rhesus monkey fed three food fats. Atherosclerosis 20:303-321 (1974)
16. D. Vesselinovitch, R. W. Wissler, T. J. Schaffner, and J. Borensztajn. The effects of various diets on atherogenesis in rhesus monkeys. Atherosclerosis 35:198-207 (1980)
17. R. W. Wissler, D. Vesselinovitch, H. R. Davis, P. H. Lambert, and M. Bekermeier. A new way to look at atherosclerotic involvement of the artery wall and the functional effects. Ann. N.Y. Acad. Sci. 454:9-22 (1985)

18. R. W. Wissler, D. Vesselinovitch, and A. Komatsu. The contribution of studies of atherosclerotc lesions in young people to future research. Ann. N.Y. Acad. Sci. 598:418-434 (1990)

19. Y. Kusumi and R. W. Wissler. Aortic Lp(a) deposition in young people. FASEB J. 5:A1254 (1991)

20. T. M. A. Bocan, T. A. Schifani, and J. R. Guyton. Ultrastructure of the human aortic fibrolipid lesion: formation of the atherosclerotic lipid-rich core. Am. J. Pathol. 123:413-424 (1986)

21. A. Komatsu, R. W. Wissler, and D. Vesselinovitch. Cell populations in atheromatous lesions in young people. Arteriosclerosis 9:709a (1989)

22. R. W. Wissler and D. Vesselinovitch. The time course of atherosclerotic lesion regression in macaque monkeys, in: "Atherosclerosis and Cardiovascular Disease: 7th International Meeting," pp. 391-400. G.C. Descovitch, A. Gaddi, G.L. Magri, and S. Lenzi, eds., Kluwer Academic Publishers, Dordrecht (1990)

MICROSCOPIC AND ULTRAMICROSCOPIC METHODS OF IDENTIFYING AND QUANTITATING

CELLS IN DIFFUSE FIBROUS ARTERIAL THICKENINGS AND ATHEROMATOUS PLAQUE

G.R. CAMPBELL[1] and J.H. CAMPBELL[2]

[1]Department of Anatomy,
University of Melbourne,
Grattan Street,
Parkville, Victoria, 3052
Australia

[2]Baker Medical Research
Institute,
Commercial Road,
Prahran, Victoria, 3181
Australia

INTRODUCTION

Identification of the cellular components of atheroma and their distribution within lesions can provide important information concerning pathogenesis of the disease. However, to understand how and why the disease develops, these observations cannot be limited to a single time frame but must be extended over the complete period of development, with particular emphasis on changes in childhood and early adults such as in the PDAY studies described by Professor Robert Wissler (this volume).

Just to identify the cellular components through a series of windows of time will still not answer all the questions we need to know. In the last few decades more and more evidence has accumulated which suggests that with time and development of the disease, cells change their behaviour and/or function. Thus to determine the exact role played by a particular cell type in the etiology of atherosclerosis, we may need to follow that cell type throughout development of the lesions and in progressively more complex stages. As well, since changes in the form and function (phenotype) of a specific cell type may be triggered by a different cell population, any alterations to individual cells should be monitored in conjunction with concomitant data on changes to other cell populations. While many of the changes in cell populations can be visualized by a qualitative examination, more subtle changes often require a morphometric approach. These data can then be analysed using the full range of statistical methodologies and definitive conclusions drawn.

This article reviews some of the more recent approaches to identify cellular components of atherosclerosis and their distribution. It also discusses how changes in phenotype of these cells (usually as the result of interactions with other cell types) could lead to errors in assessment.

IDENTIFICATION OF DIFFERENT CELL TYPES IN ATHEROSCLEROSIS

Numerous studies have established, by various criteria, that the major cell types present in or around the established atheromatous plaque are smooth muscle cells, macrophages, endothelial cells, lymphocytes, platelets and foam cells. The methods used for identification usually fall into one of three categories: morphological criteria, histochemical techniques and immunohistochemical techniques.

Atherosclerotic Plaques, Edited by R.W. Wissler *et al.*
Plenum Press, New York, 1991

a)   Morphological criteria

The criteria used to identify the different cell types in atheroma and examples of their usage at the light and electron microscope level have been reviewed extensively (Haust and More, 1963; Ghidoni and O'Neal, 1967; Stary and Strong, 1967; Geer and Haust, 1972; McGill, 1974; Haust, 1983; Ross et al., 1984; Mosse et al., 1985, 1986; Stary, 1989). Recently the dissociation of fixed human specimens into single cells by the use of alcoholic alkaline solutions has allowed quantitation of the cell population of normal and atherosclerotic aortic intima. Apart from the cells of hematogenous origin, the population can be divided into four groups on the basis of shape: elongated bipolar cells, elongated cells with side processes, stellate cells and irregularly shaped cells (Orekhov et al., 1984; Orekhov et al., 1986). These four groups all appear to be differing phenotypes of smooth muscle (Orekhov et al., 1986; Babaev et al., 1988; Chazov et al., 1986).

b)   Histochemical criteria

A variety of histochemical markers such as non-specific esterase (Fritz et al., 1980; Gerrity, 1981) cytochrome oxidase (Adams and Bayliss, 1976), peroxidase (Gerrity, 1981; Schaefer, 1981), acid lipase (Schaefer, 1981; Schaffner et al., 1980; Davis et al., 1984), acid phosphatase (Cookson, 1971), acid esterase (Gaton and Wolman, 1977) and purine nucleoside phosphorylase (Verheyen et al., 1988) have been used to identify monocytes and macrophages and to determine the origin of foam cells, particularly in atherosclerotic lesions of experimental animals. Fc and C3 receptor activity has also been used for the same purpose (Schaffner et al., 1980; Fowler et al., 1979; 1980). Unfortunately all these methods are limited in both sensitivity and specifity.

c)   Immunohistochemical techniques

Polyclonal antibodies against contractile proteins were first used to establish the presence of smooth muscle cells in atheroma (Knieriem et al., 1967; Becker and Murphy, 1969). More recently they have been used to establish the existence of smooth muscle cells of different phenotype in lesions (Campbell and Campbell, 1987; Kocher and Gabbiani, 1988; Benzonana et al., 1988).

Monoclonal antibody technology has provided tools for identification of cell types using antibodies directed against cell lineage-specific antigens. Some of the monoclonal antibodies used to identify smooth muscle cells in atheromatous plaques are summarized in Table 1.

WHAT HAVE THESE TECHNIQUES TOLD US ABOUT THE CELLULAR COMPOSITION OF THE ATHEROMATOUS PLAQUE?

Macrophages

Macrophages often predominate in the cellular area immediately surrounding the necrotic core of the lesion. The majority of foam cells in the core are derived from macrophages. The studies of Jonasson et al. (1986) are summarized in Fig. 1. These agree with other immunocytochemical studies (Aqel et al., 1985; Klurfeld, 1985; Watanabe et al., 1985; Gown et al., 1986; Tsukada et al., 1986; Glukhova et al., 1987; Roessner et al., 1987) and the morphological study of Stary (1989).

Lymphocytes

B cells and different subsets of T cells (Fig. 1) are present in atheromatous plaques (Jonasson et al., 1986; Emeson and Robertson, 1988;

DESIGNATION	ANTIGEN	REFERENCE	
		ORIGIN	USAGE
CGA 7	α and γ SMOOTH MUSCLE ACTIN	Gown et al., 1985	Gown et al., 1986
HHF 35	α MUSCLE ACTIN α and γ SMOOTH MUSCLE ACTIN	Tsukada et al., 1987	Gown et al., 1986 Tsukada et al., 1986
	CHICKEN GIZZARD DESMIN	Kocher et al., 1984	Jonasson et al., 1986
YPC 1/3.12		Finan et al., 1982	Agel et al., 1985
3-Lena	Gangliosides GM3,GD3,GD1a, GT1b	Orekhov et al., 1986	Orekhov et al., 1986
IIG10	Surface antigen	Glukhova et al., 1985	Glukhova et al., 1987
2P1A2		Lamaziere et al., 1988	Lamaziere et al., 1988
1PC1		Lamaziere et al., 1988	Lamaziere et al., 1988
10F3	90 kd SURFACE ANTIGEN	Printseva et al., 1989	Printseva et al., 1989
DEB5	DESMIN	Debus et al., 1984 (Amersham, Boehringer)	Osborn et al., 1987
V9	VIMENTIN	Osborn et al., 1984 (Amersham, Boehringer)	Osborn et al., 1987
Anti-αSM-1	α SMOOTH MUSCLE ACTIN	Skalli et al., 1986	Benzonana et al., 1988

Hansson et al., 1988). T cells are particularly numerous in the fibrous cap where they constitute almost 20% of the cell population.

Smooth Muscle Cells

The predominant cell type in the intimal thickening adjacent to the plaque (~ 87%, Mosse et al., 1985) and in the fibrous cap is the smooth muscle cell (Ross et al., 1984; Gown et al., 1986; Stary, 1989). Smooth muscle cells also contribute to the foam cell population.

Jonasson et al. (1986) quantitated the number of desmin positive staining cells as a measure of smooth muscle. However, they found that while the smooth muscle cells in the adjacent intima were largely desmin negative, those within the lesion were desmin positive. This finding has been more recently substantiated by the study of Osborn et al. (1987). Thus we must be careful to avoid ambiguities when viewing the desmin staining results of Jonasson et al. (1986).

Gown et al. (1986) who were in a better position to quantitate the number of smooth muscle cells present in atherosclerosis with their use of more specific antibodies did not do so because, they considered it a particularly thorny problem. "Owing largely to the great variation from lesion to lesion and from region to region within plaques, quantification schemes are difficult to employ. Nonetheless, because this is a persistent question, it should be pursued by using three-dimensional reconstructive methods coupled with immunocytochemistry performed on serial sections; counting could be performed with a slide-based computer-assisted quantitative microscopy system".

Thus the papers of Jonasson et al. (1986) and Gown et al. (1986) raise two important issues:

1) A quantitative analysis of the number of smooth muscle cells present in different regions of atherosclerotic plaques still needs to be performed, and

2) One must be particularly careful with the criteria chosen to identify smooth muscle, because there is increasing evidence that these cells exist in a variety of different phenotypes in the atherosclerotic lesion.

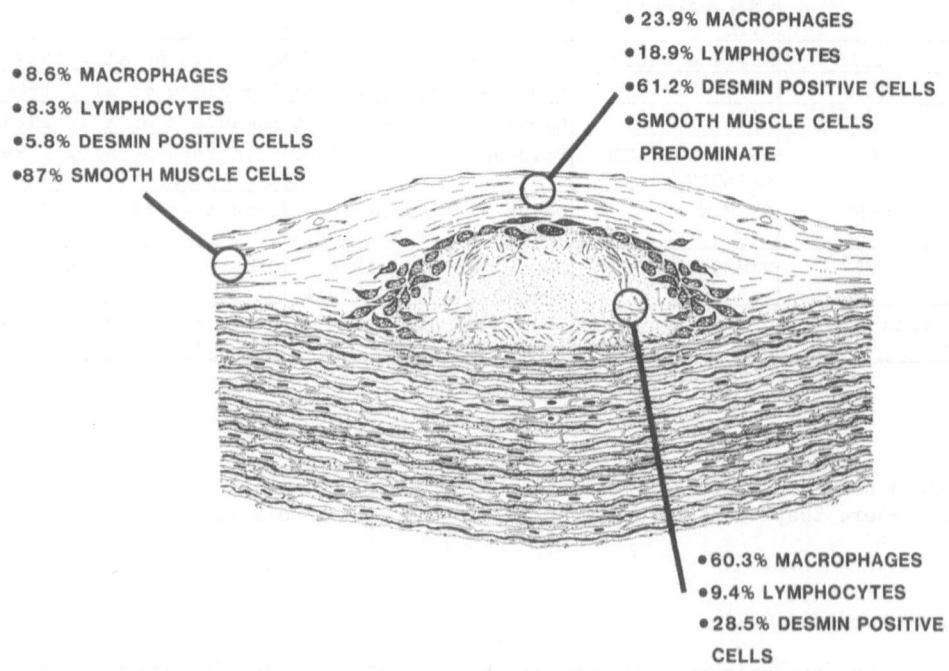

● 23.9% MACROPHAGES
● 18.9% LYMPHOCYTES
● 61.2% DESMIN POSITIVE CELLS
● SMOOTH MUSCLE CELLS PREDOMINATE

● 8.6% MACROPHAGES
● 8.3% LYMPHOCYTES
● 5.8% DESMIN POSITIVE CELLS
● 87% SMOOTH MUSCLE CELLS

● 60.3% MACROPHAGES
● 9.4% LYMPHOCYTES
● 28.5% DESMIN POSITIVE CELLS

Figure 1. Percentage of cells present in the necrotic core of a developed atheromatous plaque, the fibrous cap and an area of intimal thickening adjacent to the lesion. Data from Jonasson et al., 1986, Mosse et al., 1986 and Stary 1989.

PHENOTYPES OF SMOOTH MUSCLE EXPRESSED IN HUMAN ATHEROMA

In 1866 Langhans described a population of subendothelial cells which he regarded as fibroblasts or fibrocytes (Langerhans, 1866). Since then, these cells have been described as modified smooth muscle cells (see Geer and Haust 1972), multifunctional mesenchymal cells (Wissler, 1968), differentiating or dedifferentiating smooth muscle cells (Geer, 1965), intermediate smooth muscle cells (Altschul, 1950) or mesenchymal appearing cells (Wilcox et al., 1988). Ultrastructural studies indicated that these cells are smooth muscle of altered phenotypic state (Geer and Haust, 1972; Haust, 1983; Ross et al., 1984; Mosse et al., 1985, 1986) and in recent years a wide variety of techniques have been used to demonstrate further structural and functional differences between medial smooth muscle cells and those muscle cells in or around human atheromatous lesions (see Table 2).

TABLE 2
SMOOTH MUSCLE PHENOTYPIC CHANGES IN HUMAN ATHEROMA

FEATURE	AORTIC MEDIA	AORTIC INTIMA ASSOCIATED WITH ATHEROMA	REFERENCE
CELL SHAPE	LARGELY SPINDLE OR BIPOLAR	UP TO 40% STELLATE IN SHAPE	Orekhov et al (1984) Orekhov et al (1986)
V$_V$MYO	77%	52%	Mosse et al (1985) Mosse et al (1986)
ACTIN	47.58pg/cell	21.39pg/cell	Kocher & Gabbiani (1986)
α SM-actin	62%	10%	Gabbiani et al (1984).
β actin	31%	70%	
γ actin	−	20%	
MYOSIN CHICKEN GIZZARD	+	FEW	Campbell & Campbell, (1987)
BOVINE AORTIC	+	SOME	Benzonana et al (1988)
HUMAN PLATELET	FEW	+	
TROPOMYOSIN	13.08pg/cell	4.92pg/cell	Kocher & Gabbiani (1986)
INTERMEDIATE FILAMENTS VIMENTIN	6.07pg/cell	16.49pg/cell	Kocher & Gabbiani (1986)
D+V+	MOST	FEW	Osborn et al (1987)
D−V+	FEW	ALMOST ALL	
META-VINCULIN	41%	18%	Glukhova et al (1988)
CALDESMON (150 kDa)	78%	50%	Glukhova et al (1988)
CYCLIC NUCLEOTIDES		CYCLIC GMP ↑ 1.5-2 FOLD CYCLIC AMP ↓ 2.8 FOLD	Tertov et al (1987)
90kD SURFACE ANTIGEN	−	+	Printseva et al (1989)
FIBRONECTIN (extra domain A)	−	+	Glukhova et al (1989)
MHC antigens HLA-DR	−	+ (up to 33% of cells)	Hansson et al (1986)
HLA-DQ	−	+	
DECAY-ACCELERATING FACTOR	−	+	Seifert & Hansson (1989)
PDGF mRNA A-CHAIN	3.9% (of +ve cells)	85.1% (of positive cells)	Wilcox et al (1988)
B-CHAIN	0.9% (of +ve cells)	75% (of positive cells)	

Cell Shape

As mentioned above, alcoholic alkaline dissociation of fixed
specimens has allowed quantitation of the cell population of normal and
atherosclerotic human aortic intima. The four groups of cells isolated

all appear to be differing phenotypes of smooth muscle (Orekhov et al., 1986; Babaev et al., 1988; Chazov et al., 1986). Alterations in the numbers of cells within a particular category appears to vary with specific parameters related to atherosclerosis, for example, there is a high positive correlation between increases in numbers of stellate shaped cells within the intima and increases in intimal thickening, deposition of lipid and collagen synthesis (Orekhov et al., 1986).

Volume Fraction of Myofilaments (Vymyo)

The Vymyo of smooth muscle cells in diffuse intimal thickenings of human carotid artery adjacent to atheromatous plaques differs from that in atherosclerosis-free areas of intima (52% and 75% respectively). Also, adjacent to the plaque the Vymyo of the intimal cells is significantly lower than that of the subjacent medial cells (52% and 77% respectively) (Mosse et al., 1985), but in atherosclerosis-free areas the Vymyo in smooth muscle cells from the diffuse intimal thickening is not significantly different from that of the media (75% and 79% respectively) (Mosse et al., 1986).

Actin

Six actin isoforms have been described in mammals, four of which are specific for muscle tissues, the remaining two, called cytoplasmic (ß and γ), are found in practically all cells. The four muscle actin isoforms: α-skeletal, α-cardiac, α- and γ-smooth muscle are specific for skeletal, cardiac and smooth muscle tissues respectively (Vanderkerkhove and Weber, 1978). Not only is there a dramatic drop in the amount of actin present in smooth muscle cells of human aortic fibrous plaque when compared with cells of the media (21.39 pg/cell plaque-47.58 pg/cell media) (Kocher and Gabbiani, 1986) but there are changes in the actin isoforms expressed by the cells. Smooth muscle of the media contains 62% of its actin in the α-smooth muscle form and 31% in the ß non-muscle form. Smooth muscle of the plaque contains 10% α smooth muscle actin, 70% ß actin and 20% γ actin (Gabbiani et al., 1984).

Myosin

Different myosin isoforms exist in smooth muscle (Beckers-Bleukx and Marechal, 1985; Lema et al., 1986; Rovner et al., 1986; Eddinger and Murphy, 1988; Nagai et al., 1989) and these can be differentially expressed under specific conditions (Larson et al., 1984; Rovner et al., 1986; Gaylinn et al., 1989; Seidel et al., 1989; Kumar et al., 1989). Polyclonal antibodies to human uterine myosin (Babaev et al., 1988), chicken gizzard myosin (Campbell and Campbell, 1987) and bovine aortic myosin (Benzonana et al., 1988) stain smooth muscle cells in the aortic media, but only a limited number of smooth muscle cells in the human fibrous plaque stain with chicken gizzard and bovine aortic myosin, while human uterine myosin antibodies do not stain a population of 5-33% of these smooth muscle cells. Antibodies to human platelet myosin stain a few smooth muscle cells in the media and most of the cells in the fibrous plaque (Benzonana et al., 1988). These data indicate that different isoforms of myosin are expressed in smooth muscle cells of the atheromatous plaque.

Tropomyosin

Smooth muscle cells of the human aortic fibrous plaque contain less than half (4.92 pg/cell cf 13.08 pg/cell) the amount of tropomyosin than cells of the media (Kocher and Gabbiani, 1986).

Intermediate Filaments

The intermediate filaments of vascular smooth muscle cells can contain both desmin and vimentin (i.e. D+ V+), or contain vimentin only (i.e. D-V+). The media of the normal human aorta contains few smooth muscle cells which are D-V+ and most cells are D+V+. However, smooth muscle cells within the fibrous plaque are almost all D-V+, only a few being D+V+ (Osborn et al., 1987). Earlier plaques do contain intimal cells of the D+V+ type. There is almost a three fold increase in the amount of vimentin present in cells of fibrous plaques when compared with cells of the aortic media (Kocher and Gabbiani, 1986).

Vinculin/meta-Vinculin

Vinculin is a 130,000 dalton cytoskeleton protein which is associated with microfilament-membrane association sites, including cell-cell and cell-matrix contact areas (Geiger, 1979). It has been postulated that it plays a key role in microfilament-membrane linkage and has been detected in many different cell types (Evans et al., 1984). Four isoforms have been detected (α, α^1, ß and γ) (Belkin et al., 1988).

Meta-vinculin is a 150,000 dalton cytoskeleton protein which shares similar properties to vinculin (Siliciano and Craig, 1987). It is located in F-actin-membrane attachment sites or dense bodies and appears to be specific for smooth muscle (Glukhova et al., 1986). Meta-vinculin can exist in two isoforms, α, and ß-meta-vinculin (Belkin et al., 1988).

In the media of normal aorta, meta-vinculin accounts for 41% of total immunoreactive vinculin (meta-vinculin + vinculin), while the total fractional meta-vinculin content of normal intima is 39%. However, in the total intima containing atheroma the fractional meta-vinculin content drops to 17.9% (Glukhova et al., 1988).

Caldesmon

Caldesmon is a major component of the contractile apparatus of smooth muscle. It is believed to be involved in a Ca^{++}- dependent control mechanism modulating actin-myosin interaction, and thus contraction (Fürst et al., 1986). It is present on some of the thin filaments of smooth muscle (Lehman et al., 1987) and binds to myosin (Ikebe and Reardon, 1988). Two different species of caldesmon exist, and in vascular smooth muscle a 150kDa form is predominant (Fürst et al., 1986). Platelets, lymphocytes and peritoneal macrophages contain a lower molecular weight form of about 70kDa (Owada et al., 1984).

In normal aortic media 150kDa caldesmon constitutes 79% of the total caldesmon and 75% of the normal total intima. However, in intima containing atheroma 150kDa caldesmon constitutes only 50.5% of the total caldesmon (Glukhova et al., 1988).

Cyclic nucleotides

Cyclic nucleotides play important regulatory roles in mediating hormonal effects on cells. Cyclic AMP content in fatty streaks and atherosclerotic plaques is 3-5 fold lower than uninvolved human aortic intima. Cyclic GMP levels in atherosclerotic plaques are 3-fold higher than in grossly normal areas. Basal activity of adenylate cyclase in fatty streaks and plaques is 2-6 fold lower than in unaffected intima (Tertov et al., 1987a,b).

Fibronectin

Fibronectin is a 500 kDa glycoprotein found in extracellular matrix and blood plasma. It consists of two subunit chains linked by disulphide bonds. Each subunit is divided into domains which specifically bind cell surface components, collagen, heparin, and fibrinogen/fibrin (Hynes, 1985). Thus, by means of these domains, fibronectin mediates the attachment and spreading of cells on a variety of substrata and influences their migration, growth and differentiation (Yamada et al., 1985). The differences in the primary structures of fibronectin synthesized by various cells are due to alternative splicing of the RNA transcript of a single fibronectin gene. Sequence variations in humans can occur at three different points of the fibronectin subunit: extra domain A, extra domain B and IIICS (Hynes, 1985). Extra domain A fibronectin is not present in the tunica media of the human aorta. It is however present in diffuse intimal thickenings and atherosclerotic plaques of human aorta (Glukhova et al., 1989).

Platelet derived growth factor (PDGF)

PDGF can be produced by many cell types, including macrophages, endothelial cells and arterial smooth muscle cells *in vitro* (Ross, 1986). Smooth muscle cells *in situ* within the human aortic media produce little PDGF A or B chain, but do produce significant amounts within atherosclerotic plaques (Wilcox et al., 1988; Barrett and Benditt, 1988).

Decay-Accelerating Factor (DAF)

DAF is a constitutively expressed plasma membrane glycoprotein that inhibits cell surface C3/C5 convertase formation, thus inhibiting complement activation and protecting cells from lysis by the terminal complement components. Seifert and Hansson (1989) have recently shown that while DAF is not present in normal arterial smooth muscle, 20-60% of muscle cells from human atherosclerotic lesions stain positively with monoclonal antibodies to DAF.

Class II antigens of the major histocompatibility complex (MHC)

The class II MHC antigens are involved in communication between cells which regulate the immune response. Functionally, these antigens termed HLA-DR, HLA-DP and HLA-DQ, participate in the presentation of foreign antigens to T-lymphocytes (Hansson et al., 1986), and therefore are normally only expressed by cells of the immune system. However, many smooth muscle cells of the human atherosclerotic plaque express HLA-DR and HLA-DQ (Hansson et al., 1986; Jonasson et al., 1985) demonstrating another form of phenotypic expression of smooth muscle in lesions. It is interesting to note that in fibrous plaques 93% of all HLA-DR positive staining cells are desmin positive (Hansson et al., 1988).

WHAT IS THE SIGNIFICANCE OF THE PHENOTYPICALLY ALTERED SMOOTH MUSCLE CELLS TO THE DEVELOPMENT OF ATHEROSCLEROSIS?

To date few studies have attempted to address this question. Some indication may be derived from studies of smooth muscle in cell culture which under specific conditions expresses similar phenotypes to those observed in human atheroma (see Table 3).

In primary cell culture, aortic medial smooth muscle cells which have been enzyme-dispersed and seeded at densities below confluence undergo similar changes in phenotypic expression to a low V_{vmyo} (similar to those observed in intimal thickenings adjacent to atheromatous lesions - Mosse et al., 1985, 1986). These changes are accompanied by distinct alterations in biology with the cells gaining the ability to proliferate

220

TABLE 3

Some Phenotypic Changes of Smooth Muscle Cells in Culture	
1. Changes in V$_{V}$myo and amount of myofilaments.	Chamley et al 1977, Chamley-Campbell et al 1979, Thyberg et al 1983, Campbell et al 1989
2. Alteration in the pattern of actin isoforms expressed.	Gabbiani et al 1984, Campbell et al 1989, Owens et al 1986, Kocher & Gabbiani 1987
3. Alteration in the pattern of myosin heavy chains present.	Gröschel-Stewart et al 1975, Larson et al 1984, Rovner et al 1986, Kawamoto and Adelstein, 1987, Seidel et al 1989
4. Increase in cells containing vimentin only. Decrease in vimentin plus desmin containing cells.	Skalli et al 1986
5. Decreases in the amounts of γ-vinculin and meta-vinculin expressed.	Herman et al 1987, Belkin et al 1988 Glukhova et al 1986
6. Alteration in the form of caldesmon expressed.	Ueki et al 1987, Glukhova et al 1987 Glukhova et al 1988
7. Different forms of fibronectin expressed.	Glukhova et al 1989
8. Class II MHC gene expresssion stimulated by interferon γ.	Hansson et al 1988, Warner et al 1989
9. PDGF-A and PDGF-B genes expressed.	Sjolünd et al 1988, Majesky et al 1988, Libby et al 1988,Valente et al 1988, Birinyi et al 1989
10. Expression of decay-accelerating factor.	Seifert and Hansson, 1989

logarithmically in response to mitogens (Chamley-Campbell et al., 1979), to migrate readily, to synthesize 25-45 fold the amount of collagen (Ang et al., 1990) and to accumulate 7-fold the amount of lipid upon exposure to ß-VLDL (Campbell et al., 1985), all significant features of atherogenesis.

CONCLUSIONS

To be able to determine the precise role of a specific cell population in atherogenesis (in particular the smooth muscle cell), there is need to quantitate the cells within these lesions during different stages of development. The use of specific monoclonal antibodies with computer-assisted quantitative microscopy appears the simplest approach. However, the fact that smooth muscle cells can dramatically alter their phenotype in response to many, as yet unknown, stimuli coupled with the possibility that there may be distinct subpopulations of smooth muscle in human arteries, makes the choice of monoclonal antibodies to be used for identification purposes critical.

ACKNOWLEDGEMENTS

This study was supported by grants from the National Heart Foundation of Australia and the N.H.&M.R.C. The secretarial assistance of Ann Best is gratefully acknowledged.

REFERENCES

Adams, C. W. & O. B. Bayliss, 1976. Detection of macrophages in atherosclerotic lesions with cytochrome oxidase. Brit. J. Exp. Pathol. 57:30-36.

Altschul, R. 1950. Selected studies on Arteriosclerosis. Charles C. Thomas, Springfield.

Ang, A.H., G. Tachas, J.H. Campbell, J.F. Bateman & G.R. Campbell. 1990. Collagen synthesis by cultured rabbit aortic smooth muscle cells: alteration with phenotype. Biochem. J. 265:461469.

Aqel, N. M., R. Y., Ball, H. Waldmann, & M. J. Mitchinson, 1985. Identification of macrophages and smooth muscle cells in human atherosclerosis using monoclonal antibodies. J. Pathol. 146:197-204.

Babaev, V. R., A. S. Antonov, O. S. Zacharova, Y. A. Romanov, A. V. Krushinsky, V. P. Tsibulsky, V.P. Shirinsky, V. S. Repin & V.N. Smirnov. 1988. Identification of intimal subendothelial cells from human aorta in primary culture. Atherosclerosis 71:45-56.

Barrett, T. B. & E. P. Benditt. 1988. Platelet-derived growth factor gene expression in human atherosclerotic plaques and normal artery wall. Proc. Natl. Acad. Sci. USA 85:2810-2814.

Becker, C. G. & G. E. Murphy. 1969. Demonstration of contractile protein in endothelium and cells of heart valves, endocardium, intima, arteriosclerotic plaques, and Aschoff bodies of rheumatic heart disease. Amer. J. Pathol. 55:1-37.

Beckers-Bleukx, G. & G. Maréchal. 1985. Detection and distribution of myosin isozymes in vertebrate smooth muscle. Eur. J. Biochem. 152:207-211.

Belkin, A. M., O.I. Ornatsky, A. E. Kabakov, M. A. Glukhova & V. E. Koteliansky. 1988. Diversity of Vinculin/meta-Vinculin in human tissues and cultivated cells. Expression of muscle specific variants of vinculin in human aorta smooth muscle cells. J. Biol. Chem. 263:6631-6635.

Benzonana, G., O. Skalli, & G. Gabbiani. 1988. Correlation between the distribution of smooth muscle or non-muscle myosins and α-smooth muscle actin in normal and pathological soft tissues. Cell Motil. Cytoskeleton. 11:260-274.

Birinyi, L. K., S. J. C. Warner, R. N. Salomon, A. D. Callow & P. Libby. 1989. Observations on human smooth muscle cell cultures from hyperplastic lesions of prosthetic bypass grafts - Production of platelet-derived growth factor like mitogen and expression of a gene for a platelet-derived growth factor receptor - A preliminary study. J. Vasc. Surg. 10:157-165.

Campbell G. R. & J. H. Campbell. 1987. Smooth muscle cells. In: "Atherosclerosis: Biology and Clinical Science." A.G. Olsson. ed: 105-115. Churchill Livingstone Inc., New York.

Campbell, J. H., M. F. Reardon, G. R. Campbell & P. J. Nestel. 1985. Metabolism of atherogenic lipoproteins by smooth muscle cells of different phenotype in culture. Arteriosclerosis. 5:318-328.

Campbell, J. H., O. Kocher, O. Skalli, G. Gabbiani & G. R. Campbell. 1989. Cytodifferentiation and expression of alpha-smooth muscle actin mRNA and protein during primary culture of aortic smooth muscle cells. Correlation with cell density and proliferative state. Arteriosclerosis. 9:633-643.

Chamley, J. H., G. R. Campbell, J. D. McConnell & U. Gröschel-Stewart. 1977. Comparison of vascular smooth muscle cells from adult human, monkey and rabbit in primary culture and in subculture. Cell Tiss. Res. 177:503-522.

Chamley-Campbell, J. H., G. R. Campbell and R. Ross, 1979. The smooth muscle cell in culture. Physiol. Rev. 59:1-61.

Chazov, E. I., V.S. Repin, A. N. Orekhov, A. S. Antonov, S. N. Preobrazhensky, E. L. Soboleva & V. N. Smirnov. 1986.

Cookson, F. B. (1971) The origin of foam cells in atherosclerosis. <u>Brit. J. Exp. Pathol.</u> 52:62-69.

Davis, H. R., D. Vesselinovitch, & R. W. Wissler, 1984. Histochemical detection and quantification of macrophages in rhesus and cynomolgus monkey atherosclerotic lesions. <u>J. Histochem. Cytochem.</u> 32:1319-1327.

Debus, E., K. Weber, & M. Osborn, 1983. Monoclonal antibodies to desmin, the muscle-specific intermediate filament protein. <u>EMBO J.</u> 2:2305-2312.

Eddinger, T. J. & R. A. Murphy. 1988. Two smooth muscle myosin heavy chains differ in their light meromyosin fragment. <u>Biochem.</u> 27:3807-3811.

Emeson, E. E. & A. L. Robertson, Jr. 1988. T lymphocytes in aortic and coronary intimas. Their potential role in atherogenesis. <u>Amer. J. Pathol.</u> 130:369-376.

Evans, R. R., R. M. Robson & M. H. Stromer. 1984. Properties of smooth muscle vinculin. <u>J. Biol. Chem.</u> 259:3916-3924.

Finan, P. J., R. M. Grant, C. De Mattos, F. Takei, P. J. Berry, E. S. Lennox, N. M. Blechan, 1982. Immunohistochemical techniques in the early screening of monoclonal antibodies to human colonic epithelium. <u>Brit. J. Cancer</u> 46:9-17.

Fowler, S., P. A. Berberian, S. Goldfischer & H. Wolinksy. 1980. Characterization of cell populations isolated from aortas of rhesus monkeys with experimental atherosclerosis. <u>Circ. Res.</u> 46:520-530.

Fowler, S., H. Shio, & N.J. Haley. 1979. Characterization of lipid-laden aortic cells from cholesterol-fed rabbits: IV Investigation of macrophage-like properties of aortic cell populations. <u>Lab. Invest.</u> 41:372-378.

Fritz, K. E., Daoud, A. S., & J. Jarmolych. 1980. Non-specific esterase activity during regression of swine aortic atherosclerosis. <u>Artery.</u> 7:352-366.

Fürst, D. O., R. A. Cross, J. DeMay and J. V. Small. 1986. Caldesmon is an elongated, flexible molecule localized in the actomyosin domain of smooth muscle. <u>EMBO J.</u> 5:251-257.

Gabbiani, G., O. Kocher, W. S. Bloom, J. Vandekerckhove & K. Weber. 1984. Actin expression in smooth muscle cells of rat aortic intimal thickening, human atheromatous plaque and cultured rat aortic media. <u>J. Clin. Invest.</u> 73:148-152.

Gaton, E. & M. Wolman. 1977. The role of smooth muscle cells and hematogenous macrophages in atheroma. <u>J. Pathol.</u> 123:123-128.

Gaylinn, B.D., T.J. Eddinger, P.A. Martino, P.L. Monical, D.F. Hunt, & R.A. Murphy. 1989. Expression of nonmuscle myosin heavy and light chains in smooth muscle. <u>Amer. J. Physiol.</u> 257:C997-C1004.

Geer, J. C. 1965. Fine structure of human aortic intimal thickening and fatty streaks <u>Lab. Invest.</u> 14:1764-1783.

Geer, J. C. & Haust, M. D. 1972. Smooth muscle cells in atherosclerosis: <u>In</u> Monographs on Atherosclerosis Vol. 2. Ed. Pollack, O. J., Simms, H. S. & Kirk, S. E., Basel, S. Karger A.G.

Geiger, B. 1979. A 130K protein from chicken gizzard: its localization at the termini of microfilament bundles in cultured chicken cells. <u>Cell</u> 18:193-205.

Gerrity, R. G. 1981. The role of the monocyte in atherogenesis: I. Transition of blood-borne monocytes into foam cells in fatty lesions. <u>Amer. J. Pathol.</u> 103:181-190.

Ghidoni, J. J. & R. M. O'Neal. 1967. Recent advances in molecular pathology: A review: Ultrastructure of human atheroma. <u>Exp. Mol. Pathol.</u> 7:378-406.

Glukhova, M. A., M. G. Frid, B. V. Shekhonin, T. D. Vasilevskaya, J. Grünwald, M. Saginati & V. E. Koteliansky. 1989. Expression of extra domain A fibronectin sequence in vascular smooth muscle cells is phenotype dependent. <u>J. Cell Biol.</u> 109:357-366.

Glukhova, M. A., A. E. Kabakov, A. M. Belkin, M. G. Frid, O. I. Ornatsky, N. I. Zhidkova & V.E. Koteliansky. 1986. Meta-vinculin distribution in adult human tissues and cultured cells. FEBS Lett. 207:139-141.

Glukhova, M. A., A. E. Kabakov, M. G. Frid, O. I. Ornatsky, A. M. Belkin, D. N. Mukhin, A. N. Orekhov, V. E. Koteliansky & V. N. Smirnov. 1988. Modulation of human aorta smooth muscle cell phenotype: A study of muscle-specific variants of vinculin, caldesmon, and actin expression. Proc. Natl. Acad. Sci. USA, 85:9542-9546.

Glukhova, M. A., A. E. Kabakov, O. I. Ornatsky, M. G. Frid, & V. N. Smirnov. 1985. Monoclonal antibodies that distinguish between human aorta smooth muscle and endothelial cells. FEBS Lett. 189:291-295.

Glukhova, M. A., A. E. Kabakov, O. I. Ornatsky, T. D. Vasilevskaya, V. E. Koteliansky & V. N. Smirnov. 1987. Immunoreactive forms of caldesmon in cultivated human vascular smooth muscle cells. FEBS Lett. 218:292-294.

Glukhova, M. A., O. I. Ornatsky, M. G. Frid, A. E. Kabakov, R. R. Adany, L. Muszbek, & V. N. Smirnov. 1987. Identification of smooth muscle-derived foam cells in the atherosclerotic plaque of human aorta with monoclonal antibody IIG10. Tissue and Cell 19:657-663.

Gown, A. M., T. Tsukada & R. Ross. 1986. Human atherosclerosis. II. Immunocytochemical analysis of the cellular composition of human atherosclerotic lesions. Amer. J. Pathol. 125:191-207.

Gown, A. M., A. M. Vogel, D. Gordon, & P. L. Lu. 1985. A smooth muscle-specific antibody recognizes smooth muscle actin isozymes. J. Cell Biol. 100:807-813.

Gröschel-Stewart, U., J. H. Chamley, J. D. McConnell & G. Burnstock. 1975. Comparison of the reaction of cultured smooth and cardiac muscle cells and fibroblasts to specific antibodies to myosin. Histochem. 43:215-224.

Hansson, G. K., L. Jonasson, J. Holm & L. Claesson-Welsh. 1986. Class II MHC antigen expression in the atherosclerotic plaque: smooth muscle cells express HLA-DR, HLA-DQ and the invariant gamma chain. Clin. Exp. Immunol. 64:261-2 68.

Hansson, G. K., L. Jonasson, J. Holm, M. M. Clowes & A. W. Clowes. 1988. γ-Interferon regulates vascular smooth muscle proliferation and Ia antigen expression in vitro and in vivo. Circ. Res. 63:712-719.

Hansson, G. K., L. Jonasson, B. Lojsthed, S. Stemme, O. Kocher, & G. Gabbiani. 1988. Localization of T lymphocytes and macrophages in fibrous and complicated human atherosclerotic plaques. Atherosclerosis. 72:135-141.

Haust, M. D. 1983. Atherosclerotic lesions and sequelae. In: Cardiovascular Pathology, Silver, M. D. ed., New York, Churchill Livingstone, pp. 191-315.

Haust, M. D. and More, R. H. 1963. Significance of the smooth muscle cell in atherogenesis. In: Evolution of the atherosclerotic Plaque. Jones, R. J. ed., Chicago, University of Chicago Press. pp. 51-64.

Herman, B., M. W. Roe, C. Harris, B. Wray & D. Clemmons. 1987. Platelet-derived growth factor-induced alterations in vinculin distribution in porcine vascular smooth muscle cells. Cell Motil. Cytoskel. 8:91-105.

Hynes, R. O. 1985. Molecular biology of fibronectin. Annu. Rev. Cell Biol. 1:67-90.

Ikebe, M. & S. Reardon. 1988. Binding of caldesmon to smooth muscle myosin. J. Biol. Chem. 263:3055-3058.

Jonasson, L., J. Holm, O. Skalli, G. Bondjers, & G. K. Hansson. 1986. Regional accumulations of T cells, macrophages, and smooth muscle cells in the human atherosclerotic plaque. Arteriosclerosis 6:131-138.

Jonasson, L., J. Holm, O. Skalli, G. Gabbiani & G. K. Hansson. 1985. Expression of class II transplantation antigen on vascular smooth muscle cells in human atherosclerosis. J. Clin. Invest. 76:125-131.

Kawamoto, S. & R. S. Adelstein. 1987. Characterization of myosin heavy chains in cultured aorta smooth muscle cells. A comparative study. J. Biol. Chem. 262:7282-7288.

Klurfeld, D. M. 1985. Identification of foam cells in human atherosclerotic lesions as macrophages using monoclonal antibodies. Arch. Pathol. Lab. Med. 109:445-449.

Knieriem, H. J., V. C. Y. Kao, R. W. Wissler. 1967. Actomyosin and myosin and the deposition of lipids and serum lipoproteins. Arch. Pathol. Lab. Med. 84:118-129.

Kocher, O. & G. Gabbiani. 1986. Cytoskeletal features of normal and atheromatous human arterial smooth muscle cells. Human Pathol. 17:875-880.

Kocher, O. & G. Gabbiani. 1987. Analysis of α-smooth-muscle actin mRNA expression in rat aortic smooth-muscle cells using a specific cDNA probe. Differentiation. 34:201-209.

Kocher, O. & G. Gabbiani. 1988. Cytoskeletal features of normal and atheromatous human arterial smooth muscle cells. Human Pathol. 17:875-880.

Kocher, O., O. Skalli, W. S. Bloom & G. Gabbiani. 1984. Cytoskeleton of rat aortic smooth muscle cells. Normal conditions and experimental intimal thickening. Lab. Invest. 50:645-651.

Kumar, C. C., S. R. Mohan, P. J. Zavodny, S. K. Narula and P. J. Leibowitz. 1989. Characterization and differential expression of human vascular smooth muscle myosin light chain 2 isoform in non-muscle cells. Biochem. 28:4027-4035.

Lamaziere, J-M. D., A. Desmouliere, M. Pascal & J. Larrue. 1988. Detection of atherosclerotic plaque with two monoclonal antibodies. 2P1A2 monoclonal antibody is specific for smooth muscle cells in atherosclerotic plaque. Atherosclerosis 74:115-126.

Langhans, Th. 1866. Beiträge zur normalen und pathologischen Anatomie der Arterien. Arch. Pathol. Anat. Physiol. Klin. Med. 36:187-226.

Larson, D. M., K. Fujiwara, R. W. Alexander & M. A. Gimbrone Jr. 1984. Myosin in cultured vascular smooth muscle cells: Immunofluorescence and immunochemical studies of alterations in antigenic expression. J. Cell Biol. 99:1582-1589.

Lehman, W., A. Sheldon and W. Madonia. 1987. Diversity in smooth muscle filament composition. Biochem. Biophys. Acta. 914:35-39.

Lema, M. J., E. D. Pagani, R. Shemin & F. J. Julian. 1986. Myosin isozymes in rabbit and human smooth muscles. Circ. Res. 59:115-123.

Libby, P., S. J. C. Warner, R. N. Salomon & L. K. Birinyi. 1988. Production of platelet-derived growth factor-like mitogen by smooth-muscle cells from human atheroma. New Engl. J. Med. 318:1493-1498.

Majesky, M., E. P. Benditt & S. M. Schwartz. 1988. Expression and developmental control of platelet-derived growth factor A-chain and B-chain/Sis genes in rat aortic smooth muscle cells. Proc. Natl. Acad. Sci. USA. 85:1524-1528.

McGill, H. C. Jr. 1974. The lesion In: Atherosclerosis III. Shettler, G. & Weizel, A., eds. Berlin, Springer-Verlag, pp. 27-38.

Mosse, P. R. L., G. R. Campbell & J. H. Campbell. 1986. Smooth muscle phenotypic expression in human carotid arteries. II. Atherosclerosis-free diffuse intimal thickenings compared with the media. Arteriosclerosis, 6:664-670.

Mosse, P. R. L., G. R. Campbell, Z-L. Wang & J. H. Campbell. 1985. Smooth muscle phenotypic expression in human carotid arteries. I. Comparison of cells from diffuse intimal thickenings adjacent to atheromatous plaques with those of the media, Lab. Invest. 53:556-562.

Nagai, R., M. Kuro-o, P. Babij & M. Periasamy. 1989. Identification of two types of smooth muscle myosin heavy chain isoforms by cDNA cloning and immunoblot analysis. J. Biol. Chem. 264:9734-9737.

Orekhov, A. N., E. R. Andreeva, A. V. Krushinsky, I. D. Novikov, V. V. Tertov, G. V. Nestaiko, Kh. A. Khashimov, V. S. Repin, & V. N.

Smirnov. 1986. Intimal cells and atherosclerosis. Relationship between the number of intimal cells and major manifestations of atherosclerosis in the human aorta. Amer. J. Pathol. 125:402-415.

Orekhov, A. N., G. F. Kalantarov, E. R. Andreeva, N. W. Prokazova, I. N. Trakht, L. D. Bergelson, & V. N. Smirnov. 1986. Monoclonal antibody reveals heterogeneity in human aortic intima: Detection of a ganglioside antigen associated with a subpopulation of intimal cells. Amer. J. Pathol. 122:370-385.

Orekhov, A. M., I. I. Karpova, V. V. Tertov, S. A. Rudchenko, E. R. Andreeva, A. V. Krushinsky & V. N. Smirnov. 1984. Cellular composition of atherosclerotic and uninvolved human aortic subendothelial intima. Light microscopic study of dissociated aortic cells. Amer. J. Pathol., 115:17-24.

Osborn, M., Caselitz, K., Püschel & K. Weber. 1987. Intermediate filament expression in human vascular smooth muscle and in arteriosclerotic plaques, Virchows Arch. A., 411:449-458.

Osborn, M., E. Debus & K. Weber. 1984. Monoclonal antibodies specific for vimentin. Eur. J. Cell Biol. 34:137-143.

Owada, M. K., A. Hakura, K. Iida, I. Yahara, K. Sobue & S. Kakiuchi. 1984. Occurrence of caldesmon (a calmodulin-binding protein) in cultured cells: Comparison of normal and transformed cells. Proc. Natl. Acad. Sci. USA 81:3133-3137.

Owens, G. K., A. Loeb, D. Gordon, & M. M. Thompson. 1986. Expression of smooth muscle - specific α-isoactin in cultured vascular smooth muscle cells: Relationship between growth and cytodifferentiation. J. Cell Biol. 102:343-352.

Printseva, O. Ju., M. M. Peclo, A. V. Tjurmin, A. I. Faerman, S. M. Danilov, V. S. Repin & V. N. Smirnov. 1989. A 90-Kd surface antigen from a subpopulation of smooth muscle cells from human atherosclerotic lesions. Amer. J. Pathol. 134:305-313.

Roessner, A., A. Herrera, H. J. Honing, E. Vollmer, G. Zwaldo, R. Schurmann, C. Sorg & E. Grundmann. 1987. Identification of macrophages and smooth muscle cells with monoclonal antibodies in the human atherosclerotic plaque. Virchows Archiv. A. 412:169-174.

Ross, R. 1986. The pathogenesis of atherosclerosis - an update. N. Engl. J. Med. 314:488-500.

Ross R., T. N. Wight, E. Strandness, & B. Thiele. 1984. Human atherosclerosis. I. Cell constitution and characteristics of advanced lesions of the superficial femoral artery. Amer. J. Pathol. 114:79-93.

Rovner, A. S., R. A. Murphy and G. K. Owens. 1986. Expression of smooth muscle and non-muscle myosin heavy chains in cultured vascular smooth muscle cells. J. Biol. Chem. 261:14740-14745.

Rovner, A. S., M. M. Thompson & R. A. Murphy. 1986. Two different heavy chains are found in smooth muscle myosin. Amer. J. Physiol. 250:C861-C870.

Schaefer, H. E. 1981. The role of macrophages in atherosclerosis, In: Hematology and Blood Transfusion Vol. 27. Schmalzl, F., Hukn, D. and Schaefer, H. E. eds., New York. Springer-Verlag pp. 137-142.

Schaffner, T., K. Taylor, E.J. Bartucci, K. Fischer-Dzoga, J.H. Beeson, S. Glagov & R.W. Wissler. 1980. Arterial foam cells with distinctive immunomorphologic and histochemical features of macrophages. Amer. J. Pathol. 100:57-80.

Seidel, C.L., C.L. Wallace, D.K. Dennison & J.C. Allen. 1989. Vascular myosin expression during cytokinesis, attachment, and hypertrophy. Amer. J. Physiol. 256:C793-C798.

Seifert, R. & G.K. Hansson. 1989. Decay-accelerating factor is expressed on vascular smooth muscle cells in human atherosclerotic lesions. J. Clin. Invest. 84:597-604.

Siliciano, J. D. & S. W. Craig. 1987. Properties of smooth muscle meta-vinculin. J. Cell Biol. 104:473-482.

Sjolünd, M., U. Hedin, T. Sejersen, C-H. Heldin & J. Thyberg. 1988. Arterial smooth muscle cells express platelet-derived growth factor

(PDGF) A chain mRNA, secrete a PDGF-like mitogen, and bind exogenous PDGF in a phenotype- and growth state-dependent manner. J. Cell Biol. 106:403-413.

Skalli, O., W. S. Bloom, P. Ropraz, B. Azzarone & G. Gabbiani. 1986. Cytoskeletal remodelling of rat aortic smooth muscle cells in vitro: relationships to culture conditions and analogies to in vivo situations. J. Submicrosc. Cytol. 18:481-493.

Skalli, O., P. Ropraz, A. Trzeciak, G. Benzonana, D. Gillessen & G. Gabbiani. 1986. A monoclonal antibody against α-smooth muscle actin: A new probe for smooth muscle differentiation. J. Cell Biol. 103:2787-2796.

Stary, H. C. 1989. Evolution and progression of atherosclerotic lesions in coronary arteries of children and young adults. Arteriosclerosis 9:I19-I32.

Stary, H. C. & J. P. Strong. 1967. The fine structure of non-atherosclerotic intimal thickening, of developing, and of regressing atherosclerotic lesions at the bifurcation of left coronary artery. Adv. Exp. Med. Biol. 1:89-108.

Tertov, V. V., A. N. Orekhov, G. Yu. Grigorian, G. S. Kurennaya, S. A. Kudryashov, V. A. Tkachuk & V. N. Smirnov. 1987. Disorders in the system of cyclic nucleotides in atherosclerosis: cyclic AMP and cyclic GMP content and activity of related enzymes in human aorta. Tissue and Cell. 19:21-28.

Tertov, V. V., A. N. Orekhov, S. A. Kudryashov, A. L. Klibanov, N. N. Ivanov, V. P. Torchilin & V. N. Smirnov. 1987. Cyclic nucleotides and atherosclerosis: Studies in primary culture of human aortic cells. Exp. Mol. Pathol. 47:377-389.

Thyberg, J., L. Palmberg, J. Nilsson, T. Ksiazek & M. Sjölund. 1983. Phenotype modulation in primary cultures of arterial smooth muscle cells. On the role of platelet derived growth factor. Differentation. 25:156-167.

Tsukada, T., M. Rosenfeld, R. Ross & A. M. Gown. 1986. Immunocytochemical analysis of cellular components in atherosclerotic lesions. Use of monoclonal antibodies with the Watanabe and fat-fed rabbit. Arteriosclerosis 6:601-613.

Tsukada, T., D. Tippeus, D. Gordon, R. Ross & A. Gown. 1987. HHF35, a muscle-specific monoclonal antibody. I. Immunocytochemical and biochemical characterization. Amer. J. Pathol. 126:51-60.

Ueki, N., K. Sobue, K. Kanda, T. Hada & K. Higashino. 1987. Expression of high and low molecular weight caldesmons during phenotypic modulation of smooth muscle cells. Proc. Natl. Acad. Sci. USA. 84:9049-9053.

Valente, A. J., R. Delgado, J. D. Metter, C. Cho, E.A. Sprague, C. J. Schwartz & D. T. Graves. 1988. Cultured primate aortic smooth muscle cells express both the PDGF-A and PDGF-B genes but do not secrete mitogenic activity or dimeric platelet-derived growth factor protein. J. Cell Physiol. 136:479-485.

Vandekerkhove, J. & K. Weber. 1978. At least six different actins are expressed in higher mammal: An analysis based on the amino acid sequence of the amino-terminal tryptic peptide. J. Mol. Biol. 126:783-802.

Verheyen, A. K., E. M. Vlaminckx, F. M. Lauwers, M. L. Saint-Guillain & M. J. Borgers. 1988. Identification of macrophages in intimal thickening of rat carotid arteries by cytochemical localization of purine nucleoside phosphorylase. Arteriosclerosis. 8:759-767.

Warner, S. J. C., G. B. Friedman & P. Libby. 1989. Regulation of major histocompatibility gene expression in human vascular smooth muscle cells. Arteriosclerosis 9:279-288.

Watanabe, T., M. Hirata, Y. Yoshikawa, Y. Nagafuchi, H. Toyoshima & T. Watanabe. 1985. Role of macrophages in atherosclerosis. Sequential observations of cholesterol-induced rabbit aortic lesion by the immunoperoxidase technique using monoclonal antimacrophage antibody. Lab. Invest. 53:80-90.

Wilcox, J. N., K. M. Smith, L. T. Williams, S.M. Schwartz & D. Gordon. 1988. Platelet-derived growth factor mRNA detected in human atherosclerotic plaques by in situ hybridisation. *J. Clin. Invest.* 82:1134-1143.

Wissler, R.W. 1968. The arterial medial cells, smooth muscle or multifunctional mesenchyme? *J. Arteriosclerosis.* 8:201-213.

Yamada, K.M., S.K. Akiyama, T. Hasegawa, E. Hasegawa, M.J. Humphries, D.W. Kennedy, K. Nagara, H. Urushihara, K. Olden & W-T. Chen. 1985. Recent advances in research on fibronectin and other cell attachment proteins. *J. Cell Biochem.* 28:79-97.

THE QUANTITIVE ANALYSIS OF CELL MOTILITY IN CULTURES OF SMOOTH MUSCLE CELLS, ENDOTHELIAL CELLS AND MONOCYTE/MACROPHAGES IN INDIVIDUAL AND CO-CULTURE SYSTEMS, USING TIME-LAPSE VIDEO-MICROSCOPY IN CORRELATION WITH PROGRESSION OF ATHEROSCLEROSIS

J. Grünwald[1,2], U. Bongartz[1], R. Bloom[1], P. Wülfroth[1], C. C. Haudenschild[3]

[1] Institut for Arteriosclerosis Research, University of Münster, Federal Republic of Germany
[2] Lichtwer Pharma GmbH, Berlin
[3] Mallory Institute for Pathology, Boston University Boston, Mass USA

SUMMARY

Time-lapse video-microscopy was used to analyse smooth muscle cell migration, proliferation and morphology. While earlier experiments with smooth muscle cells obtained from acute hypertensive animals had shown activated cell migration and proliferation, longer duration of 6 weeks hypertension resulted in a reduction of cellular proliferation and a normalisation of migration. The cells became larger and their metabolism may have increased. It is proposed that vascular wall cells are activated during the early phase of atherogenesis in their migratory and proliferative behaviour during a short phase of up to 3 weeks, while longer duration results in an activation of their metabolism.

In addition, the interaction of leucocytes and endothelial cells was analysed in a co-culture system. Isolated granulocytes or monocytes/macrophages were added to confluent endothelial cell cultures. The migratory behavior of the blood cells was subsequently analysed using video direct visualization and morphometry. Using this technology the active migration of blood cells through the confluent endothelial layer in both directions could be shown. All monocytes migrated from the top of the endothelial layer underneath the endothelial cells and remained there. Granulocytes showed a differentiated migration pattern. One third remained on top of the endothelium, about 50 % passed through the endothelium and remained there, the rest changed sides several times, up to 5 times per hour. The migratory speed of granulocytes was 1166 µm/h, about twice as fast as the speed of monocytes at 608 µm/h. The differentiation between the migratory speed of granulocytes on top or underneath the endothelial cells revealed a marked acceleration underneath the endothelial cells with a speed of

1519 μm/h compared to 671 μm/h on top of the endothelium. These results could be interpreted to mean that special extracellular matrix components produced by the endothelial cells activate the migratory behavior of blood cells.

Key words: smooth muscle cells, endothelial cell migration, granulocytes, monocytes/ macrophages

INTRODUCTION

In our earlier studies, investigating the effects of short term intimal injury[1,2] acute DOC-salt hypertension[3], short term renal hypertension[4] or in spontaneously hypertensive (SHR) rats[5], activated smooth muscle cell migration and proliferation were found. This study was designed to determine the effect of a longer duration (6 weeks) of renal hypertension. Time-lapse video microscopy was used to analyse individual cell motility as well as cell interdivision time and morphology[6].

During the early phase of atherogenesis, blood-borne cells like granulocytes and monocytes migrate through the endothelial barrier[7]. They may contribute to the migration and proliferation of medial smooth muscle cells by their production of growth factors. This investigation was designed to study the interaction of leucocytes and endothelial cells in a co-culture system using time-lapse video-microscopy. Using this technology, the active motility of blood cells could be studied, analyzing their speed of migration and their change between the upper and lower side of the endothelial layer under controlled cell culture conditions.

METHODS

Cellophane-perinephritis-hypertension according to Page was induced in male Wistar rats with a mean body weight of 200 - 250 g. After 1 - 2 weeks the normal blood pressure of 80 - 100 mmHg was raised to 180 - 200 mmHg. 6 weeks after stabilisation of high blood pressure values, the animals were killed. Medial explants were used from the aorta thoracica and the investigation was performed directly using smooth muscle cells migrating from these explants in primary culture.

The second set of experiments was performed with human umbilical vein endothelial cells grown to confluency and human isolated granulocytes or monocytes. The blood borne cells were isolated according to the plastic adherence method. The isolated cells were then transferred to confluent endothelial cell cultures and the motility was analysed using time-lapse video-microscopy for a period of up to 10 hours.

The time-lapse video-microscopy apparatus consisted of an inverted microscope (Nikon Diaphot) equipped with a plexiglas chamber. The temperature in the chamber is kept exactly at 37 °C by means of a recirculator heater. A video camera (Hammamatsu) is attached to the microscope and the video images are stored at a rate of 1 frame/min on a Panasonic 8050 time-lapse video recorder. The video recorder has a built-in time-date-generator, which marks the video

image with the exact date, hour, minute and second of
recording. The cell culture flasks are gassed with air
containing 5 % CO_2 and then placed under the microscope. The
video recording can be performed for a period of up to 48
hours. Three different parameters can be analysed from time-
lapse video recordings: 1. cell motility, 2. cell
proliferation as interdivision time and 3. cell area and
cell shape. The distance measurements and shape and size
calculations of the cells were performed with a semi-
automatic morphometry system (Leitz ASM).

RESULTS

Effect of long term hypertension on smooth muscle cell migration, proliferation and morphology

Smooth muscle cells grown from primary aortic explants
removed from either normotensive rats or from rats after 6
weeks with high blood pressure showed a small, non
significant activation of cell migration by 14 %, a mean
increase from 23.9 to 27.3 µm/h in hypertension. In contrast,
the cell proliferation time was prolonged from an
interdivision time of 11.0 hours in cells from normotensive
animals to 16.2 hours in cells from hypertensive animals, an
increase of 47 % (p < 0.001). At the same time, the cell area
had increased from 821 to 1308 µm² in smooth muscle cells
from hypertensive compared to normotensive animals. This
increase of 59 % was highly significant (p < 0.001). Also the
in vitro cell shape was altered. The cells of hypertensive
animals became more round as indicated by the form factor,
which increased by 21 % (p < 0.01).

These data indicate that the longer duration of high
blood pressure slowed down the proliferative activity below
that of cells from normotensive rats while the migratory
activity of the smooth muscle cells from the hypertensive rat
aortas has returned to approximately the normal level (table
1).

Table 1

	Control Culture Culture (n = 145)	Hypertensive Culture (n = 111)	Change in %	
Proliferation IDT x (h)	11.2 ± 0.2	16.18 ± 0.6	+ 47	p<0.001
Migration x (µm/h)	23.93 ± 0.9	27.28 ± 1.1	+ 14	n.s.
Area x (µm²)	821.59 ± 27	1308.65 ± 80	+ 59	p<0.001
Form x	0.203 ± 0.001	0.245 ± 0.01	+ 21	p<0.01

Co-culture of leucocytes and endothelial cells

The migration of granulocytes on plain plastic dishes was 842 µm/h for monocytes and 301 µm/h for granulocytes (figure 1). A co-culture of both cell types resulted in a mean speed of 475 µm/h.

In the co-culture system between leucocytes and endothelial cells, the video movies revealed that blood borne cells migrate through the endothelial layer in both directions. In contrast the monocytes pass through the endothelium just once and remain underneath the endothelium. Granulocytes have a different behavior. 34 % of the granulocytes remain on top of the endothelium, 54 % pass once through the endothelium and remain underneath, while 13 % pass through the endothelium up to 5 times during the first hour (table 2).

Table 2.   Migration-speed of Leucocytes on Plastic and in Co-Culture with Endothelial Cells

	Monocytes	Granulocytes	Co-cultured Monocytes and Granulocytes
	x ± SEM (µm/h)	x ± SEM (µm/h)	x ± SEM (µm/h)
Motility on plastic	300.95 ± 28	842.28 ± 20	474.85 ± 20
Motility in co-culture with endothelial cells	608.49 ± 31	1166.03 ± 29	723.81 ± 26
Motility on endothelial surface	---	671.80 ± 23	595.96 ± 22
Motility under-neath endothelial cell layer	608.49 ± 31	1519.41 ± 45	946.89 ± 51

The analysis of the migration speed of leucocytes in co-culture with endothelial cells revealed an acceleration of cellular speed for both cell types compared to plain plastic. Monocytes had a speed of 608 µm/h and granulocytes of 1166 µm/h in co-culture with endothelial cells. In co-culture of both cell types with the endothelium, a mean speed of 724 µm/h was found (figure 2).

When the migration speed of granulocytes was compared on the surface of the endothelial layer and underneath the endothelial layer, it became clear that cell motility on top of the endothelium was much slower (672 µm/h) than underneath the endothelium (1519µm/h) (figure 3).

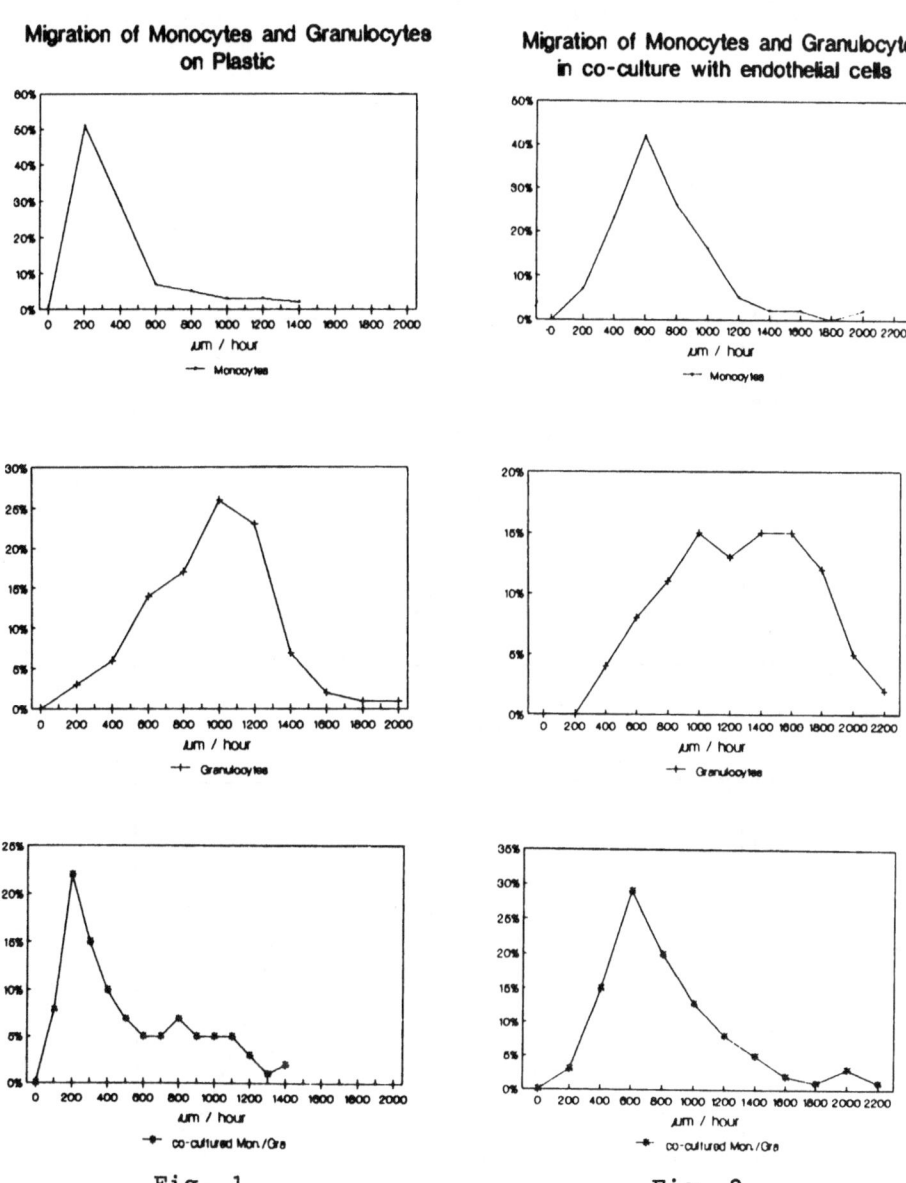

Fig. 1   Fig. 2

Figure 1

Migration of monocytes (top), macrophages (bottom) and both
cell types (middle) on plastic: Granulocytes show a faster
motility. Co-culture of both cell types reduced the fast
motility of granulocytes

Figure 2

Migration of monocytes (top), granulocytes (bottom) and both
cell types (middle) in co-culture with endothelial cells: As
on plane plastic, granulocytes show a higher motility also on
endothelial cells as compared to monocytes. The co-culture of
both cell types reduces the speed of the granulocytes.

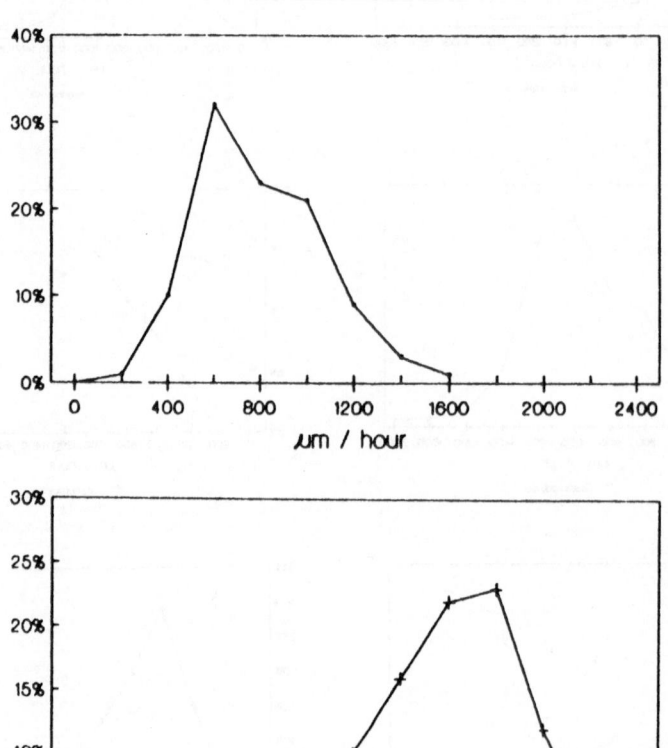

Figure 3

Migration of granulocytes on surface (top) of and underneath
(bottom) an endothelial layer: Granulocytes show a faster
motility underneath the endothelium.

Summarizing, these results have shown, that granulocytes are more active in cellular motility especially those migrating through the endothelium 5 times per hour, while monocytes pass through the endothelium and remain underneath the endothelial layer (table 3).

Table 3.   Passages through Endothelial Layer

Number of passages (in first hour after endothelial contact)	Granulocytes	Monocytes
0	34 %	---
1	54 %	100 %
2	5 %	---
3	6 %	---
4	---	---
5	2 %	---

DISCUSSION

During the early stages of atherogenesis, granulocyte and monocyte migration through the endothelial layer and subsequent migration of medial smooth muscle cells[7] are important cellular phaenomena. Isolated cells in tissue culture make it possible to study these phenomena under controlled conditions. Time-lapse video microscopy permits the analysis of individual cell behavior[6] in individual and co-culture systems. Our earlier work with acute irritations like balloon injury[1,2], DOC-salt hypertension[3], renal hypertension[4] or in spontaneously hypertensive rats (SHR)[5], has shown that smooth muscle cells were highly activated as compared to cells from control animals. This study revealed that the longer duration of hypertension (6 weeks) resulted in a normalisation of cell motility and in prolonged proliferation time.

These data suggest that cell activation during the first 2 - 3 weeks consists mainly of a migratory and proliferative response of smooth muscle cells, while a longer duration of the stimulus normalizes or even reduces those phenomena, while the cell metabolism might be accelerated, producing more extra- cellular matrix material as shown in other investigations[8,9].

A recent investigation of human smooth muscle cells cultured from atherectomized primary and restenotic plaques analysed the motility of those 2 cell groups[10]. It was found that the average migration of smooth muscle cells from primary stenosing lesions was 14.0 μm/h whereas in restenotic plaques it was increased to 37.5 μm/h. While the primary plaque probably progressed for a long time till atherectomy was performed and therefore migration had already slowed down, restenotic plaques develop much more rapidly, triggered perhaps by the atherectomy process.

The speed of monocytes and granulocytes in co-culture with endothelial cells was analysed in the second set of experiments. It was shown that most but not all granulocytes pass through the endothelium and are also able to return to the cell surface afterwards. Monocytes, at least in this system, all passed through the endothelium and remained underneath the endothelium. The speed of both cell types was activated when they had contact with endothelial cells. Granulocytes were further speeded up underneath the endothelium. This indicates an activation of the cells by extracellular matrix material laid down by the endothelial cells.

REFERENCES

1. J. Grünwald and C. C. Haudenschild, Intimal injury in vivo activates vascular smooth muscle cell migration and explant outgrowth in vitro, Arteriosclerosis 3: 183 - 189 (1984).
2. C. C. Haudenschild, J. Grünwald, Proliferative heterogeneity of vascular smooth muscle cells and its alteration by injury, Exp Cell Res 157: 364 - 370 (1985).
3. C. C. Haudenschild, J. Grünwald, A. V. Chobanian, Effects of DOC/salt hypertension on migration and proliferation of smooth muscle cells in culture, Hypertension 7 (Suppl. I): 101 - 104 (1985).
4. J. Grünwald, W. Schäper, J. Mey, W. H. Hauss, Special characteristics of cultured smooth muscle cell subtypes of hypertensive and diabetic rats, Artery 11: 1 - 14 (1982).
5. J. Grünwald, A. V. Chobanian, C. C. Haudenschild, Smooth muscle cell migration and proliferation: atherogenic mechanisms in hypertension. Atherosclerosis 67: 215 - 221 (1987).
6. J. Grünwald, Time lapse video microscopy of cultured cells and its use in cytopathology and pharmacology, Biotechniques 5: 680 - 687 (1987).
7. J. Grünwald, H. Robenek, J. Mey, W. H. Hauss, In vivo and in vitro cellular changes in experimental hypertension, Exp Mol Path 36: 164 - 176 (1982).
8. A. Schmidt, J. Grünwald, E. Buddecke, (^{35}S) proteoglycan metabolism of arterial smooth muscle cells cultured from normotensive and hypertensive rats, Atherosclerosis 45: 299 - 310 (1982).
9. J. Grünwald, J. Fingerle, H. Hämmerle, E. Betz, C. C. Haudenschild, Cytocontractile structures and proteins of smooth muscle cells during the formation of experimental lesions, Exp Mol Path 46: 78 - 88 (1987).
10. G. Bauriedel, U. Windstetter, Motility of cultivated myocytes from atherectomized primary and restenotic plaques, Eur J Clin Invest (in press), (1990).

CORRELATION OF THE MATRIX-DEGRADING ACTIVITY OF MACROPHAGES WITH CHANGES

IN SMOOTH MUSCLE CELL BIOLOGY IN ATHEROGENESIS

Julie H. Campbell[1], Robyn R. Rennick[1,2]
and Gordon R. Campbell[3]

[1]Baker Medical Research Institute, Prahran, Victoria,
Australia; [2]University College London, U.K.
[3]Department of Anatomy, University of Melbourne, Victoria,
Australia

CELL MATRIX INTERACTIONS

Studies by Bissell et al.[1,2] have stressed the importance of the
extracellular matrix surrounding each cell as an integral part of the
cellular functional unit. The cell, dependent on its phenotypic state,
produces a particular matrix which via interactions with membrane receptors
and cytoskeletal components affects gene expression. This in turn,
influences many morphological and functional properties of the cell.
Studies with many cell systems including fibroblasts, smooth muscle cells
(SMC), and endothelial and epithelial cells have shown that matrix
components regulate functions such as adhesion, shape, migration, proliferation, biosynthetic and degradative processes, morphogenesis and
differentiation[3,4].

Cell-associated heparan sulphate proteoglycans occur ubiquitously as
membrane-intercalated glycoproteins where the core protein is anchored in
the lipid interior of the plasma membrane, and the heparan sulphate chains
bind to specific sites on collagen, laminin and fibronectin[5]. One of the
functions of the proteoglycan-mediated interaction is to promote the
organisation of actin filaments in the cell which may also have the effect
of stabilizing the cell's phenotype[1]. In primary culture, we have shown
that an extract of heparan sulphate glycosaminoglycan from the aortic
intima plus inner media maintains sparsely-seeded SMC in a high $V_v$myo
"contractile" state, and that a similar effect occurs with the closely
related glycosaminoglycan heparin[6,7]. SMC in primary culture can also be
maintained in the contractile state by seeding the freshly-dispersed cells
at confluent density, or by placing sparsely-seeded cells with a spatially
separated feeder layer of confluent contractile SMC or endothelial cells[7]
which produce large amounts of an antiproliferative heparan sulphate
species[8]. Thus the presence of heparin-like glycosaminoglycans is an
important determinant of the phenotype that the smooth muscle expresses,
and high levels of this glycosaminoglycan species maintain the cells in a
contractile (high $V_v$myo) state. Furthermore, SMC which have been seeded
sparsely onto a layer of type IV collagen or basement membrane Matrigel
(a solubilized extract of EHS tumour basement membrane containing collagen
type IV, laminin, heparan sulphate proteoglycan and entactin) do not
undergo a change in phenotype, nor do isolated SMC which have been

completely embedded in a gel of collagen type I. This indicates that replacement of certain components of the basal lamina, or providing a microenvironment in which the basal lamina can be rapidly reconstituted, encourages maintenance of the contractile state[9].

External influences, and perhaps the cells themselves, must be able to modify the cell matrix contacts in a regulated manner. Mechanisms by which this might be accomplished include regulation of the amount of ligands (e.g. heparan sulphate proteoglycan) by destruction with metallo-proteinases such as the gelatinases and stromelysins and/or by endo or exoglycosidases such as heparanase, heparinase or heparitinase[10]. Protein-ases are present focally at adhesion sites in some cells actively modula-ting their actin cytoskeleton and attachments to the substrate[11].

MACROPHAGES AND ATHEROGENESIS

SMC in the intima of human arteries involved in atherogenesis are phenotypically different from those of the underlying media and express a decreased volume fraction of myofilaments ($V_V$myo), amongst other features (see Campbell and Campbell, this volume). In primary cell culture, medial SMC which have been enzyme-dispersed and seeded at densities below con-fluence undergo similar changes in phenotypic expression to a low $V_V$myo "synthetic" state accompanied by distinct alterations in biology, including gaining the ability to proliferate logarithmically in response to mitogens, to migrate readily, to synthesize 25-45 fold the amount of collagen and to accumulate 7-fold the amount of lipid upon exposure to β-VLDL[12]. This suggests that change in smooth muscle phenotype may be an important initial event in the development of atherosclerosis, which is characterized by focal proliferation of SMC and their enhanced synthesis of collagen and accumulation of lipid.

The atherosclerotic plaque has a variable cellular composition depending on its stage of development, but the macrophage is always present in significant numbers[13] (see also Campbell and Campbell, this volume). These cells function primarily as scavengers, accumulating large amounts of lipid to become the classic foam cell[14]. However, in culture the macrophage also produces a potent stimulator of cellular proliferation. This factor resembles the platelet-derived growth factor (PDGF) in that it competes with ^{125}I-PDGF for binding to receptors and is mitogenic[15]. Macrophages also secrete β-transforming growth factor (β-TGF), as well as vasoactive agents and matrix-degrading enzymes[16,17].

Thus the macrophage may play a multiplicity of roles in the initiation and development of the atheromatous plaque. We have recently demonstrated that peritoneal macrophages grown in co-culture with a confluent monolayer of SMC induce a significant decrease in the $V_V$myo of the SMC after three days as compared with both the freshly isolated SMC and those grown for three days in the absence of macrophages[18]. Since invasion of the artery wall by monocytes (which then differentiate into macrophages) is one of the earliest cellular events in experimental atherogenesis[13] we have postulated that it may be through the influence of these cells that smooth muscle phenotypic change is induced in the initial stages of atherogenesis[19] In support of this notion is the recent work of Prescott et al.[20], showing that leucocyte invasion of the vessel wall in response to the implantation of an endotoxin-soaked cotton thread in the adventitia induces phenotypic changes in medial SMC and the formation of a myointimal thickening. This occurs in the absence of hyperlipidaemia or detectable endothelial injury.

Macrophages are the prominent cells in host defense mechanisms characteristic of chronic inflammatory responses. As such they produce a vast array of secretory products including neutral metalloproteinases and heparan sulphate degrading enzymes[21]. Heparan sulphate degrading enzymes have also been described in platelets[22], T-lymphocytes[21], neutrophils[23] and tumour cells[24,25]. Indeed, the heparan sulphate degrading activity of tunour cells has been directly related to their metastatic potential, suggesting that degradation of heparan sulphate in extracellular matrix facilitates invasion of the vessel wall by normal and malignant cells[24,25]. It also raises the possibility that degradation of SMC-associated heparan sulphate by monocyte/macrophages and other blood-borne cells may be a process central to atheroma.

To determine whether macrophage initiation of the change in smooth muscle phenotypic expression could be correlated with degradation of heparan sulphate proteoglycans, we set up an assay for heparan sulphate degrading enzymes[21]. Bovine aortic endothelial cells or rabbit aortic SMC were seeded into 30 mm plastic culture dishes in the presence of 60 µCi $Na_2[^{35}S]O_4$. After 7 days the cells were removed by Triton X-100, leaving a layer of ^{35}S-labelled extracellular matrix proteoglycan (mainly heparan sulphate proteoglycan) on the bottom of the dish. The factor to be tested for heparan sulphate-degrading activity was added to the washed matrix for 24 hours at 37°C at neutral pH, then an aliquot of the supernatant passed through a Sepharose 6B column and the fractions counted by liquid scintillation. Living macrophages completely degraded the ^{35}S-labelled components of endothelial and smooth muscle cell-produced extracellular matrix into small molecular fragments which eluted with a K_{av} of 0.84 on Sepharose 6B, similar to that of free $[^{35}S]O_4^{2-}$ (K_{av} = 0.86). A lysate of whole macrophages produced degradation peaks at K_{av} 0.60 ($M_r \sim 10,000$ daltons) and 0.84. Both macrophage lysomal lysate at neutral pH and heparinase (10 units/ml) degraded the ^{35}S-labelled matrix components into fragments which eluted at K_{av} 0.63, and which were identified as heparan sulphate chains by their complete degradation in the presence of low pH nitrous acid and resistance to chondroitin ABC lyase. At acid pH, the macrophage lysosomal lysate produced a second peak eluting at K_{av} 0.84, indicating that the enzymes responsible for the complete degradation of the heparan sulphate chains were present in the lysosomes and only active at acid pH. Only a small amount of heparan sulphate degrading enzyme was released into the incubation medium by living macrophages, and there was no activity on isolated plasma membranes of macrophages, although proteolytic enzymes were evident in both instances. Furthermore, when confluent, high $V_v$myo rabbit aortic SMC 8 days in primary culture were exposed to macrophage lysosomal lysate, heparinase (10 units/ml), chondroitin ABC lyase (10 units/ml) or trypsin (10 µg/ml), only the macrophage lysosomal lysate and heparinase induced a decrease in the $V_v$myo of the smooth muscle cells, similar to that previously observed in the presence of living macrophages.

In order to demonstrate a more direct relationship between degradation of ^{35}S-heparan sulphate in the basal lamina of SMC and initiation of SMC phenotypic change, we seeded freshly isolated rabbit aortic SMC at confluent density (8 x 10⁵ cells/dish) in 30 mm plastic dishes and after 7 days in primary culture added 60 µCi $Na_2[^{35}S]O_4$. Over a 24 hour period, this ^{35}S was incorporated into the sulphated proteoglycans of the SMC basal lamina. Eighty-seven percent of the incorporated ^{35}S was shown to be cell-associated (pericellular) and only 13% in the extracellular matrix. Of the pericellular (basal lamina) incorporated ^{35}S, 41-44% was in heparan sulphate proteoglycan, with the majority of the remainder in chondroitin sulphate proteoglycan. To this washed monolayer of ^{35}S-labelled high $V_v$myo "contractile" SMC, was added an equivalent number of rabbit peritoneal

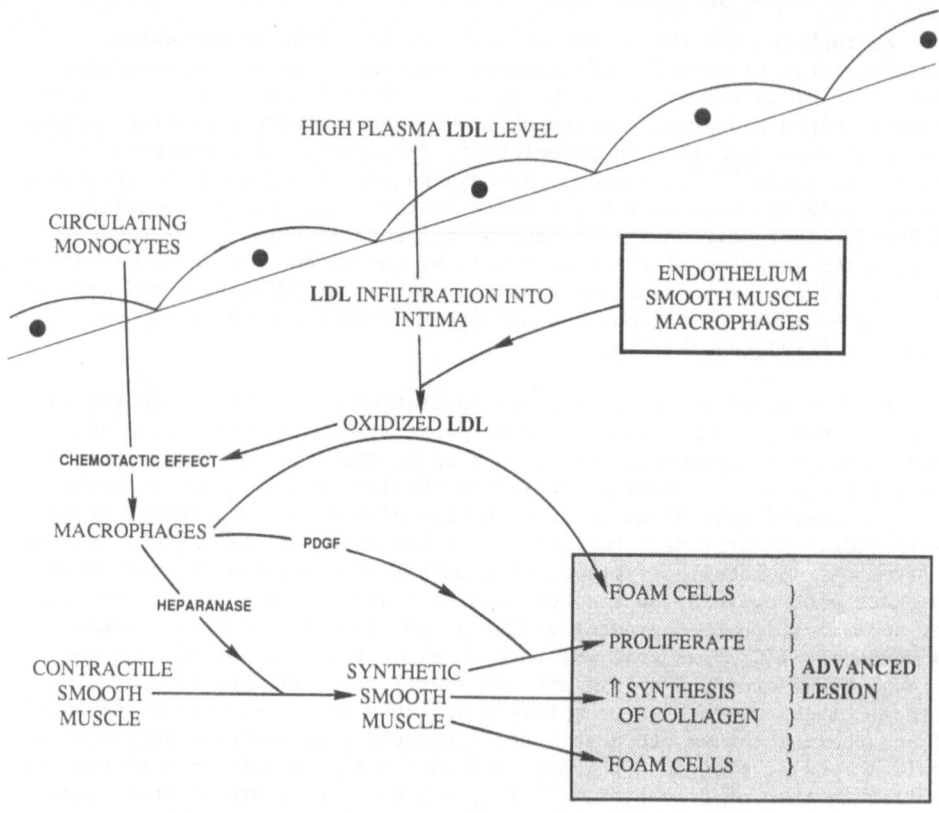

HIGH PLASMA **LDL** LEVEL

CIRCULATING
MONOCYTES

LDL INFILTRATION INTO
INTIMA

ENDOTHELIUM
SMOOTH MUSCLE
MACROPHAGES

OXIDIZED **LDL**

CHEMOTACTIC EFFECT

MACROPHAGES

PDGF

HEPARANASE

CONTRACTILE
SMOOTH
MUSCLE

SYNTHETIC
SMOOTH
MUSCLE

FOAM CELLS }
}
PROLIFERATE }
} **ADVANCED**
⇑ SYNTHESIS } **LESION**
OF COLLAGEN }
}
FOAM CELLS }

Fig.1. Schema of monocyte entry into the artery wall in hyperlipidaemic states and their subsequent role in the
formation of atheroma. In hypercholesterolaemia, there is
enhanced adhesion of monocytes to the endothelium. Monocytes are chemo-attracted into the wall by LDL which has
been oxidized by endothelium, smooth muscle and macrophages.
Once in the wall, the monocytes differentiate into macrophages which oxidize more LDL. This, in turn, attracts
additional monocytes into the vessel wall. The macrophages
readily take up the oxidized lipoprotein to become "foam
cells". Macrophages also take up and degrade the heparan
sulphate proteoglycans in the basal lamina of SMC, which
triggers change in smooth muscle phenotype to a state
whereby they are capable of proliferation in response to
mitogens from the macrophages and other sources, synthesis
of greatly increased amounts of matrix particularly collagen
type I, and accumulation of large amounts of lipid.

macrophages. After 24 hours it was shown that low molecular weight (<1,000
daltons) degraded products of the ^{35}S-labelled proteoglycans appeared in
the supernatant and the $V_V$myo of the SMC decreased significantly. In
addition, it was shown that the amount of heparan sulphate degradation
products appearing in the supernatant increased with increasing numbers of
macrophages to reach a plateau at a macrophage to SMC ratio of 1:3. That
is, one macrophage degraded all the removable sulphated glycosaminoglycans

from the basal lamina of three SMC. However, this study is complicated by the fact that even in the absence of macrophages there is some degradation of the ^{35}S-proteoglycans of the SMC basal lamina (see zero point Fig.1). Indeed, it is known that heparan sulphate in the basal lamina of SMC is constantly being internalized, degraded and resynthesized by the SMC themselves, and for subcultured (low $V_v$myo "synthetic" state) SMC, its half-life is in the region of 4 hours[26]. In some cell systems it has been demonstrated that a small fraction of the heparan sulphate enriched in the rare 2-0 sulphate glucuronate units is transported to the cell nucleus where it is implicated in cell growth control[27], but whether this is also the mechanism by which heparan sulphate/heparin affects SMC phenotypic expression is unknown.

Based on the studies reported here, we suggest one possible scenario in relation to the genesis of atherosclerosis: monocyte/macrophages which have entered the subendothelium in response to hyperlipidaemia, endothelial injury or other stimuli, release heparan sulphate proteoglycans from the surface of SMC by the action of proteinases either secreted or present on the plasma membrane. The proteoglycans are phagocytosed by the macrophages and the heparan sulphate chains completely degraded in the lysosomes, temporarily removing all heparan sulphate from the surface of the SMC. This, by an unknown pathway, initiates the process of phenotypic modulation to a "synthetic" state in which the SMC are capable of proliferation, synthesis of large amounts of collagen, and accumulation of large amounts of lipid to become foam cells (Fig.1).

Thus quantitation of the levels and activity of heparan sulphate-degrading enzymes in cells which invade or release their products into the vessel wall (such as monocyte/macrophages, platelets, T-lymphocytes, and to a lesser extent, basinophils and neutrophils), may act as an indicator of their potential to induce phenotypic changes in SMC in the early stages of the atherogenic process.

ACKNOWLEDGEMENTS

This work was supported by the National Heart Foundation of Australia and the National Health and Medical Research Council. The excellent technical assistance of Silvia Kalevitch is gratefully acknowledged.

REFERENCES

1. M.J. Bissell and M.H. Barcellos-Hoff, The influence of extracellular matrix on gene expression: Is structure the message? J. Cell Sci. 8(Suppl):327 (1987).
2. M.J. Bissell, H.G. Hall and G. Parry, How does the extracellular matrix direct gene expression? J. Theoret. Biol. 99:31 (1982).
3. E.D. Hay, ed., Cell Biology of the extracellular matrix, Plenum Press, New York, London (1981).
4. G. Parry, B. Cullen, C.S. Kaetzel, R. Kramer and L. Moss, Regulation of differentiation and polarized secretion in mammary epithelial cells maintained in culture: Extracellular matrix and membrane polarity influences, J. Cell Biol. 105:2043 (1987).
5. S. Saunders and M. Bernfield, Cell surface proteoglycan binds mouse mammary epithelial cells to fibronectin and behaves as a receptor for interstitial matrix. J. Cell Biol. 106:423 (1988).
6. J.H. Chamley-Campbell and G.R. Campbell, What controls smooth muscle phenotype? Atherosclerosis 40:347 (1981).

7. J.H. Campbell and G.R. Campbell, Cellular interactions in the artery wall, in: "The Peripheral Circulation," S. Hunyor, J. Ludbrook, J. Shaw, M. McGrath, ed., Elsevier, New York (1984).

8. L.M. Fritze, C.F. Reilly and R.D. Rosenberg, An antiproliferative heparan sulphate species produced by post-confluence smooth muscle cells, J. Cell Biol. 100:1041 (1985).

9. E. Stadler, J.H. Campbell and G.R. Campbell, Do cultured vascular smooth muscle cells resemble those of the artery wall? If not, why not? J. Cardiovasc. Pharmacol. 14(Suppl.6):S1 (1989).

10. L.A. Liotta, C.N. Rao and U.M. Wewer, Biochemical interactions of tumor cells with the basement membrane, Ann. Rev. Biochem. 55: 1037 (1986).

11. J. Pöllänen, K. Hedman, L.S. Nielsen, K. Dano and A. Vaheri, Ultrastructural localization of plasma membrane-associated urokinase-type plasminogen activator at focal contacts, J. Cell Biol. 106: 87 (1988).

12. G.R. Campbell and J.H. Campbell, Phenotypic modulation of smooth muscle cells in primary culture, in: "Vascular Smooth Muscle In Culture," J.H. Campbell, G.R. Campbell, eds., CRC Press, Boca Raton (1987).

13. L. Jonasson, J. Holm, O. Skalli, G. Bondjers and G.K. Hansson, The human atherosclerotic plaque: Regional accumulations of T cells, macrophages and smooth muscle cells. Arteriosclerosis 6:131 (1986).

14. S. Fowler, H. Shio and N.J. Haley, Characterization of lipid-laden aortic cells from cholesterol fed rabbits. IV. Investigation of macrophage-like properties of aortic cell populations, Lab. Invest. 41:372 (1979).

15. K. Shimokado, E.W. Raines, D.K. Madtes, T.B. Barnett, E.R. Benditt and R. Ross, A significant part of macrophage-derived growth factor consists of at least two forms of PDGF, Cell 43:277 (1985).

16. M.B. Sporn and A.B. Roberts, Peptide growth factors and inflammation, tissue repair and cancer, J. Clin. Invest. 78:329 (1986).

17. R.C. Page, P. Davies and A.C. Allison, The macrophage as a secretory cell, Int. Rev. Cytol. 52:119 (1978).

18. R.E. Rennick, J.H. Campbell and G.R. Campbell, Vascular smooth muscle phenotype and growth behaviour can be influenced by macrophages in vitro. Atherosclerosis 71:35 (1988).

19. J.H. Campbell and G.R. Campbell, Potential role of heparanase in atherosclerosis, News In Physiol. Sci. 4:9 (1989).

20. M.F. Prescott, C.K. McBride and M. Court, Development of intimal lesions after leukocyte migration into the vascular wall, Am. J. Pathol. 135:835 (1989).

21. N. Savion, I. Vlodavsky and Z. Fuks, T-lymphocytes and macrophages interaction with cultured vascular endothelial cells: Attachment, invasion and subsequent degradation of the subendothelial extracellular matrix, J. Cell Physiol. 118:169 (1984).

22. A. Wasteson, B. Glimelius, C. Busch, B. Westermark, C.H. Heldin and B. Norling, Effect of a platelet endoglycosidase on cell surface associated heparan sulphate of human cultured endothelial and glial cells, Thrombosis Res. 11:309 (1977).

23. Y. Matzner, M. Bar-Ner, J. Yahalom, R. Ishai-Michaeli, Z. Fuks and I. Vlodavsky, Degradation of heparan sulphate in the subendothelial extracellular matrix by a readily released heparanase from human neutrophils. Possible role in invasion through basement membranes, J. Clin. Invest. 76:1306 (1985).

24. M. Nakajima, T. Irimura, D. Di Ferrante, N. Di Ferrante and G.L. Nicholson, Heparan sulphate degradation: relation to tumor invasion and metastatic properties of mouse B16 melanoma sublines, Science 220:611 (1983).

25. I. Vlodavsky, Z. Fuks, M. Bar-Ner, Y. Ariav and V. Schirrmacher, Lymphoma cell-mediated degradation of sulphated proteoglycans in the subendothelial extracellular matrix: relationship to tumor cell metastasis, Cancer Res. 43:2704 (1983).
26. A. Schmidt and E. Buddecke, Cell-associated proteoheparan sulfate from bovine arterial smooth muscle cells, Exp. Cell. Res. 178: 242 (1988).
27. N.S. Fedarko and H.E. Conrad, A unique heparan sulfate in the nuclei of hepatocytes: structural changes with the growth state of the cells, J. Cell Biol. 102:587 (1986).

Burnstock, who was chairing the session, and Siegel opened the
discussion of G. Campbell's presentation indicating that since contractile
smooth muscle cells in atheroma have 1.5 to 2x more HcGMP than those of the
media one should perhaps look for changes in vascular tone since this decrease
in HcGMP (associated with the change from a contractile to a synthetic state)
could mean that the vessels cannot relax as well as normal arteries. Campbell
said that he could not answer this question at the moment, and that further
work was in progress on this subject. Burnstock indicated that some of these
questions about vascular tone in atherogenesis may be answered during session
number seven.

Bassenge suggested that some of the components in the lesions get there
by contamination with endothelial cells or other cells, for instance that of
secreting fibronectin, and that one has to be careful about preparations in
which some endothelial cells may remain. G. Campbell indicated that he
believed there was little possibility of contamination by endothelial cells in
the preparations he was using.

The discussion following Grünwald's presentation started with comments
by Burnstock. He stated that he and his colleagues had made similar
observations when the interaction of lymphocytes with human pancreatic tumour
cells was examined in culture and that when fibroblasts were added to the
system, the interaction of lymphocytes with the tumor cells no longer
occurred, and that the lymphocytes preferentially patrolled the fibroblasts.
Burnstock then enquired whether Grünwald had examined the effect of adding
fibroblasts or a third cell type to his system and Grünwald replied that he
thought it would be a good idea. Bond asked whether endothelial cells develop
the tight junctions in vitro and Grünwald said that they really do not have
much evidence for that because the culture, while confluent, was not yet as
mature as it might be later on. He indicated that other studies in the
literature did show that tight junctions develop with these types of in vitro
conditions.

Bond then asked whether one can estimate the amount of time it takes
once the monocyte has marginated on the endothelial surface for passage into
or through the endothelium to occur. Grünwald said that it is very fast, that
it takes about two minutes, and that the cells stop at the border between the
endothelial cells for a few seconds and then there appears to be some kind of
enzymatic action which opens up the border and within five to six seconds they
continue migrating. Really they appear to enter the endothelium after they
have migrated for some distance. Grünwald also indicated that he believed
that all of the cells that enter his endothelial preparations enter through
junction areas and do not go through the transport vesicles of the endothelial
cell. Wissler then asked whether Grünwald had utilized hyperlipidemic serum
or LDL from hyperlipidemic serum in this system and Grünwald said that so far
this had not been done. Wissler then asked whether anyone had utilized
cycline, the nickname for the cellular proliferation nuclear antigen (PCNA) to
study the atherosclerotic process. Grünwald responded that as far as he knew

this had not yet been utilized to identify and quantify the proliferating cells in atherosclerotic lesions. Burnstock commented that after X-irradiation of blood vessels there was an increase in the number of intimal smooth muscle cells present. He wondered whether the trigger for this is similar to the trigger for cell migration in the model that Grünwald had just described. Grünwald said that as far as he knew this had not been studied in a system similar to the one that he is using.

In the question and answer period following J. Campbell's presentation Weber asked whether arterial constriction is important and Campbell responded that the cells were probably returning to a more primitive phenotype, normally expressed during development. In developing embryos or in very young animals most of the arterial medial smooth muscle cells are rich in organelles involved in protein synthesis. Very few smooth muscle cells with prominent myofilament bundles are present. The major function of these developing cells of the arterial system is proliferation and production of matrix. When the animals become adult the function of the smooth muscle cells changes so that their major function is then contraction or constriction. During repair or regeneration of an injured artery the smooth muscle cells modulate their phenotypes back to one which can repair the defective or injured artery wall. The fact that the cell population can go back and forth in phenotype was the reason for using the term modulation instead of dedifferentiation. The latter was usually considered to be an irreversible process. Skeletal muscle on the other hand cannot undergo this type of phenotypic modulation. Some other connective tissue cells such as chrondrocytes can also alter their phenotype in response to various stimuli.

Cornhill complimented J. Campbell on her presentation and indicated that he was particularly impressed by the importance of the microenvironment to the smooth muscle cells, which her studies emphasized. He wondered whether they had looked at cells undergoing cyclical stretching and relaxation as they do in the artery wall during the cardiac cycle. He also enquired as to whether the stimuli for phenotypic modulation were active in the same way under these in vitro conditions. J. Campbell responded that Shirinsky from Smirnov's institute in Moscow had been working with them in Melbourne recently and had used Glagov's University of Chicago system of growing the cells on a stretchable membrane. Under these circumstances the cells did not appear to undergo any further phenotypic modulation. However, they increased collagen production considerably. The question of whether the cells were already in a phenotypically modulated state during these studies was raised and J. Campbell indicated that, yes, the cells had already undergone their change in phenotype.

Wissler then indicated that he was intensely interested in the work that both Campbells are doing on heparinase as a controlling enzyme for cell proliferation and perhaps as an important enzyme in phenotypic modulation. He pointed out that in the PDAY study one of the big problems is to find one, two, or three additional markers that indicate that atherogenesis is beginning and he wondered if the heparinase system might be used as a marker in vivo to help identify the areas in which the atherosclerotic plaque is being initiated. J. Campbell indicated that that was exactly what they were working on at the present time. They are currently using immunological approaches to find out whether they can localize heparinase in developing plaques. Hay also indicated that it might be the chondroitin sulfate that is released or altered in the absence of heparin to which the smooth muscle cells were responding. He wondered if the signal for smooth muscle cells to react might be engendered by the presence of an excess of small molecules released by heparinase activity. J. Campbell said it was very difficult to comment on this question at present because they have no idea of exactly how heparan sulfate maintained the smooth muscle contractile phenotype. Perhaps the protein core controls the transport of heparan sulfate through the plasma membrane in the same region where the actin filaments insert so that their removal affects the cytoskeleton. This in turn may influence or control gene expression. In view of the fact that heparan sulfate is being constantly internalized by smooth muscle cells and then degraded (as appears to be true in a number of other cell systems) this might influence the effect of heparan sulfate on the gene expression. What needs to be determined is how heparan sulfate influences the phenotype of the smooth muscle cell at the molecular level. This was the big challenge. Liu also added his compliments to the presentation that J. Campbell made. He suggested that it is particularly exciting and important work because sodium heparin can reverse the atherosclerotic process. He wondered whether there are any ideas as to the potential mechanism by which heparin controls the process of cell proliferation? Are the free radical scavengers important in this process? J. Campbell responded that they have studied the effects of free radical scavengers on their system and they found no effects whatsoever. Regarding heparin and how it works, they are continuing their studies at the molecular level and hope to have some additional evidence as to how heparan sulfate reacts in the next few months. She pointed out that heparin and heparan sulfate are just different parts of the same species of compounds and that many heparan sulfates have large segments identical to the heparin molecule. She hoped that the differences in the functions of these molecules could be defined in their current studies.

The general discussion of the session then began and Wissler pointed out that G. Campbell's diagrams always showed advanced plaques whereas the PDAY study of lesions in youth was concentrating on the differences between lesion-prone and lesion-resistant areas along with the differences between diffuse fibrous thickening and early atherosclerosis (Professor Wissler is a principal investigator and program director of these studies involving cellular reactions, in conjunction with Cornhill and several other investigators). The lesion-prone areas show largely smooth muscle cell accumulations with abundant intracellular or intracytoplasmic lipid. In other words, these relatively early fatty plaques show mostly smooth muscle cells which have undergone phenotypic modulation. He noted that the studies that he and Kusumi had been doing indicate that the fatty plaques in young people show quite a different localization of Lp(a) as compared to their own observations and to the reports in the literature of the localization of Lp(a) in advanced plaques in older individuals. He noted that it would be particularly valuable if the change of the cells towards phenotypic modulation could be used as an additional indicator of plaque progression in a quantitative way to add an additional definition of the development of atherosclerosis over and above the presence of intracellular lipid in the lesion.

Wissler pointed out that one of the main problems in the microscopic parts of the PDAY study is that so far only the fat stains help as a more or less definitive guide and indicator of the development of atherosclerosis as differentiated from the diffuse intimal thickening and/or the focal cushion lesions that have generally been defined as being distinct from atherosclerosis. G. Campbell responded that the scientific community was hoping that the PDAY study would answer exactly those kinds of questions in a quantitative way. In other words, it is hoped that this study will define once and for all the main indicators one can use to identify and to measure the inception and the progression of true atherosclerosis as contrasted to the many other responses of the artery wall. Wissler indicated his hope that before the PDAY study is completed a number of selected cases can be studied at the ultrastructural level by both Campbells so that their superior experience in defining the state of the developing plaque relative to phenotypic modulation of smooth muscle cells can be applied using the background of the standardized sampling of arteries from young people where many of the risk factors have been identified and a great deal is known about the size, lipid content, cellular population, and lipoprotein populations of the lesions.

Heistad then questioned Wissler about the extent of endothelial damage that occurs in his experience in both human and experimental animal atherosclerosis and stated that he was surprised that Wissler had indicated that there might be extensive endothelial damage over monkey lesions. Wissler indicated that the rhesus monkey lesions that he was speaking of are really quite advanced atherosclerotic plaques with necrotic centers and fibrous caps and that they occupy between one third and two thirds of the arterial lumen even after pressure perfusion fixation. Since they were produced with a coconut oil and butter fat diet with 2% cholesterol, they are really very florid lesions like the ones that we sometimes see in heterozygous FH patients in their twenties or thirties. They almost always show extensive mico-ulcers and endothelial cell loss. He indicated that he really wasn't sure what happens to the endothelial lining in lesions that are produced more slowly and with somewhat gentler atherogenic regimens.

F. Dincer indicated that she appreciated G. Campbell's presentation very much because of the insight that it provided about differentiating diffuse fibrous arterial thickening from the development of atherosclerosis in the carotid artery where, following carotid endarterectomy, secondary fibrosis and restenosis may develop. F. Dincer hoped that the methodologies that he had described might be helpful in the microscopic and ultramicroscopic studies that are done on endarterectomy specimens following restenosis of the internal carotid artery. Campbell pointed out that they had not yet looked at restenotic lesions from the human carotid artery endarterectomy patients, but certainly in experimental animals they had found that the same kinds of changes occur. Thus the same differential parameters they have been using in human carotid arteries appear applicable to lesions that occur after extensive endothelial injury.

Bini pointed out that she had been able to study some of the cynomolgus monkey lesions at the Oregon Regional Primate Center which Malinow had utilized and she agreed with Wissler that these probably should be called atheroarteritis because they are very different from the lesions that she has studied in usual human atherosclerosis. She felt that the cynomolgus monkey lesions were quite different no matter whether one looks at the cerebral arteries in the circle of Willis, or the arteries to the testes. Unfortunately, she did not have the opportunity to study the surface of these arteries with scanning EM. Bond pointed out that he has now studied over 1000 nonhuman primates used for atherosclerosis experiments focusing largely on the aorta, the carotid arteries, and the coronary arteries. In fact Lewis has not found the kind of damage to the endothelium that Ross reported, or that Wissler has studied with Weber, but the ensuing discussion indicated that the diets that were used to produce these lesions at Bowman Grey were quite different in relation to the types of food fats utilized and the percentage of cholesterol in the diet. In other words, the University of Chicago rations were designed to produce very severe atherosclerosis in a relatively short period of time. They had succeeded in mimicking the advanced human lesion in almost all respects.

Bond then asked Wissler whether he had expected to see advanced plaques in the aorta and coronary arteries from the PDAY subjects and Wissler replied that they did, unfortunately, see them more frequently than they had anticipated. There ensued an extensive discussion of whether the arterial lesions that had been published in Egyptian mummies were really atherosclerosis or some other kind of degenerative arterial disease such as Mönkeberg's sclerosis. Paulin then requested that Wissler expand his discussion of concentric and transmural lesions as being a hallmark of the atheroarteritis which occurs in people who have circulating immune complexes. Wissler pointed out that in almost all of the published studies of human atherosclerosis the coronary arteries most frequently show eccentric and quite typical intimal plaques that usually do not involve more than one third to one half of the arterial circumferance and relatively little inflammation. He also pointed out that some of the studies which Glagov and Zarins have reported from the University of Chicago generally show that whenever an artery is going around a curve the lesions develop in the areas of turbulence or lowered shear stress and that this generally results in eccentric plaques in most muscular arteries. In fact, if one looks at the several dozen illustrations which Roberts, the chief of pathology at the National Heart, Lung, and Blood Institute on the Bethesda, Maryland campus, has published, one sees that almost all of the atherosclerotic lesions of which he has published photomicrographs are eccentric. This appears to be especially true in the coronary arteries. At the present time, in studies of both MIRU patients' coronary arteries and those that have been evaluated thus far in PDAY, the concentric transmural coronary artery lesions are unusual, probably representing less then 10% of the total lesions studied. In general, the correlations between concentric transmural atheroarteritic lesions in these individuals and circulating immune complexes are direct and fairly consistent. This result along with the recent evidence that autoimmunity may be developing in some individuals who have oxidized low density lipoproteins in their lesions adds to the possiblities for an injurious form of immunological reaction. Perhaps latent viruses, endotoxin injury, and other types of endothelial injury, possibly due to oxidized LDL, which have not as yet been very well documented may be responsible for some of the cases of atheroarteritis now being observed.

Paulin pointed out that he thought that concentric lesions were much more common, but maybe his evaluation was influenced by the numbers of post-balloon catheter angioplasty patients that they were asked to evaluate in their radiological practice. He also pointed out that since they rely frequently on contrast media arteriography, the tendency for the atheroarteric lesions to undergo compensatory dilatation may have influenced their quantitative estimates of how many patients with endothelial injury atheroarteritis they are seeing. Bond pointed out that in his opinion a lot of the concentric lesions that he sees in both human coronary and carotid arteries as well as in experimental animals simply represent an advanced process and not necessarily any difference in pathogenesis. He also called attention to the fact that in some hearts some of the lesions in the coronary artery are concentric and some are eccentric. Wissler agreed with this completely and pointed out that this had been true in the MIRU hearts that they had studied and, he also pointed out, in all of the immunological arteritis which he had studied. These cases of concentric and transmural atheroarteritis usually had been found to be segmental in localization so that the affected areas occurred at intervals throughout the arterial length. It would be logical, he pointed out, that the intervening areas would have a more usual localization of the atherosclerotic plaque.

Gerrity brought the discussion back to the question of endothelial damage and reported that he found not a shred of evidence in the literature which implicated endothelial damage as an initiating factor in early atherosclerotic plaques in experimental animals. Wissler agreed with this statement and pointed out that the various risk factors that appear to have endothelial damage as a part of their early pathogenesis probably are confined to a small percentage of lesions in the experimental animal and the human where circulating immune complexes, endotoxins, homocystine, and other endothelial-toxic factors play a major role. Gerrity also pointed out that when the cholesterol levels were high enough, as they are in some of their more recent studies, one begins to see definite endothelial damage in 12-15 weeks. This experimental set of conditions is probably very similar to that which has been used in the rhesus monkey studies that <u>Wissler</u> described. <u>Wissler</u> was offered the last word in this discussion. He indicated that the role of endothelial damage in atherogenesis probably depends on how one defines endothelial damage. If it is defined as the result of factors which lead to monocyte sticking or mononuclear cells crossing the endothelial barrier, then certain kinds of diets and a number of other conditions might be said to be causing endothelial damage even though the endothelium is not ulcerated and substantial numbers of endothelial cells are not being lost. <u>Gerrity</u> agreed that one has to define the endothelial damage before one can make general statements about how much of a factor it is in the pathogenesis of atherosclerosis.

CONSTRICTION AND DILATATION IN

ATHEROSCLEROTIC AND HYPERTENSIVE ARTERIES

Donald D. Heistad, J. Antonio G. Lopez, Frank M. Faraci,
and Mark L. Armstrong

Department of Internal Medicine, VA Medical Center and
University of Iowa College of Medicine, Iowa City, Iowa

INTRODUCTION

We will emphasize three points that pertain to approaches to quantification of changes in atherosclerotic lesions.

First, changes in responsiveness of arteries to vasoactive substances occur very early in atherosclerosis. Thus, examination of vascular reactivity may be a sensitive way to detect changes in atherosclerotic lesions. It seems likely that examination of vascular reactivity may be more sensitive than measurement of changes in vascular diameter and perhaps wall thickness in detection of early and moderately severe atherosclerosis.

Second, we will mention briefly the changes in vascular responses in chronic hypertension. Hypertension alters vascular responses, but mechanisms of the changes are quite different from those observed in atherosclerotic arteries.

Third, we will discuss effects of regression of atherosclerosis on vascular reactivity. It appears that studies of vascular responsiveness may be a sensitive approach during regression as well as progression of atherosclerosis.

In this era, which may be characterized as the dawn of effective treatment of hypercholesterolemia, a critical question is whether treatment of hypercholesterolemia has beneficial hemodynamic consequences. Perhaps the major implication of this paper is that, in detection of regression of atherosclerosis, examination of vascular reactivity may be far more sensitive than examination of structural changes by angiography.

VASCULAR RESPONSES TO PLATELETS

Several approaches indicate that atherosclerosis alters vascular reactivity. Responses to constrictor and dilator stimuli are altered in atherosclerotic arteries in vitro (1-5), in experimental animals in vivo

Atherosclerotic Plaques, Edited by R.W. Wissler *et al.*
Plenum Press, New York, 1991

(6), and in patients (7). Exaggeration of vasoconstrictor responses, combined with impairment of vasodilator responses, predispose to vasospasm, which is an important complication of atherosclerosis (8).

A major hypothesis concerning the pathophysiology of vasospasm focuses on the role of platelets (9). The hypothesis is that platelets adhere to damaged endothelium over atherosclerotic lesions, and the platelets aggregate and release their vasoactive products. We have examined effects of atherosclerosis on vascular responses to ADP, serotonin, and thromboxane, which are the three major products that are released by platelets.

When platelets aggregate in a normal artery, ex vivo, the potent vasodilator effects of adenosine diphosphate (ADP) usually mask the vasoconstrictor effects of thromboxane and the variable effects of serotonin, so that the net response is vasodilatation (10). Activation of platelets also produces vasodilatation in vivo, but we have performed several studies which indicate that atherosclerosis profoundly alters responses to vasoactive products that are released by platelets.

First, we examined vascular responses to injection of ADP, serotonin, and thromboxane. Several experimental approaches were used including studies of a limb that was perfused in vivo (6,11), measurement of blood flow with microspheres (12,13), and measurement of microvascular pressure (12). Vasodilator responses to ADP are impaired by atherosclerosis, vasodilator responses to serotonin are reversed to vasoconstriction, and vasoconstrictor responses to thromboxane are augmented (6,11). Vascular responses to these agonists are altered in atherosclerotic cynomolgus monkeys in several vascular beds: the limb (6,11), coronary arteries (12), and cerebral and ocular circulation (13). These studies indicate that vascular responses to ADP, serotonin, and thromboxane are altered by atherosclerosis in a direction that would favor augmented vasoconstriction or vasospasm when platelets aggregate.

Second, we have infused purified bovine collagen in the perfused limb of monkeys, to produce aggregation of platelets in vivo (14). Infusion of collagen produced vasodilatation in normal monkeys, presumably from release of ADP from platelets. In atherosclerotic cynomolgus monkeys, that were fed an atherogenic diet for 18 months, collagen produced marked constriction of large arteries. The constrictor effect was prevented by pretreatment of the monkeys with indomethacin. Thus, activation of platelets in vivo produces constriction of large atherosclerotic arteries. These findings support the hypothesis that, when platelets are activated in vivo, they may produce constriction or perhaps spasm of atherosclerotic arteries.

VASCULAR RESPONSES TO LEUKOCYTES

There are many leukocytes (primarily monocyte-macrophages) in atherosclerotic lesions (15). Blood-borne monocytes adhere to endothelium, and monocyte-macrophages are present within atherosclerotic lesions. A major hypothesis is that growth factors that are released by monocyte-macrophages may stimulate cellular migration and proliferation and thus play a critical role in the development and progression of the atherosclerotic lesion (15).

We have proposed a new hypothesis in relation to the role of leukocytes in atherosclerosis. The hypothesis is that leukocytes may contribute to spasm of atherosclerotic arteries.

The initial experimental evidence for this hypothesis was based on responses to injection of a peptide, f-met-leu-phe (fMLP), which activates leukocytes and releases their vasoactive products. Injection of fMLP had little effect in the limb of normal monkeys. In striking contrast, fMLP produced marked vasoconstriction in atherosclerotic monkeys (16). Thus, we speculate that activation of leukocytes within or on atherosclerotic arteries is capable of initiating constriction or perhaps spasm of atherosclerotic arteries.

Several vasoactive substances are released when leukocytes are activated. Oxygen-derived free radicals and several arachidonate metabolites, including thromboxane, prostaglandin E_2, and leukotrienes, are released by leukocytes. Our evidence suggests that prostaglandin E_2, which normally is a vasodilator, constricts large arteries in atherosclerotic monkeys (16), and thus may contribute to leukocyte-induced vasoconstriction. Oxygen-derived free radicals and thromboxane also may contribute to this response.

EFFECTS OF EARLY LESIONS

Most of our studies have been performed in monkeys that were fed an atherogenic diet for 18 months, and had moderately severe atherosclerotic lesions. At this stage of atherosclerosis, vascular responses are altered profoundly (6,11-13).

We have examined vascular responses after shorter periods of hypercholesterolemia. When monkeys are fed an atherogenic diet for 3-4 months they have pronounced hypercholesterolemia but they rarely have atherosclerotic lesions in peripheral arteries. At this stage, with hypercholesterolemia but before peripheral lesions develop, we have not been able to detect altered vascular responses (6,11).

When monkeys are fed an atherogenic diet for 8-10 months, they have very early atherosclerotic lesions in peripheral arteries (11). We found that vasodilator responses to ADP are impaired by early lesions, and vasoconstrictor responses to serotonin are potentiated. Thus, even early atherosclerotic lesions alter vascular responses in a direction that would favor augmented vasoconstriction or even vasospasm.

The finding that early atherosclerosis alters vascular responses provides strong evidence for the sensitivity of this approach in detection of lesions that almost certainly would not be detectable by angiography.

LIMITATIONS OF ANGIOGRAPHIC APPROACHES

Angiography clearly is effective at detection of focal vascular stenoses. Advances in quantitative angiography allow good quantitation of progression or regression of stenotic lesions.

Unfortunately, a major theoretical and practical limitation in quantitative angiography has emerged in the past decade. The concept that atherosclerotic arteries undergo "remodeling" presents a major, and perhaps insurmountable, obstacle to quantitation of atherosclerosis with angiography.

As originally demonstrated by Bond and colleagues (17), atherosclerotic lesions are displaced abluminally by remodeling of the vessel wall, so that the vascular lumen is preserved despite the presence of moderately severe lesions. This concept has received strong support in primates (18) and humans (19, 20). Thus, measurement of lumenal diameter even with quantitative angiography may grossly

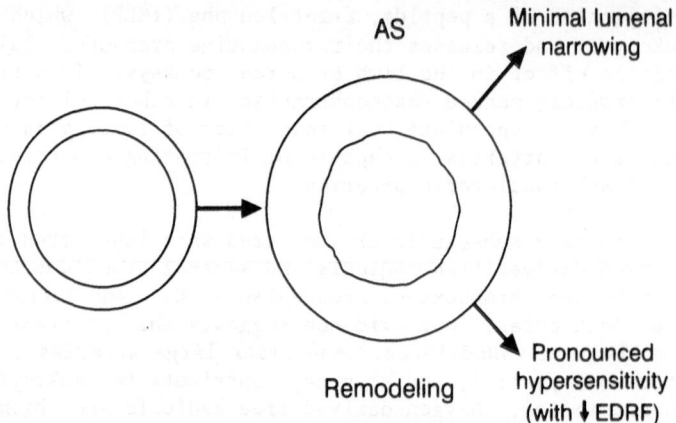

AS

Minimal lumenal
narrowing

Remodeling

Pronounced
hypersensitivity
(with ↓EDRF)

Figure 1. Atherosclerotic arteries undergo "remodeling",
as the vessel wall is displaced abluminally. Thus, there
may be minimal lumenal narrowing despite moderately severe
atherosclerotic lesions. Atherosclerotic arteries
manifest pronounced hypersensitivity to several stimuli,
which is related in part to decreased release of
endothelium-derived relaxing factor (EDRF).

underestimate the severity of atherosclerosis, because remodeling tends
to preserve the lumenal diameter despite moderately severe
atherosclerosis (Fig. 1).

It is likely that further remodeling occurs during regression of
atherosclerotic lesions, and thus compromises quantitation of regression
of atherosclerosis. This speculation is not yet well-supported by
experimental data. Nevertheless, it is clear that remodeling presents a
formidable problem in quantitation of progression and regression of
atherosclerosis with angiographic approaches.

MECHANISMS OF ALTERED VASCULAR REACTIVITY

A few years ago, several groups (including ours) proposed that
atherosclerosis produces endothelial dysfunction and thereby alters
vascular responses (1-4). A wide variety of vasoactive stimuli,
including ADP, serotonin, PGE$_2$, and platelets, release an endothelium-
derived relaxing factor (EDRF) in normal arteries. These stimuli fail
to produce relaxation, or may produce contraction, when endothelium is
removed from normal arteries.

In atherosclerotic arteries, endothelium is present but
endothelium-dependent relaxation is greatly impaired (1-4). Intimal
proliferation may present a barrier to diffusion of EDRF from
endothelium to vascular muscle. In addition, impairment of endothelium-
dependent relaxation by atherosclerosis may be the result primarily of
impaired release of EDRF from endothelium.

It is likely that impaired release of EDRF, which has been
demonstrated in vitro by bioassay (21), contributes to potentiation of
vasoconstrictor responses that we have observed in atherosclerotic
arteries in vivo. For example, impaired release of EDRF may result in
vasoconstrictor responses, instead of vasodilator responses, to
serotonin or aggregation of platelets by collagen in atherosclerotic
arteries. Although endothelial dysfunction almost certainly contributes
to alteration of vascular responses in atherosclerotic arteries in vivo,

we have not excluded the possibility that other mechanisms also play a major role. For example, an endothelium-derived contracting factor (EDCF) may be released by atherosclerotic arteries, or metabolism of vasoconstrictor agonists may be impaired by atherosclerosis.

Studies in patients suggest that endothelial function is abnormal in atherosclerotic arteries (7). Acetycholine produces coronary vasodilatation in patients whose vessels appear relatively normal. In contrast, acetylcholine produces coronary vasoconstriction in patients with stenotic lesions (7). These abnormal responses probably are related to endothelial dysfunction. It is of interest that patients with variant angina are especially likely to develop coronary vasospasm in response to acetylcholine (22). This hypersensitivity probably is related to endothelial dysfunction.

VASCULAR CHANGES IN CHRONIC HYPERTENSION

Chronic hypertension produces vascular changes which in some ways mimic those that occur in atherosclerosis. There are fundamental differences, however, in the vascular changes in chronic hypertension and atherosclerosis.

We have proposed that there is remodeling of hypertensive, as well as atherosclerotic, vessels (23). It is well-established that maximal vasodilator responses are impaired by chronic hypertension. Impairment of maximal vasodilatation has been attributed to vascular hypertrophy, with encroachment on the lumen. A puzzling finding, however, is that the increase in cross-sectional area of hypertensive vessels (i.e., the extent of vascular hypertrophy) is not sufficient to account for the reduction in area of the vascular lumen.

This observation led us to propose that a reduction in external diameter of blood vessels may play a major role in encroachment on the vascular lumen in chronic hypertension. We found that external diameter of cerebral arterioles is significantly less in stroke-prone spontaneously hypertensive rats (SHRSP) than in normotensive Wistar-Kyoto (WKY) rats (23). We calculated that the amount of hypertrophy accounts for less than one-fourth of the encroachment on the lumen, and reduction in external diameter accounts for more than three-fourths.

We have characterized reduction in external diameter of cerebral arterioles in SHRSP as "remodeling". Vascular remodeling results in reduction of the vascular lumen in chronic hypertension, and preservation of the lumen in atherosclerosis. In both disease states, however, vascular remodeling may be an adaptive and protective mechanism. In chronic hypertension, reduction in arteriolar diameter by remodeling tends to protect the distal vessels against elevated pressure. In atherosclerosis, preservation of arterial diameter by remodeling attenuates decreases in dilator capacity of the vessel.

There are functional as well as structural vascular changes in chronic hypertension. Vasodilator responses to endothelium-dependent agonists are impaired by chronic hypertension as well as by atherosclerosis. Luscher and Vanhoutte (24) demonstrated that the aorta of spontaneously hypertensive rats (SHR) releases an endothelium-derived contracting factor (EDCF). This factor is blocked by cyclooxygenase inhibitors, which suggests that it is either a prostanoid or an oxygen-derived radical that is a product of the cyclooxygenase pathway. Endothelium-dependent relaxation is impaired in the aorta of SHR, and responses are restored to normal by pretreatment with cyclooxygenase inhibitors (24).

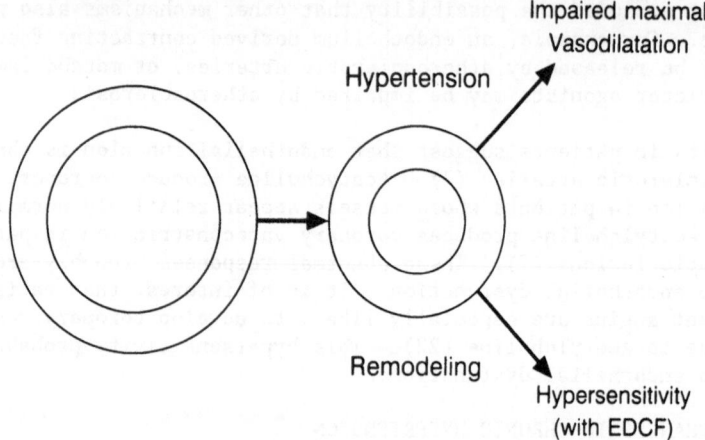

Impaired maximal
Vasodilatation

Hypertension

Remodeling

Hypersensitivity
(with EDCF)

Figure 2. In chronic hypertension, there is "remodeling"
of blood vessels, as the outer diameter of the vessel is
reduced. Remodeling and vascular hypertrophy lead to
encroachment on the vascular lumen, with impairment of
maximal vasodilatation. Hypertensive vessels also
manifest hypersensitivity to several stimuli, which is
related in part to release of an endothelium-derived
contracting factor (EDCF).

In the cerebral microcirculation of SHRSP, there is profound
impairment of vasodilator responses to endothelium-dependent agonists.
Dilator responses of cerebral arterioles to acetylcholine, ADP, and
serotonin, which are endothelium-dependent agonists, are profoundly
impaired in SHRSP (25,26). In contrast, dilator responses to adenosine
and nitroglycerin, which act directly on vascular muscle, are normal in
SHRSP. Indomethacin largely restores endothelium-dependent
vasodilatation to normal in SHRSP, which is consonant with the concept
that endothelium of SHRSP may release an EDCF (24,26)(Fig. 2).

Thus, responses to endothelium-dependent vasodilators are impaired
in both chronic hypertension and atherosclerosis. Mechanisms of
impairment, however, differ in hypertension and atherosclerosis. In
chronic hypertension, it appears that the primary mechanism by which
endothelium-dependent vasodilatation is impaired involves release of a
contracting factor (EDCF). In contrast, the primary mechanism by which
endothelium-dependent vasodilatation is impaired in atherosclerosis
probably involves impairment of release of EDRF.

REGRESSION OF ATHEROSCLEROSIS

A critical question is whether treatment of hypercholesterolemia is
beneficial. There are several types of answers to that question.

First, morphological evidence in primates provides strong evidence
for regression of atherosclerosis, with resorption of lipid from the
intima and reduction of intimal mass.

Second, epidemiological evidence indicates that treatment of
hypercholesterolemia in patients is beneficial.

Third, angiographic studies provide evidence that treatment of hypercholesterolemia impairs the progression, or may produce regression, of atherosclerotic lesions. In general, however, the magnitude of regression that has been demonstrated by angiographic studies is disappointingly small.

Fourth, we have examined maximal vasodilator responses after regression of atherosclerosis in primates. Despite clear morphological evidence of regression, characterized by decreased thickness of intima, there was no consistent improvement in maximal vasodilator capacity (27). Vascular fibrosis during regression probably compromises the recovery of maximal vasodilator capacity (28). This finding may have important functional implications. We speculate that exercise-induced angina and intermittent claudication, which are the result of impaired maximal vasodilatation, may not improve consistently despite regression of atherosclerosis.

Fifth, regression of atherosclerosis in primates has profound effects on vascular reactivity. Hyperresponsiveness to serotonin is abolished (29) and impaired vasodilator responses to ADP are restored to normal by regression of atherosclerosis. Regression of atherosclerosis also restores endothelium-dependent relaxation of vessels in vitro to normal (30). In light of the findings that augmented responses to vasoconstrictor stimuli are abolished by regression of atherosclerosis, we are optimistic that vasospastic disorders will improve during regression of lesions.

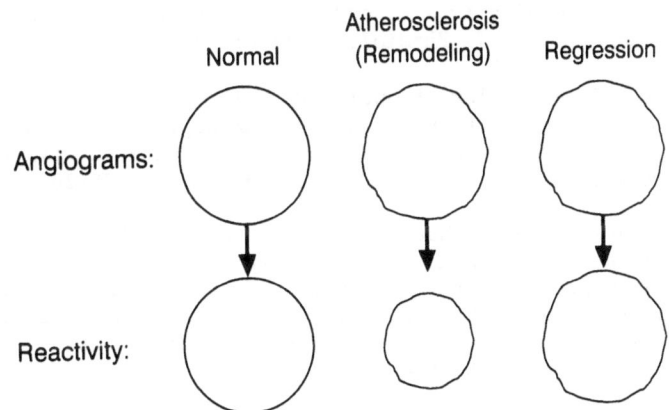

Figure 3. Schematic diagram of effects of atherosclerosis and regression on the arterial lumen. Remodeling and alterations in vascular reactivity have important implicatons for detection of atherosclerosis and regression. Remodeling tends to preserve the arterial lumen despite moderately severe atherosclerosis, and thus compromise the sensitivity of angiography in evaluation of severity of atherosclerosis and, presumably, regression of lesions. In contrast, vascular reactivity is altered even by early atherosclerosis, and may return to normal after regression. Thus, vascular reactivity may be a useful approach in evaluation of atherosclerosis and regression.

CONCLUSIONS

Atherosclerosis produces profound alteration of vascular responses. These changes in vascular reactivity result in striking potentiation of vasoconstrictor responses to some agonists. Alteration of vascular responses occurs early in the atherosclerotic process, and subsides with regression of atherosclerosis.

We speculate that examination of vascular reactivity may be a useful approach in evaluation of regression of atherosclerosis. The usefulness of angiographic approaches in evaluation of progression and regression of atherosclerosis is seriously compromised by vascular remodeling. We speculate that studies of vascular reactivity may be more sensitive and useful than angiographic approaches in evaluation of regression of atherosclerosis (Fig. 3)

ACKNOWLEDGMENTS

We thank Ms. Marge Keaough for typing the manuscript, and Mr. Donald Piegors, Keith Breese, and Ms. Pam Tomkins for technical assistance with the original studies described in this paper. Original studies were supported by a Medical Investigator Award, Associate Investigator Award, and research funds from the Veterans Administration, and by National Institutes of Health Grants HL 14230, NS 24621, HL 14388, and HL 16066.

REFERENCES

1. R.L. Jayakody, M.P.J. Senaratne, A.B.R. Thomson, C.T. Kappagoda, Cholesterol feeding impairs endothelium-dependent relaxation of rabbit aorta, *Can. J. Physiol. Pharmacol* 63:1206-1209 (1985).

2. J.B. Habib, C. Bossaller, S. Well, C. Willliams, J.D. Morrisett, P.D. Henry, Preservation of endothelium-dependent vascular relaxation in cholesterol-fed rabbits by treatment with the calcium blocker PN 200110. *Circulation Res* 58:305-309 (1986).

3. T.J. Verbeuren, F.H. Jordaens, L.L. Zonnekeyn, C.E. Van Hove, M.C. Coene, A.G. Herman, Effect of hypercholesterolemia on vascular reactivity in the rabbit. I. Endothelium-dependent and endothelium-independent contractions and relaxations in isolated arteries of control and hypercholesterolemic rabbits. *Circulation Res* 58:552-564 (1986).

4. P.C. Freiman, G.G. Mitchell, D.D. Heistad, M.L. Armstrong, and D.G. Harrison, Atherosclerosis impairs endothelium-dependent vascular relaxation to acetylcholine and thrombin in primates, *Circ Res* 58:783-789 (1986).

5. U. Förstermann, A. Mügge, U. Alheid, A. Haverich, and J.C. Frölich, Selective attenuation of endothelium-mediated vasodilation in atherosclerotic human coronary arteries, *Circ Res* 62:185-190 (1988).

6. D.D. Heistad, M.L. Armstrong, M. Marcus, D.J. Piegors, and A.L. Mark, Augmented responses to vasoconstrictor stimuli in hypercholesterolemic and atherosclerotic monkeys, *Circ Res* 54:711-718 (1984).

7. P.L. Ludmer, A.P. Selwyn, T.L. Shook, R.R. Wayne, G.H. Mudge, R.W. Alexander, and P. Ganz, Paradoxical vasoconstriction induced by acetylcholine in atherosclerotic coronary arteries, *N Engl J Med* 315:1046-1051 (1986).

8. A. Maseri, A. L'Abbate, G. Baroldi, S. Chierchia, M. Marzilli, A.M. Ballestra, S. Severi, O. Parodi, A. Biagini, A. Distante, and A. Pesola, Coronary vasospasm as a possible cause of myocardial infarction, *N Engl J Med* 299:1271-1277 (1978).

9. J. Willerson, D. Hillis, M. Winniford, and L. Buja, Speculation regarding mechanisms responsible for acute ischemic heart disease syndrome, *J Am Coll Cardiol* 8:245-250 (1986).

10 D.S. Houston, J.T. Shepherd, and P.M. Vanhoutte, Aggregating human platelets cause direct contraction and endothelium-dependent relaxation of isolated canine coronary arteries, *J Clin Invest* 78:539-544 (1986).

11 J.A.G. Lopez, M. Armstrong, D. Piegors, and D.D. Heistad, Effect of early and advanced atherosclerosis on vascular responses to serotonin, thromboxane A_2, and ADP, *Circulation* 79:698-705 (1989).

12 W.M. Chilian, K.C. Dellsperger, S.M. Layne, C.L. Eastham, M.A. Armstrong, M.L. Marcus, and D.D. Heistad, Effects of atherosclerosis on the coronary circulation, *Am J Physiol:Heart* 27:H529-539 (1990).

13 J.K. Williams, G.L. Baumbach, M.L. Armstrong, D.D. Heistad, Hypothesis: Vasoconstriction contributes to amaurosis fugax, *J Cereb Blood Flow Metab* 9:111-116 (1989).

14. J.A.G. Lopez, J.C. Hoak, M.L. Armstrong, D.J. Piegors, and D.D. Heistad, Effect of intravascular collagen in atherosclerotic primates, *J Am Coll Cardiol* (Abstract) 15:12A (1990).

15. R.G. Gerrity, The role of the monocyte in atherogenesis. Transition of blood-borne monocytes into foam cells in fatty lesions, *Am J Pathol* 103:181-190 (1981).

16. J.A.G. Lopez, M.L. Armstrong, D.G. Harrison, D.J. Piegors, and D.D. Heistad, Vascular responses to leukocyte products in atherosclerotic primates, *Circ Res* 65;1078-1086 (1989).

17. M.G. Bond, M.R. Adams, and B.C. Bullock, Complicating factors in evaluating coronary artery atherosclerosis, *Artery* 9:21-29 (1981).

18. M.L. Armstrong, D.D. Heistad, M.L. Marcus, M.B. Megan, and D.J. Piegors, Structural and hemodynamic responses of peripheral arteries of macaque monkeys to atherogenic diet, *Arteriosclerosis* 5:336-346 (1985).

19. S. Glagov, E. Weisenberg, C.K. Zarins, R. Stankunavicius, and G.J. Kolettis, Compensatory enlargement of human atherosclerotic coronary arteries, *N Engl J Med* 316:1371-1375 (1987).

20. D.D. McPherson, L.F. Hiratzka, W.C. Lamberth, B. Brandt, M. Hunt, R. A. Kieso, M.L. Marcus, and R.E. Kerber, Delineation of the extent of coronary atherosclerosis by high frequency epicardial echocardiography, *N Engl J Med* 316:304-309 (1987).

21. R. Guerra, Jr., A F.A. Brotherton, P.J. Goodwin, C.R. Clark, M.L. Armstrong, D.G. Harrison, Mechanisms of abnormal endothelium-dependent vascular relaxation in atherosclerosis: implications for altered autocrine and paracrine functions of EDRF, *Blood Vessels* 26:300-314 (1989).

22. H. Yasue, Y. Horio, N. Nakamura, H. Fujii, N. Imoto, R. Sonoda, K. Kugiyama, K. Obata, Y. Morikami, and T. Kimura, Induction of coronary artery spasm by acetylcholine in patients with variant angina: possible role of the parasympathetic nervous system in the pathogenesis of coronary artery spasm, *Circulation* 74:955-963 (1986).

23. G.L. Baumbach and D.D. Heistad, Remodeling of cerebral arterioles in chronic hypertension, *Hypertension* 13:968-972 (1989).

24. T.F. Luscher and P.M. Vanhoutte, Endothelium-dependent contractions to acetylcholine in the aorta of the spontaneously hypertensive rat, *Hypertension* 8:334-348 (1986).

25. W.G. Mayhan, F.M. Faraci, and D.D. Heistad, Impairment of endothelium-dependent responses of cerebral arterioles in chronic hypertension, *Am J Physiol: Heart Circ Physiol* 22:H1435-H1440 (1987).

26. W.G. Mayhan, F.M. Faraci, and D.D. Heistad, Responses of cerebral arterioles to adenosine 5'-diphosphate, serotonin, and the thromboxane analogue U-46619 during chronic hypertension, *Hypertension* 12:556-561 (1988).

27. M. Armstrong, D. Heistad, M. Marcus, D.J. Piegors, and F.M. Abboud, Hemodynamic sequelae of regression of experimental atherosclerosis, *J Clin Invest* 71:104-113 (1983).

28. D. Vesselinovitch and R.W. Wissler, Reversal of atherosclerosis: comparison of nonhuman primate models. In: "Atherosclerosis V," Gotto AM Jr., Smith LC and Allen B, eds., Springer-Verlag, New York (1980).

29. D.D. Heistad, A.L. Mark, M.L. Marcus, D.J. Piegors, and M.L. Armstrong, Dietary treatment of atherosclerosis abolishes hyperresponsiveness to serotonin: Implications for vasospasm, *Circ Res* 61:346-351 (1987).

30. D.G. Harrison, M.L. Armstrong, P.C. Freiman, and D.D. Heistad, Restoration of endothelium-dependent relaxation by dietary treatment of atherosclerosis, *J Clin Invest* 80:1808-1811 (1987).

Günter Siegel[1], Kirsten Rückborn[2], Axel Walter[1], Frank Schnalke[1], and Günter Stock[3]

[1] Institute of Physiology, Biophysical Research Group, The Free University of Berlin, 1000 Berlin 33, Germany
[2] Institute of Physiology, The University of Rostock, 2500 Rostock 1, Germany
[3] Cardiovascular Pharmacology, Research Laboratories of Schering, 1000 Berlin 65, Germany

INTRODUCTION

A variety of local or systemic influences regulate peripheral organ perfusion, e.g. K^+ ions, pH value, noradrenaline, prostacyclin, endothelial factors (1). With the multiplicity of effectors, and since several can be changed at the same time, the question of mechanism arises. To refer to Sherrington (2), it is important to find the "final common pathway" of their integration, even in the vascular smooth muscle cell. Electrophysiology opens up one approach to this problem. Nevertheless, biochemical processes in the cell membrane and in the cell interior have a part to play, particularly when the transmembrane passage of ions is modulated by the known intracellular second messengers like Ca^{2+}, cAMP, cGMP, GTP-binding proteins, protein kinase C and ATP (3). This study deals mainly with the regulation of smooth muscle tone by the membrane potential with voltage-gated channels predominating.

ELECTROMECHANICAL COUPLING AND VASODILATATION

Recording, for example, the membrane potential and tension as a function of the extracellular H^+ concentration, one can eliminate the effector parameter H^+ concentration and plot the developed tension against the membrane potential (4). When executing this procedure for a variety of effector influences, one arrives at the stationary activation curve (Fig. 1). We have used isolated segments of the canine common carotid artery in our studies. The sigmoid activation curve shows the resting potential of the vascular smooth muscle cells of about -60 mV. The depolarized portion of the curve between -60 and -40 mV is linear. This range can be obtained by application of noradrenaline, an increased extracellular K^+ concentration or a shift of the pH value of the blood substitute solution to the alkaline side. From the activation curve and the measured values it is quite clear that the same change in tone occurs with a defined change in membrane potential, no matter from which effector influence the latter originates (5). Thus, this curve serves as a strong indication for the existence of electromechanical coupling in vascular smooth muscle. We will deal only with the hyperpolarized part of

Atherosclerotic Plaques, Edited by R.W. Wissler *et al.*
Plenum Press, New York, 1991

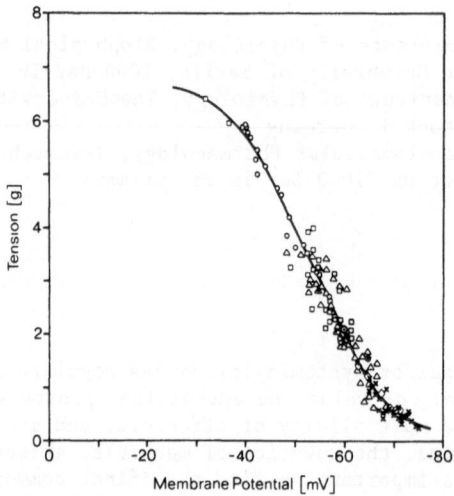

Fig. 1   Dependency of mechanical tension on the membrane potential in isolated carotid arteries (stationary activation curve). The membrane potential was changed by varying the extracellular concentration of H^+ (Δ), K^+ (□), Ca^{2+} (●), norepinephrine (o), or prostacyclin (◊) or by lowering the oxygen tension (x). The marked point on the curve (⊙) indicates membrane potential and mechanical force under control conditions.

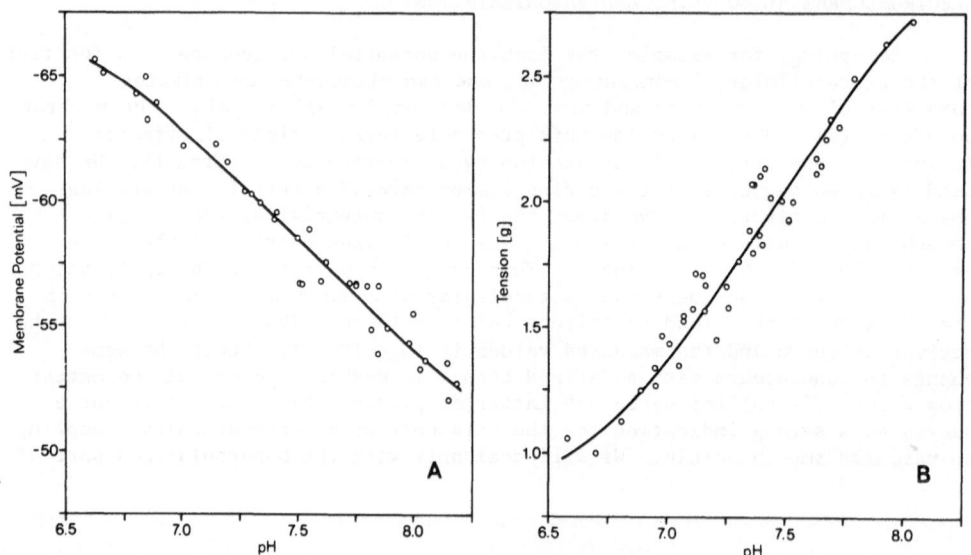

Fig. 2   (A) Membrane potential of vascular smooth muscle in relation to the external pH value of the Krebs solution. (B) Tension developed in isolated carotid segments as a function of the extracellular H^+ concentration.

262

the activation curve, in which vasodilatation occurs (6).

It is of clinical interest whether a membrane physiological correlate exists to the well-known vasodilatation with acidosis and vasoconstriction with alkalosis. The reason for these mechanical changes is a hyperpolarization with acidosis as well as a depolarization with alkalosis (Fig. 2). The voltage changes during acidification or alkalinization of the blood substitute solution are attributed to an increase in passive K^+ permeability and a simultaneous decrease in Na^+ permeability with acidosis (5), and inverse effects with alkalosis.

Prostacyclin (PGI_2), the main but unstable metabolite of arachidonic acid in vascular tissue, is often considered to be a vasorelaxing autacoid in hypoxic dilatation. In our studies we were interested to see whether the observed vasodilatation has an electrophysiologic correlation. Because of the extreme chemical instability of natural PGI_2, we used iloprost, a stable prostacyclin analogue. How a muscle additionally contracted by noradrenaline reacts to an application of iloprost is of particular interest to us. Fig. 3

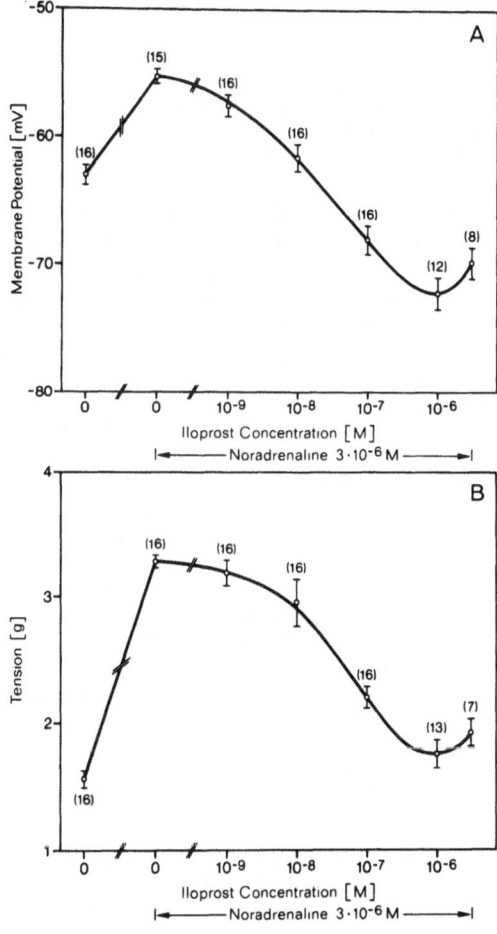

Fig. 3   Membrane potential (A) and mechanical force development (B) of noradrenaline-depolarized and contracted vascular strips of the canine carotid artery as a function of the iloprost concentration in the Krebs solution. The preparation was incubated for 10 minutes at each iloprost concentration step.

shows the effect iloprost has on the membrane potential depolarized by noradrenaline. After a noradrenaline application the potential was -55.2 mV. Iloprost repolarized and hyperpolarized the resting membrane by 20 mV maximally in a concentration-dependent manner (7). The depolarization is combined with contraction, the hyperpolarization with relaxation. The application of noradrenaline leads to a strong contraction which is abolished step by step as the iloprost concentrations increase. The initial tone, without noradrenaline, is almost attained.

A reduction of the oxygen partial pressure in general leads to vasodilatation in the systemic circulation. In our vessel strip preparations of the canine carotid artery, the lowering of O_2 partial pressure in the incubation medium with normal CO_2 partial pressure leads to membrane hyperpolarization and a decrease in tone of the smooth muscle cells as soon as values lower than 150 mm Hg are reached (Fig. 4A). Maximum values of both alterations are obtained at oxygen partial pressures around 35 mm Hg (8). A further decrease of P_{O2} below 30 mm Hg induces a relative depolarization of the cell membrane and a contraction of smooth musculature. Products of the arachidonic acid metabolism are considered to be possible mediators of the observed cell reactions. In order to elucidate the importance of eicosanoids for the P_{O2}-dependent changes in potential and tone of the vascular muscle cells, comparable investigations were carried out following inhibition of cyclooxygenase by indomethacin (10^{-5} mol/l), after complete removal of the endothelium or after destruction of the adrenergic nerve endings by 6-hydroxydopamine (1.8 x 10^{-3} mol/l).

Fig. 4 illustrates the results under control conditions (a), in indomethacin-treated (b), deendothelialized (c), and in 6-hydroxydopamine-preincubated preparations (d). The following quantitative conclusions can be drawn from the steady state changes in voltage and tone in the carbogen Krebs solution, and from the alterations of the courses of the curves at variable P_{O2} about the participation of the different vasodilatory and vasoconstricting factors. In the basal release, and also in the changes in direction of membrane hyperpolarization and vasorelaxation at variable P_{O2} prostacyclin appears to take effect at 20-30%, the endothelial dilator EDHF at 70-80% (8, 9). The share of EDHF may be underestimated by a few percent because the hyperpolarization and the relaxation seen in the curves (c) reflect the release of PGI_2 from vascular smooth muscle cells. Moreover, we must consider that the endogenous release of noradrenaline, which steadily increases with falling oxygen tension, prevents an even more pronounced membrane hyperpolarization and vasorelaxation than demonstrated in curve (a). Below P_{O2} levels of 35 mm Hg, the effect of noradrenaline is quite distinct and is decisively involved in the reversal of the voltage and tension curve (10). Under these O_2 partial pressures, endothelin and/or products of the cytochrome P-450 pathway may also have a part to play, as the depolarization and contraction observed could not be completely abolished by an α-receptor blockade (regitine 5 x 10^{-4} mol/l) or by the application of 6-hydroxydopamine. It may be concluded that the response of vascular smooth musculature to a decline in the oxygen tension represents a balanced interplay between hyperpolarizing-vasodilatory (PGI_2/EDHF) and depolarizing-vasoconstrictory factors (noradrenaline, endothelin, 12-HETE). The same holds true for the adjustment of muscle tone under stationary resting conditions (P_{O2} = 535 mm Hg) because all these compounds have a basal release.

Whether this concept of hypoxia-induced vascular reactions can be transferred to humans, and in which way it has to be modified in pathological conditions, was examined by experiments using human blood vessels. In Fig. 5 one recognizes how the lowering of O_2 partial pressure influences membrane potential and tension of vascular smooth muscle cells in coronary arteries taken from heart transplant patients. Circles represent the results of

264

control experiments and squares the results of atherosclerotic vessel segments. Voltage and tension as a function of P_{O2} show courses similar to those which we have already described in the canine carotid. There is a continuous hyperpolarization and relaxation with a reduction of P_{O2} from 535 mm Hg to 35 mm Hg and a depolarization and contraction between 35 and 0 mm Hg. It is striking that in the case of atherosclerosis, vascular smooth muscle cells are more depolarized and have more tone. This is true for all O_2 tensions. The endothelial function is possibly limited in this tissue. Iloprost, in a concentration of 10^{-7} mol/l, is able to induce additional hyperpolarization and relaxation at all O_2 partial pressures, even with maximal hyperpolarization and dilatation at about 35 mm Hg P_{O2} (7, 9). In

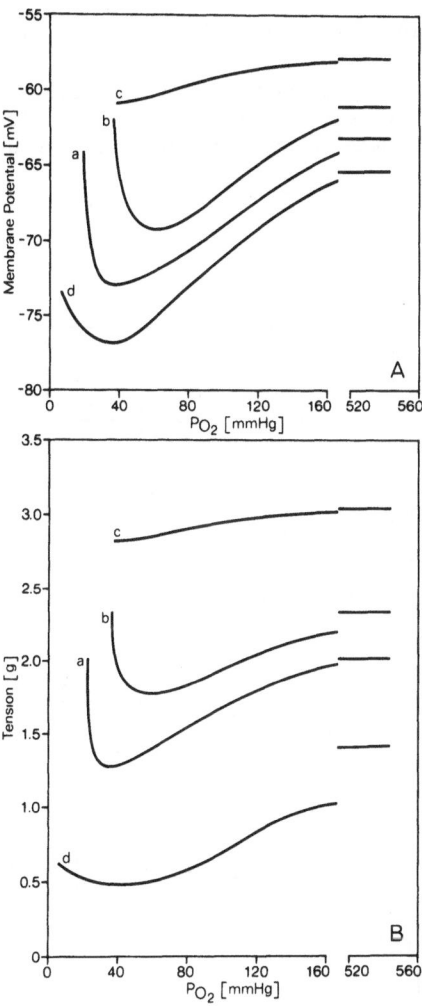

Fig. 4   Membrane potential (A) and tension (B) in isolated vascular strips of the A. carotis communis of the dog in dependency on the oxygen partial pressure of the Krebs solution. Mean values from 28 experiments. a: normal Krebs solution; b: Krebs solution with indomethacin (10^{-5} mol/l); c: normal Krebs solution, endothelial layer of the carotid segments removed; d: normal Krebs solution, preparations pretreated by 6-hydroxydopamine (1.8×10^{-3} mol/l).

normal and in atherosclerotic blood vessels, the hypoxic depolarization and
contraction with oxygen pressure below 35 mm Hg is prevented by iloprost. A
quantitative examination between normal and arteriosclerotic coronary arteries
gives the following results. When the P_{O2} is reduced from 535 to 35 mm Hg,
the relaxation in arteriosclerotic vessels is diminished by 51.2% in
comparison to normal vessels. Under the same conditions, but with the
addition of prostacyclin (iloprost 10^{-7} mol/l), this reduction is only 38.7%.
It is possible that the PGI_2 production and release in arteriosclerotic
arteries is decreased with hypoxia. Thus prostacyclin would imply a
protective effect. This is supported by the findings that in the control
experiments an overrelaxation of 62.3% occurs when the P_{O2} is reduced from 535
to 35 mm Hg and iloprost is also applied. This overrelaxation amounts to
103.6% with arteriosclerotic vessels in the test series.

K^+ CHANNEL OPENING AND VASORELAXATION

In the preceeding paragraph physiologically relevant vasodilators were
cited. To determine whether each of these factors has its own mechanism
leading to a membrane potential change in the direction of hyperpolarization,

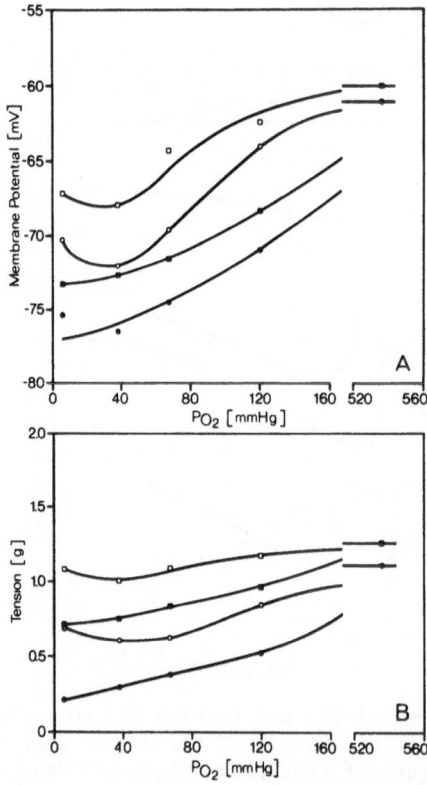

Fig. 5   Membrane potential (A) and tension (B) in isolated vascular strips
of human coronary arteries dependent on the oxygen partial
pressure of the Krebs solution. Mean values from 5 experiments
each. (o) normal coronary arteries with intact endothelium, (•) +
iloprost 10^{-7} mol/l; (□) atherosclerotic coronary arteries, (■) +
iloprost 10^{-7} mol/l.

we first used classical membrane physiology. We started with the investigation of mass fluxes to single channel analysis, the application of the Ussing-Teorell's flux ratio (11, 12) via the equations of Hodgkin, Huxley, and Katz (13) to the Goldman relationship (14).

The observed vasorelaxation with acidification, exogenous application of prostacyclin, or decrease in O_2 partial pressure are preceded by membrane hyperpolarization of the vascular smooth muscle cells. Hyperpolarization can be effected by an increase in K^+ permeability of the cell membrane, a decrease in Na^+ permeability or a stimulation of active, electrogenic Na^+ outward transport. Fig. 6 is a semilogarithmic plot of the $^{42}K^+$ efflux curves of segments of a basilar artery at pH steps 6.8, 7.3, and 7.8. The flux curves have a regularly graded pH-dependent course. The bold curves represent the optimal functions calculated by computer. In the process of fitting, the three amplitudes and time constants of the e-functions were computed and utilized in a detailed compartment model for flux determination. Close inspection of the flux curves reveals that the slowest exchange (phase 3) occurs with almost identical time constant at all pH steps, whereas exchange phase 2 has the smallest time constant at pH 6.8, the largest at pH 7.8 (left inset). In addition, the amplitude falls regularly with increasing pH, which likewise indicates a flux reduction with alkalinization.

It was possible to draw conclusions about corresponding changes of K^+ current and permeability from the pH-dependent alterations of individual compartments and kinetic coefficients. K^+ current and permeability increase with acidification and decrease with alkalinization, while Na^+ ions show the inverse behavior (Table 1). This indicates that membrane hyperpolarization of vascular smooth muscle cells under acidosis is causally due to a rise in passive K^+ permeability with simultaneous fall in passive Na^+ permeability (15).

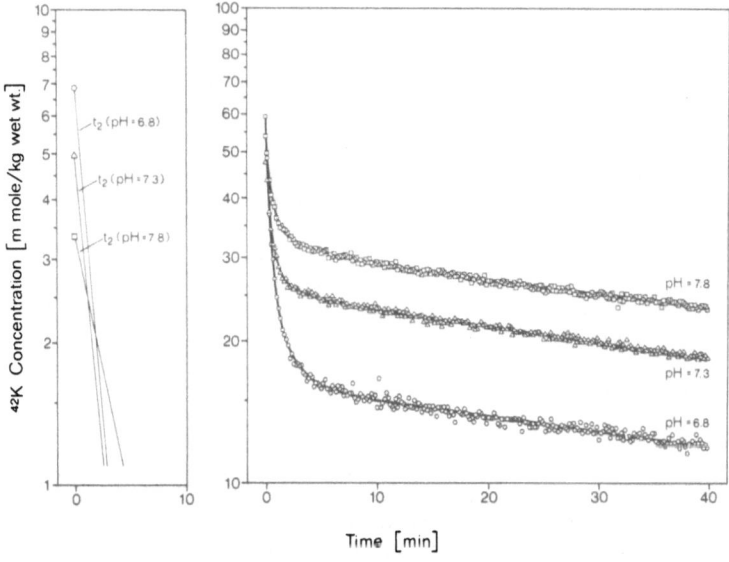

Time [min]

Fig. 6 $^{42}K^+$ efflux in the basilar artery of the dog according to the direct method in Krebs solutions with pH 6.8 (o), 7.3 (Δ), and 7.8 (□). The graph shows the time course of radioactive K^+ decrease within the preparations at intervals of 10 s in single experiments. The superimposed lines represent the optimal triple-exponential functions found by computer fitting. In the left inset the pH-dependent exchange phases 2 are represented separately.

Table 1.   Effects of external pH changes on ionic current (I) and permeability (P) in vascular smooth muscle of the basilar artery of the dog.

	pH = 6.8	pH = 7.3	pH = 7.8
I_{Na} [$\mu A/cm^2$]	-0.28	-0.52	-0.62
P_{Na} [cm/s x 10^{-9}]	8.80	18.32	23.41
I_K [$\mu A/cm^2$]	3.69	2.13	1.69
P_K [cm/s x 10^{-6}]	1.00	0.56	0.40
$P_K : P_{Na}$	113.8	30.5	17.3

Table 2.   Membrane potentials (V), equilibrium potentials (E), ionic currents (I), and permeabilities (P) in canine carotid vascular smooth muscle

	Control	+Iloprost (10^{-6} mol/1)
V [mV]	-63.4 ± 0.6 (19)	-70.8 ± 0.9 (16)
E_{Na} [mV]	+35.5	+38.6
E_K [mV]	-86.3	-85.3
I_{Na} [$\mu A/cm^2$]	- 1.29	- 2.00
P_{Na} [cm/s x 10^{-8}]	3.48	4.89
I_K [$\mu A/cm^2$]	0.87	2.23
P_K [cm/s x 10^{-6}]	0.54	2.40
$P_K : P_{Na}$	15.6	49.2

These results led to the question of how prostacyclin effects hyperpolarization of the cell membrane. $^{24}Na^+/^{42}K^+$ efflux experiments carried out by double tracer techniques (7) and patch-clamp investigations in the whole cell configuration (16), substantiated the finding of an increased open state probability of K^+ channels under the influence of iloprost (Table 2). There were no changes in intracellular concentrations of Na^+ and K^+ ions and their equilibrium potentials, but transmembrane Na^+ current and permeability were slightly increased. However, K^+ current and permeability were markedly increased (7, 16). The rise in Na^+ permeability by 40% and in K^+ permeability by 340% with iloprost demonstrates that following treatment with this drug the permeability of the cell membrane increases drastically and almost selectively for K^+ ions (9). The resulting membrane hyperpolarization could effect relaxation via T-type Ca^{2+} channels that were recently discovered by means of patch-clamp techniques (17). The open state probability of these Ca^{2+} channels, the activation curve of which lies between -80 mV and -40 mV decreases voltage-dependently with hyperpolarization. The Ca^{2+} inward current which elicits contraction or which triggers the release of calcium from internal storage sites is suppressed. The consequence would be a fall in intracellular Ca^{2+} activity and thus vasodilatation.

CATION BINDING IN VASCULAR CONNECTIVE TISSUE

What we have discussed up to now as an explanation for the membrane potential changes which is documented in Tables 1 and 2 is based on the application of classical membrane physiological concepts. In an organ whose cells are surrounded by closely meshed connective tissue structures, it is questionable whether the ion concentrations in the tiny crevices on both sides of the cell membrane can be considered as stationary over time, especially with changes of physical state functions, e.g., the pH value, or with rhythmically active tissues (5). So, diffusion problems may play an important role. This even more, since at the barriers which surround these spaces and in the compartments themselves a reversible binding of ions takes place. We know that not only in the basement membrane, but also in the cell membrane,

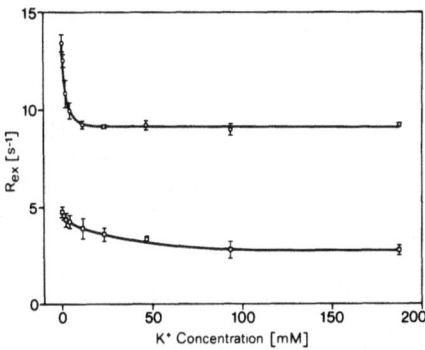

Fig. 7 $^{23}Na^+$ excess transverse (o) and longitudinal relaxation rates (□) for titration of native vascular connective tissue with KCl in Krebs solution (pH 7.3). The K^+ concentration at the start of the titration was 0.2 mmol/l.

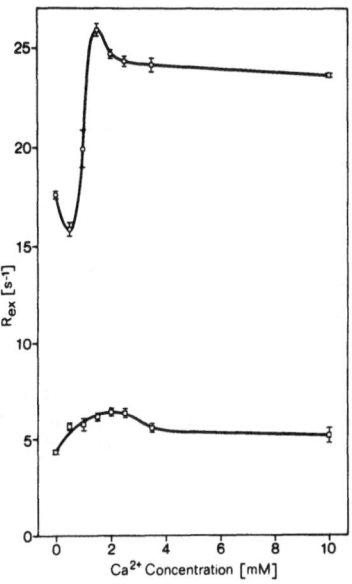

Fig. 8 $^{23}Na^+$ excess longitudinal (□) and transverse relaxation rates (O), R_{1ex} and R_{2ex} in dependence on different Ca^{2+} concentrations of a normal Krebs solution ($[Na^+]_o = 151.2$ mmol/l) containing native vascular connective tissue at pH 7.3. For 0.5 mmol/l $< [Ca^{2+}]_o <$ 1.5 mmol/l the ratio R_{1ex}/R_{2ex} is indicative of a conformational transition in the connective tissue polyanions. In addition, the initial rise of the longitudinal relaxation rate signifies allosteric, cooperative Na^+ binding to the matrix macromolecules.

269

polyanionic macromolecules, namely the proteoglycans, interact permanently with small cations. Therefore, we have tried to address these problems with a new approach, the nuclear magnetic resonance technique.

In Fig. 7 the excess longitudinal (R_1) and the transverse relaxation rates (R_2) of $^{23}Na^+$ nuclear magnetic resonance spectra of adventitial connective tissue are shown as a function of increasing K^+ concentrations. In this competition experiment, the 'Na$^+$ salt' of the glycosaminoglycans bound to their natural protein component, as they are in native vascular connective tissue, can be studied under in vivo conditions. With increasing K^+ concentration, Na^+ ions are displaced from their binding sites by K^+ ions according to the mass action law and released into the blood substitute solution (18). As the relaxation rates, in our case of Na^+ ions ($^{23}Na^+$ - NMR), are a measure for the ratio of bound to free ions, both rates decrease with increasing K^+ concentrations as an expression of a falling bound Na^+ fraction. In extreme cases R_1 and R_2 go down to the relaxation rates of free Na^+ ions.

Fig. 8 shows another competition experiment, however, with Ca^{2+} ions as the counterion species. As with K^+ ions, the transverse relaxation rate decreases to 0.5 mmol/l Ca^{2+} but then increases steeply with further additions of $CaCl_2$ to 1.5 mmol/l. In contrast to the K^+ competition experiment, R_1 already increases with the first additions of Ca^{2+}. Calculating the correlation times from the ratio of the relaxation rates leads to an abrupt increase for small Ca^{2+} concentrations in the range between 0.5 and 1.5 mmol/l (Fig. 9). This means reduced local mobility of the Na^+ ions which is due to a

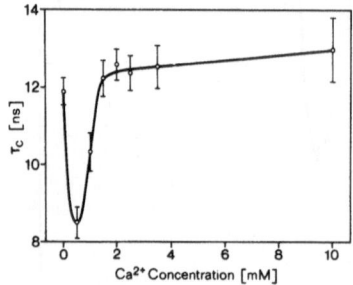

Fig. 9   Correlation time for sodium ions bound to native vascular connective tissue as a function of the Ca^{2+} concentration of a Krebs solution at pH 7.3. The ratio R_{1ex}/R_{2ex} was used in the calculation of τ_c.

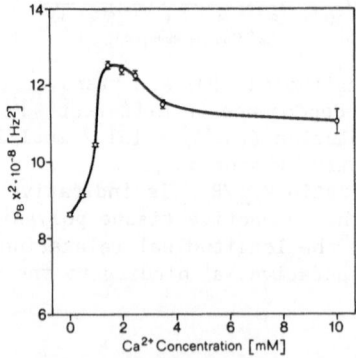

Fig. 10 $p_B x^2$, the product of the fraction of bound Na^+ and the squared quadrupolar coupling constant, as a function of the Ca^{2+} concentration of a 151.2 mmol/l Na^+ Krebs solution containing native vascular connective tissue at pH 7.3.

conformational transition of the connective tissue polyanions (19). The half-maximal conformational change is observed with 1.15 mmol/l Ca^{2+}, i.e., in the physiologically relevant range, considering that half of the serum Ca^{2+} of 2.5 mmol/l is bound to proteins.

The static contribution to relaxation, i.e., the Na^+ binding, may be calculated using both relaxation rates and correlation times (Fig. 10). The bound Na^+ fraction increases at once and reaches a maximal augmentation of 50% with 1.5 mmol/l Ca^{2+} concentration. Therefore, the elevation of the Ca^{2+} concentration in the blood substitute solution does not effect an expulsion of Na^+ ions from their binding sites, but on the contrary it induces an allosteric Na^+ adsorption to the polyanionic macromolecules of vascular connective tissue (5, 18, 20).

These investigations which were carried out on proteoglycans isolated from vascular connnective tissue, on native connective tissue, and on proteoglycans, e.g., heparan sulfate derived from the cell membrane of smooth muscle, show that the microenvironment of these structures is largely determined by their ion binding properties. For example, the allosteric Na^+ binding to the polyanions of vascular connective tissue induced by Ca^{2+} ions can lead to a transient reduction of the extracellular Na^+ concentration in the narrow tissue clefts between basement membrane and cell membrane (18). The consequence would be a reduction in Na^+ equilibrium potential and thus membrane hyperpolarization with vasorelaxation.

The chemical composition of these barriers might be changed pathophysiologically, or to be more specific, pathobiochemically. Therefore, we have started to investigate changes of the ion binding of human vascular connective tissue during aging, atherosclerosis, or hypertension. The changes in the grade of sulfate addition and the affinity constant, particularly for Ca^{2+} ions, are of special importance in these cases. Thus the field is wide open for physiologically and clinically oriented basic research.

ACKNOWLEDGEMENTS

The authors thank Mrs Ch Fuhrmann and Mr H Ewald for their skillful technical assistance. We are grateful to Mrs M Krawczynski for her outstanding work in preparing the illustrations and to Mr P Holzner for the photographic work. Thanks are due to Mrs A Scheuermann for her editorial help with the manuscript.

REFERENCES

1. G. Siegel, Membranphysiologische Grundlagen der peripheren Gefäßregulation, Physiol. akt. 1:31 (1986).
2. C. S. Sherrington, Correlation of reflexes and the principle of the common path, Brit. Ass. Rep. 728 (1904).
3. N. S. Cook, The pharmacology of potassium channels and their therapeutic potential, Trends Pharmacol. Sci. 9:21 (1988).
4. G. Siegel and W. Schneider, Anions, cations, membrane potential, and relaxation, in: "Vasodilatation," P. M. Vanhoutte and I. Leusen, eds., Raven Press, New York (1981).
5. G. Siegel, A. Walter, M. Bostanjoglo, A. W. H. Jans, R. Kinne, L. Piculell, and B. Lindman, Ion transport and cation-polyanion interactions in vascular biomembranes, J. Membrane Sci. 41:353 (1989).
6. G. Siegel, M. Bostanjoglo, M. Thiel, A. Adler, A. Carl, G. Stock, and J. Grote, Membranphysiologische Mechanismen der Vasodilatation, in: "Frühveränderungen bei der Atherogenese," E. Betz, ed., W. Zuckschwerdt Verlag, München (1987).
7. G. Siegel, A. Carl, A. Adler, and G. Stock, Effect of the prostacyclin

analogue iloprost on K⁺ permeability in the smooth muscle cells of the canine carotid artery, <u>Eicosanoids</u> 2:213 (1989).

8. G. Siegel and J. Grote, P_{O2}-induced changes of membrane potential and tension in vascular smooth musculature, <u>in</u>: "Oxygen Sensing in Tissues," H. Acker, ed., Springer-Verlag, Berlin (1988).

9. G. Siegel, F. Schnalke, G. Stock, and J. Grote, Prostacyclin, endothelium-derived relaxing factor and vasodilatation, <u>Adv. Prostaglandin Thromboxane Leukotriene Res.</u> 19:267 (1989).

10. G. Siegel, J. Grote, F. Schnalke, and K. Zimmer, The significance of the endothelium for hypoxic vasodilatation, <u>Z. Kardiol.</u> 78, Suppl. 6:124 (1989).

11. H. H. Ussing, The distinction by means of tracers between active transport and diffusion, <u>Acta Physiol. Scand.</u> 19:43 (1950).

12. T. Teorell, Membrane electrophoresis in relation to bioelectrical polarization effects, <u>Arch. Sci. Physiol.</u> 3:205 (1949).

13. A. L. Hodgkin, A. F. Huxley, and B. Katz, Measurement of current-voltage relations in the membrane of the giant axon of <u>Loligo</u>, <u>J. Physiol. (Lond.)</u> 116:424 (1952).

14. D. E. Goldman, Potential, impedance, and rectification in membranes, <u>J. Gen. Physiol.</u> 27:37 (1943).

15. G. Siegel, The effect of external pH changes on Na⁺ and K⁺ permeabilities in the smooth muscle fibre membrane of canine cerebral vessels, <u>J. Physiol. (Lond.)</u> 329:56P (1982).

16. G. Siegel, J. Mironneau, F. Schnalke, G. Schröder, B.-G. Schulz, and J. Grote, Vasodilatation evoked by K⁺ channel opening, <u>Prog. Clin. Biol. Res.</u> 327:299 (1990).

17. G. Loirand, P. Pacaud, C. Mironneau, and J. Mironneau, Evidence for two distinct calcium channels in rat vascular smooth muscle cells in short-term primary culture, <u>Pflügers Arch.</u> 407:566 (1986).

18. G. Siegel, A. Walter, A. W. H. Jans, and R. Kinne, Binding of mono- and divalent cations to different components of the extracellular matrix, <u>Abhandl. Rhein.-Westf. Akad. Wissensch.</u> 82:155 (1989).

19. H. Gustavsson, G. Siegel, B. Lindman, and L.-Å. Fransson, ²³Na⁺-NMR studies of cation binding to multichain and single-chain glycosaminoglycan peptides, <u>Biochim. Biophys. Acta</u> 677:23 (1981).

20. G. Siegel, A. Walter, and B. Lindman, Cation binding to anionic biopolymers of vascular connective tissue, <u>J. Phys. (Paris)</u> 45:C2-595 (1984).

EFFECT OF NATIVE AND OXIDIZED LDL ON VASCULAR TONE

Jan Galle and Eberhard Bassenge

Department of Applied Physiology
University of Freiburg
Hermann-Herderstr.7, D-7800 Freiburg, FRG

INTRODUCTION

The atherogenic properties of low density lipoproteins (LDL) are well established, and recent evidence suggests that oxidation of LDL is an important step in atherogenesis (1). However, it remains controversial whether lipoproteins *directly* affect arterial endothelial function or smooth muscle tone. Several studies showed impairment of endothelium-mediated vasodilation in hypercholesterolemia in animals and humans (2, 3), and an arterial hyperresponsiveness to different vasoconstrictors in hypercholesterolemic animals (2, 4, 5). In in vitro investigations, it was found that both Human Native (n) LDL and Oxidized (ox) LDL can be cytotoxic to endothelial cells (6), and recently it was proposed that high concentrations of LDL inhibit endothelium-derived relaxing factor (EDRF) formation via the endothelial LDL-receptor (7).

In hypercholesterolemia, n-LDL and ox-LDL are found in the arterial wall (8), and might therefore exert direct vasomotor effects. Since the vascular tone represents a net balance between vasoconstrictor and vasodilator influences (9), we investigated the effects of LDL and its oxidized derivative on transfer and formation of EDRF, and on vascular smooth muscle tone.

MATERIAL AND METHODS

Preparation and oxidative modification of LDL

n-LDL was prepared from fresh human plasma by sequential ultracentrifugation in the presence of antioxidants and proteolysis inhibitors as recently described (10). For the oxidative modification, n-LDL was separated from the antioxidants and incubated with Cu^{++} 10 μM. The degree of oxidation was detected by increase in electrophoretic mobility, increase in diene formation (11), and apoprotein B100 fractionation (SDS-PAGE, 11). LDL was then concentrated, purified by gel filtration, and sterilized by filtration (millex, Millipore). Stock solutions of the lipoproteins were kept in the dark at 4°C for no longer than three weeks.

Drugs

Phenylephrine, indomethacin, serotonin, bradykinin, thimerosal, and verapamil were purchased from Sigma (Munich, FRG). Indomethacin was dissolved in ethanol-0.1 M NaHCO₃ (1:3) vol/vol and diluted with Tyrode's solution. Norepinephrine (Arterenol) (Hoechst, Frankfurt, FRG), diltiazem hydrochloride (Dilzem) (Goedecke, Berlin, FRG), and acetylcholine hydrochloride (Sigma, Munich, FRG) were also dissolved in Tyrode's solution. Nitrendipine (Bayer, Leverkusen, FRG) was dissolved in absolute ethanol, and further diluted with Tyrode's solution.

Bioassay experiments

Endothelial cell culture. Bovine aortic endothelial cells were isolated and cultured as described elsewhere in detail (12). Briefly, the endothelium was scraped off freshly obtained aortae and grown on standard culture dishes. For bioassay experiments with endothelium-denuded artery segments, cells were subcultured on microcarrier beads (Biosilon, Nunc-Intermed, Wiesbaden, FRG), and packed into a column. The endothelial cell column was perfused with oxygenated Tyrode's solution (pO₂ about 140 mm Hg) at a rate of 30 ml/h, and stimulated for continuous EDRF-release with thimerosal (5 uM) (13). The outflow tubing of the cell column was connected with the inflow cannula of a preconstricted artery segment which served as detector for EDRF (Fig. 1). The dilator compound released from the cell columns was characterized as EDRF as in earlier experiments (12). To investigate whether lipoproteins inactivate *released* EDRF, the lipoproteins were applied distally to the endothelial cell columns by a T-connection (Fig. 1). The perfusion rate through this branch was 1/10 of that through the endothelial cell columns, and the lipoproteins (stock solution concentration: 10 mg/ml) were administered here at a final concentration of 1 mg/ml.

While testing the inhibitory action of lipoproteins, a second detector segment not perfused with the lipoproteins served as control for continuous and stable EDRF-release. The effluent of the endothelial cell columns was perfused alternatively through the segments.

Inactivation of EDRF by the lipoproteins is expressed as percent of the vasodilations in the absence of lipoproteins.

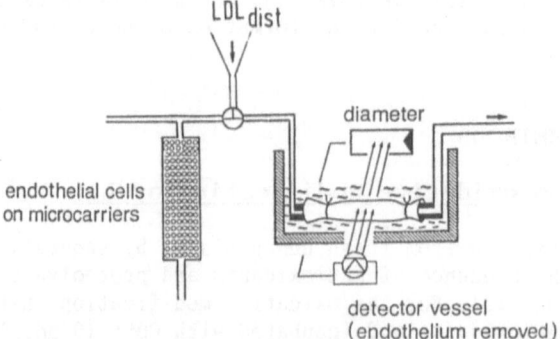

Figure 1. Experimental setup used for bioassay of EDRF released from cultured endothelial cells after stimulation with thimerosal (5 μM). A preconstricted, endothelium-denuded detector vessel was perfused either by the EDRF containing effluent of an endothelial cell column or by Tyrode's solution. Lipoproteins were administered distally to the endothelial cell column. External diameter of the detector segment was recorded by a photoelectrical device.

Vessel preparation. Intact segments of the femoral artery were obtained from rabbits of either sex (2.5-3.5 kg). For part of the experiments, the endothelium was removed mechanically. Intactness or absence of endothelium was tested as described earlier (14). The segments were fixed between two steel cannulas and placed in an organ bath (37°c) containing oxygenated Tyrode's solution (pH 7.4). The solution was perfused through the organ bath at a rate of 0.66 ml/min. In addition to organ bath perfusion the segments were perfused intraluminally (Tyrode's solution: PO_2 130 mmHg, PCO_2 28 mmHg, pH 7.38, at a rate of 0.5 ml/min). Outer vascular diameters were recorded continuously by a photoelectric device. The transmural pressure was adjusted hydrostatically to 40 mmHg (isobaric conditions). The resting diameter under these conditions was 1755 ±22 μm (n=28). Full details of this experimental set-up have been published (14). Endothelium-dependent vasodilations before and after 1 hour incubation with n-LDL or ox-LDL (1 mg/ml) were elicited by intraluminal perfusion with cumulative doses of acetylcholine (0.03 - 1 μM). For bioassay experiments, the segments were preconstricted with norepinephrine (0.1 μM) applied to the organ bath, and the effluent of the endothelial cell columns was perfused intraluminally through the endothelium-denuded segments as described above. Since ox-LDL has an enhancing effect on norepinephrine-induced vasoconstrictions (10), the norepinephrine concentration in the organ bath was lowered in the presence of ox-LDL to achieve the same level of preconstriction as under reference conditions without ox-LDL.

The effects of the lipoproteins on smooth muscle tone were tested in each experiment in one pair of vascular segments with and without endothelium mounted in two separate organ bath chambers simultaneously. n-LDL (50-500 μg), ox-LDL (50-500 μg/ml), acetylcholine (Ach, 0.5 μM), indomethacin (10 μm), verapamil (1 μM), diltiazem (10 μM) and nitrendipine (1 μM) were administered at the intimal side by adding to the intraluminal perfusate. Norepinephrine (NE, 1-100 nM), phenylephrine (PE, 0.01-1 μM), serotonin (5-HT, 0.01-1 μM) and potassium (K^+, 20-40 mM) were added to the organ bath (if not otherwise indicated). For experiments with (sub)threshold concentrations of the contractile agonists, concentrations were chosen which evoked no or minimal vasoconstrictions. Concentration-response relations of NE and PE with and without ox-LDL were performed by adding the compounds to the intraluminal perfusate.

In an additional series of experiments, we compared the influence of n-LDL and ox-LDL on endothelium-dependent vasorelaxations in arterial ring preparations with those in arterial segments. Pairs of rings and segments were prepared from the same rabbit aorta. The aortic segments and the femoral segments were investigated similarily. The aortic rings (4 mm in diameter, 3 mm wide) were mounted on a force transducer (Biegestab K 30, H. Sachs, Hugstetten, FRG) under 1.5 g resting tension, and superfused with oxygenated Tyrode's solution (95% O_2 - 5% CO_2, pH 7.4, 37 °C, 40 ml/h). After 30 min equilibration time, the rings were precontracted with norepinephrine (0.1 μM), and endothelium-dependent relaxation was elicited by 1 μM acetylcholine before and after 30 min superfusion with 1 mg/ml n-LDL, ox-LDL, or Tyrode's solution without lipoproteins (control). Relaxation is expressed as percent of precontraction.

Statistics

All data are presented as means ± SEM. Paired Student's t test was used to evaluate statistical significance of differences. For multiple comparison of data, Bonferroni's correction was performed. $p \leq 0.05$ was considered to be statistically significant.

Inactivation by n-LDL and ox-LDL of EDRF released from cultured endothelial cells

Fig. 2a illustrates the EDRF-inactivating effect of n-LDL (1 mg/ml) on a detector segment preconstricted with norepinephrine. The EDRF-mediated vasodilation of the detector segment was markedly reduced when n-LDL was added to the effluent of an endothelial cell column. The same holds true for administration of ox-LDL. Fig. 2b illustrates the time course of the EDRF-inactivation by n-LDL during continous EDRF-perfusion of a detector segment. Addition of n-LDL to the effluent caused immediate suppression of the vasodilation, which was also immmediatly reversible when the n-LDL perfusion was stopped. Addition of n-LDL reduced the vasodilations of the detector segments by 38.5 ±5.3%, and addition of ox-LDL by 55.5 ±4.6% (n=12).

Endothelium-mediated dilatation in perfused femoral segments preincubated with n-LDL and ox-LDL

Dose-response relations of preconstricted rabbit femoral arteries to acetylcholine before and after 1 hour incubation with n-LDL or ox-LDL (1 mg/ml) are shown in Fig. 3a and 3b. Throughout the whole concentration range, dilations to acetylcholine did not differ significantly between lipoprotein-incubated segments and control segments. Thus, n-LDL and ox-LDL did not impair acetylcholine induced endothelium-dependent vasodilations in perfused segments.

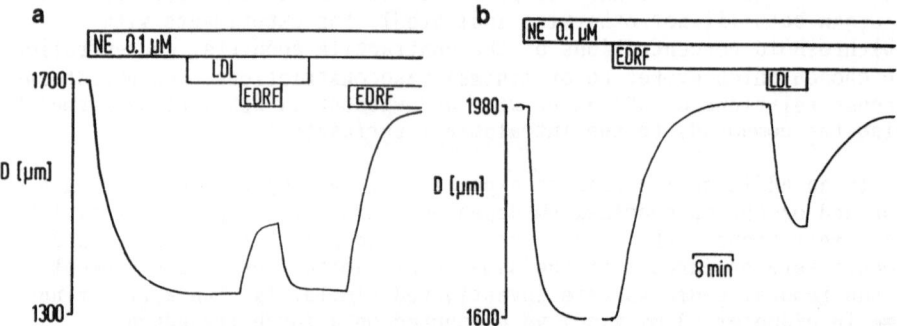

Figure 2a/2b. Diameter (D) recordings of an endothelium-denuded rabbit femoral artery segment, perfused with either Tyrode's solution or the EDRF-containing effluent from an endothelial cell column. The detector segment was preconstricted with norepinephrine 0.1 μM, and vasodilations were elicited by switching the intra-luminal perfusate from Tyrode's solution to the EDRF containing effluent from the endothelial cell column.
a) In presence of n-LDL (1 mg/ml) added to the effluent *distally* to the endothelial cell column, the EDRF-mediated vasodilation was markedly reduced.
b) Adding n-LDL to the EDRF-containing effluent caused *immediate* suppression of the vasodilation, which was also immediately reversible.

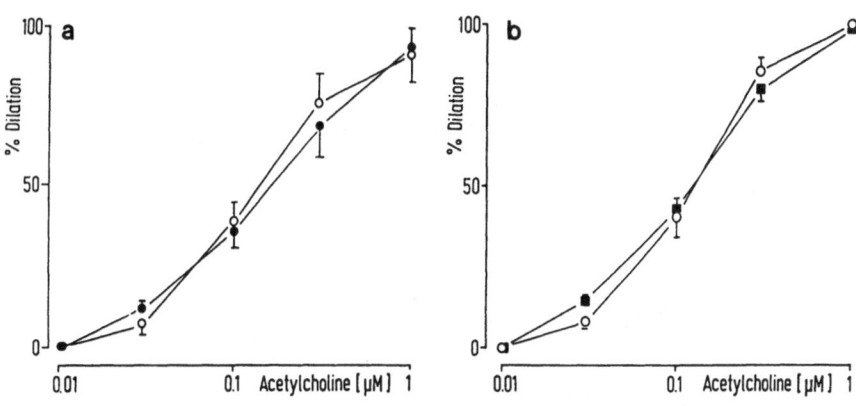

Figure 3a/3b. Vasodilations evoked by acetylcholine in intact rabbit femoral artery segments prior and after 1 h incubation with 1 mg/ml n-LDL or ox-LDL. Acetylcholine was perfused intraluminally through the segments in cumulative dosages (0.03, 0.1, 0.3, 1 µM). Vasodilations are expressed as % of preconstriction (induced by norepinephrine 0.1 µM).
a) Vasodilations before (control, -o-) and after incubation with n-LDL (-•-).
n = 7
b) Vasodilations before (control, -o-) and after incubation with ox-LDL (-■-).
n = 9
The vasodilations did not differ significantly.

Comparison of the influence of n-LDL on endothelium-dependent relaxations in aortic rings and aortic segments

As in femoral segments, vasodilations of aortic segments to acetylcholine (1 µM) were not impaired after 1 hour incubation with 1 mg/ml n-LDL: 81 ± 5% dilation before vs. 79 ± 5% dilation after incubation with n-LDL (n = 4). In contrast, relaxations of aortic rings to acetylcholine (1 µM) were significantly (p < 0.05) reduced after 30 min superfusion with 1 mg/ml n-LDL (73 ±7% vs. 44 ±9% relaxation, n = 8) or ox-LDL (82 ±7% vs. 56 ±7% relaxation, n = 6). Relaxations of control rings without incubation with lipoproteins did not change within this time interval.

Effects of n-LDL and ox-LDL upon stimulated segments

Intraluminal perfusion of unstimulated segments (no contractile agonists present in the organ bath) with n-LDL or ox-LDL caused no or only weak vasoconstrictions. However, as shown by the diameter recording in Fig. 4, ox-LDL caused markedly augmented contractile responses in the presence of the contractile agonist phenylephrine (PE), which was administered at threshold concentrations.

Similar enhancement of contractile responses was observed with the agonists norepinephrine (NE), serotonin, and potassium. n-LDL did not enhance the contractile responses to these agonists. For each agonist, the enhancement was significantly greater in endothelium-denuded than in endothelium-intact segments.

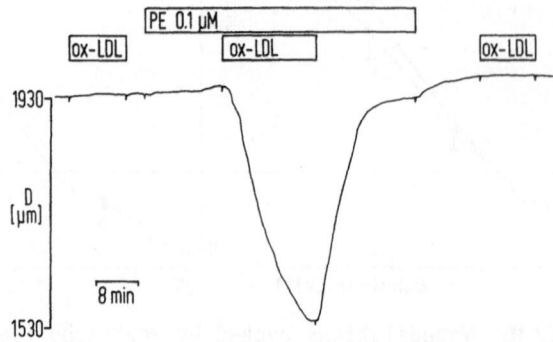

Figure 4. Diameter (D) recording of a rabbit femoral artery segment, intraluminally perfused with ox-LDL (80 µg/ml) either in absence or in presence of phenylephrine (PE) in subthreshold concentration (0.1 µM). ox-LDL caused no vasoconstriction on its own, but substantial vasoconstriction in presence of phenyl ephrine. Bars indicate the presence of ox-LDL or phenylephrine.

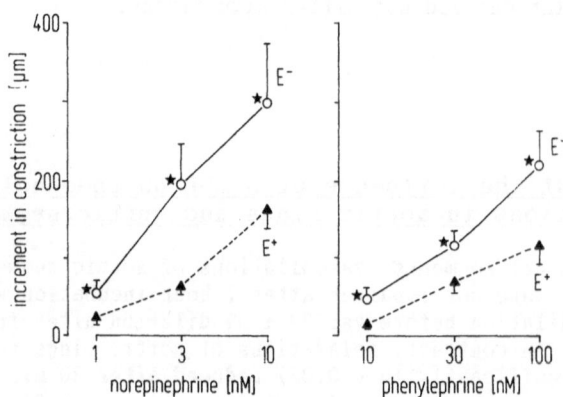

Figure 5. Increase in potency of norepinephrine (NE) and phenylephrine (PE) by ox-LDL in rabbit femoral arteries. NE (0.3-10 nM) and PE (0.3-30 nM) were administered in cumulative doses to the intraluminal perfusion, with and without ox-LDL (80 µg/ml). Triangles represent increments of contractile responses (means ± SEM) to NE (left) and PE (right) when ox-LDL was additionally administered to the intraluminal perfusion of endothelium-intact (E⁺) segments; circles represent increments of contractile responses by ox-LDL in endothelium-denuded (E⁻) segments. In segments without endothelium, the increments of contractile responses were significantly greater than in segments with endothelium. Ox-LDL alone caused no vasoconstriction.
* = $p < 0.05$

In the case of NE and PE, cumulative concentration-response relations were obtained with and without ox-LDL. As shown in Fig. 5, ox-LDL increased the potency of NE and PE in endothelium-intact and endothelium-denuded segments. Again, the enhancement of the contractile response was significantly greater in endothelium-denuded than in endothelium-intact segments.

Effects of Ca^{2+}-antagonists and indomethacin upon ox-LDL evoked vasoconstrictions

To investigate whether the ox-LDL evoked vasoconstrictions are linked to a transmembraneous Ca^{2+}-influx, we preincubated segments with three structurally different types of Ca^{2+}-channel blockers: diltiazem, verapamil and nitrendipine. As shown in Fig. 6, the ox-LDL induced vasoconstrictions were nearly equally suppressed by diltiazem, verapamil and nitrendipine in the presence of norepinephrine. These inhibitory effects were more pronounced in endothelium-denuded than in endothelium-intact segments.

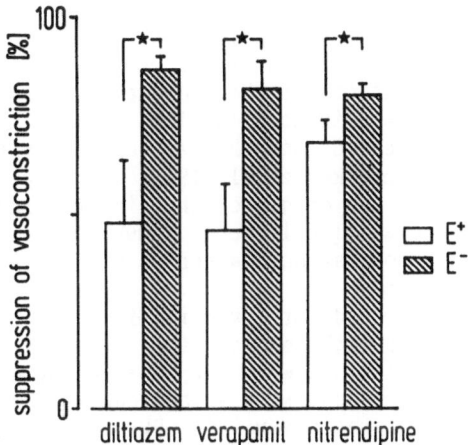

Figure 6. Suppression of ox-LDL (80 µg/ml) evoked contractile responses by the Ca^{2+}-antagonists verapamil (1 µM), diltiazem (10 µM), and nitrendipine (1 µm) in presence of norepinephrine (n = 6). Suppression is expressed in percent of the contractile response. The suppression by diltiazem, verapamil, and nitrendipine was more effective in endothelium-denuded (E$^-$) than in endothelium-intact (E$^+$) segments. * = p < 0.05.

Results similar to those obtained in the presence of norepinephrine were also found in the absence of contractile agonists. The vasoconstriction induced by ox-LDL alone was reduced by verapamil by 52 ± 4% (diltiazem: 65 ± 6%) in endothelium-intact segments, and by 71 ± 5% (diltiazem: 77 ± 5%) in endothelium-denuded segments (n = 6). When the segments were perfused with the cyclooxygenase inhibitor indomethacin (10 µM), no change in the potentiation of contractile responses to ox-LDL was detected.

DISCUSSION

The data presented in this study suggest that both n-LDL and ox-LDL inactivate EDRF after its release from endothelial cells, and that unlike native LDL, its oxidized derivatives enhance contractile responses of the isolated rabbit femoral artery to various agonists. Endothelium-dependent vasodilations were reduced only in arterial *ring* preparations, but not in *intact segments* after 1 h incubation with n-LDL and ox-LDL.

There is strong evidence suggesting that both native and oxidized LDL are present in the arterial wall in hypercholesterolemia (8). Thus, it is conceivable that the inactivation of EDRF by n-LDL and ox-LDL contributes to the impairment of endothelial function in hypercholesterolemia, as it has been observed in numerous studies (2, 4, 15). Also, the markedly reduced responsiveness of atherosclerotic arteries to EDRF/NO-superfusion (16) can be explained by this direct inactivating effect of n-LDL and ox-LDL accumulating in fatty streaks and atherosclerotic plaques. Furthermore, the increased responsiveness to vasoconstricting agents observed in arteriosclerotic human (2) and animal arteries (2, 4, 5, 15) and their increased disposition for vasospasms might be explained by the potentiating effect of ox-LDL on vascular smooth muscle contractions. However, our observation that a short exposure (1 hour) to neither n-LDL nor to ox-LDL attenuates endothelium-dependent vasodilation in intact segments, is in contrast to conclusions drawn by others. In studies performed with arterial *strip* preparations, Andrews et al (7) and Tomita et al (17) found impairment of endothelium-dependent vasodilations already after less then 30 min incubation with `native` LDL. Henry and associates observed impairment of endothelial function with ox-LDL (2 hours incubation) (18), and Vedernikov et al (19) found, dependent on the route of LDL-application and on the origin of the lipoproteins, both endothelium-dependent vasorelaxation induced by LDL and impairment of acetylcholine-induced vasodilations (after 30 min LDL-incubation).

Different techniques used for investigation of effects of the lipoproteins on vasomotion might explain the various findings. While endothelium-mediated vasodilations were not impaired by n-LDL and ox-LDL in *intact segments*, these responses were significantly reduced after incubation of arterial *ring* preparations with n-LDL or ox-LDL. Immersed in the lipoproteins-containing solution, the access of n-LDL and ox-LDL to the smooth muscle layers of the media might be much better in *ring* or *strip* preparations than in segments, where the lipoproteins initially (added from the intraluminal side) have to surmount the endothelial barrier to reach the subintimal space. The rapid infiltration of the wall would render the direct EDRF-inactivating effect of n-LDL and ox-LDL, and thus explain the attenuation of endothelium-dependent vasodilations in ring and strip preparations (7, 17, 19, 20) after relatively short exposure to lipoproteins.

In general, a comparison of the cited studies on n-LDL or ox-LDL is difficult. Absence of adequate measures against lipid peroxidation favors the development of oxidatively modified LDL. Hence, without adequate detection of the oxidative state of the LDL preparation (17, 19), the observed effects can not be attributed unequivocally to `native` LDL. In the present study, the effects of ox-LDL on endothelium-dependent vasomotion did not differ significantly from those of n-LDL. However, `oxidized LDL` is not clearly defined. During the lipid peroxidation process, a variety of partly unstable biologically active substances is formed (21). ox-LDL can be cytotoxic to endothelial cells (6), but its composition can differ depending on the plasma origin and the oxidative conditions (21). With respect to this problem, we used lipoproteins prepared following a standardized protocol in all the systems studied. A biological test for our standardization was the ability of oxidized LDL to potentiate vasoconstrictions.

The fact that EDRF-formation was not attenuated by one hour incubation with the potentially cytotoxic ox-LDL can be explained by the rather short incubation time, which must be clearly differentiated from long-term exposure. Thus, we may have missed cytotoxic effects of ox-LDL occuring after more protracted incubation.

The molecular mechanism responsible for inactivation of EDRF/NO by LDL is unknown. A possible desensitization of the vascular smooth muscle to EDRF by the lipoproteins seems unlikely. When n-LDL was added in the bioassay experiments *during* continuous EDRF-perfusion of the detector segment, vasodilations were suppressed immediately. Also, the suppression was immediately reversible by lipoprotein washout. This suggests rather a direct inactivation of EDRF by the lipoproteins than an effect on the target organ smooth muscle. The highly hydrophobic core of the LDL particle may act as a sink for EDRF/NO, which is about 8-fold more soluble in hydrophobic than in hydrophilic media (22). The NO radical could be consumed by reaction with hydrocarbonic radicals inside the LDL particle. However, the exact mechanism of NO inactivation by LDL remains to be clarified.

The mechanism of the ox-LDL-induced enhancement of contractile responses also remains to be determined. The enhancing effect was observed in endothelium-intact segments, and, even more pronounced, in endothelium-denuded segments, providing evidence that the site of action is at the smooth muscle itself rather than at the endothelium. Further evidence that the endothelium was not involved in the enhancing mechanism is based on an undisturbed production of EDRF even after 2 h incubation of the segments with ox-LDL in concentrations which already markedly augmented agonist-induced vasoconstrictions. This certainly does not rule out that ox-LDL can be cytotoxic; but if so, it would predominantly act on the smooth muscle cells. The fact that the enhancing effect of ox-LDL was more pronounced in endothelium-denuded segments might be due to the loss of basal release of EDRF (23). This enhancement of contractile responses following endothelium removal has already been described in earlier studies (9, 23).

The suppressor effect of the Ca^{2+}-antagonists on vasoconstrictions elicited by ox-LDL both in the presence and in the absence of contractile agonists suggests that ox-LDL induces predominantly an increased transmembraneous Ca^{2+}-influx. However, an additional release of Ca^{2+} from intracellular stores cannot be excluded.

The possibility that ox-LDL sensitizes the contractile apparatus to Ca^{2+} is less likely. The enhancing effect started after a few minutes, and washout also reversed the effect within ten minutes. It is not conceivable that ox-LDL enters and leaves the smooth muscle cells within this short period of time.

Since the enhancing effect is observed with various receptor binding agonists, and also with the receptor-independent K^+-depolarisation, ox-LDL seems to act distally to the receptor-coupled signal transduction cascade. One can speculate that ox-LDL modulates via stimulation of phosphatidylinositol metabolism the voltage-gated Ca^{2+}-channels and thus the transmembraneous Ca^{2+}-influxes in the plasma membrane. However, further investigation is needed to clarify the molecular mechanism.

In conclusion, our findings suggest that both native and oxidized LDL directly inactivate EDRF, and that oxidized LDL enhances agonist induced vasoconstrictions by direct interaction with vascular smooth muscle. EDRF-mediated vasodilations were suppressed only in arterial ring preparations, but not in intact segments. These mechanisms may be of particular pathophysiological relevance in regions with lipoprotein accumulation in the vessel wall and may favor the initiation of inappropriate vasoconstriction.

REFERENCES

1. Steinberg, D., Parthasarathy, S., Carew, T. E., Khoo, J. C., Witztum, J. L., Beyond cholesterol: Modifications of low-density lipoprotein that increase its atherogenicity, N. Engl. J. Med., 320:915-924 (1989)

2. Bossaller, C., Habib, G. B., Yamamoto, H., Williams, C., Wells, S., Henry, P. D., Impaired muscarinic endothelium-dependent relaxation and cyclic guanosine 5'-monophosphate formation in atherosclerotic human coronary artery and rabbit aorta, J. Clin. Invest., 79:170-174 (1987)

3. Verbeuren, T., Jordaens, F., Zonnekeyn, L., Van Hove, C., Coene, M., Herman, A., 1. Endothelium-dependent and endothelium-independent contractions and relaxations in isolated arteries of control and hypercholesterolemic rabbits, Circ. Res., 58:552-564 (1986)

4. Tomoike, H., Egashira, K., Yamamoto, Y., Nakamura, M., Enhanced responsiveness of smooth muscle, impaired endothelium-dependent relaxation and the genesis of coronary spasm, Am. J. Cardiol., 63:33E-39E (1989)

5. Heistad, D. D., Armstrong, M. L., Marcus, M. L., Piegors, D. J., Mark, A. L., Augmented responses to vasoconstrictor stimuli in hypercholesterolemic and atherosclerotic monkeys, Circ. Res., 54:711-718 (1984)

6. Hennig, B., Chow, C. K., Lipid peroxidation and endothelial cell injury: implications in atherosclerosis, Free Radical Biol. Med., 4:99-106 (1988)

7. Andrews, H. E., Bruckdorfer, K. R., Dunn, R. C., Jacobs, M., Low-density lipoproteins inhibit endothelium-dependent relaxation in rabbit aorta, Nature, 327:237-239 (1987)

8. Ylä-Herttuala, S., Palinsky, W., Rosenfeld, M. E., Parthasarathy, S., Carew, T. E., Butler, S., Witzum, J. L., Steinberg, D., Evidence for the presence of oxidatively modified low density lipoprotein in atherosclerotic lesions of rabbit and man, J. Clin. Invest., 84:1086-1095 (1989)

9. Bassenge, E., Busse, R., Endothelial modulation of coronary tone, Prog. Cardiovasc. Dis., 30:349-380 (1988)

10. Galle, J., Bassenge, E., Busse, R., Oxidized low density lipoproteins potentiate vasoconstrictions to various contractile agonists by direct interaction with vascular smooth muscle, Circ. Res., 66:1287-1293 (1990)

11. Steinbrecher, U. P., Witztum, J. L., Parthasarathy, S., Steinberg, D., Decrease in reactive amino groups during oxidation or endothelial cell modification of LDL. Correlation with changes in receptor-mediated catabolism, Arteriosclerosis, 7:135-143 (1987)

12. Lückhoff, A., Busse, R., Winter, I., Bassenge, E., Characterization of vascular relaxant factor released from cultured endothelial cells, Hypertension, 9:295-303 (1987)

13. Förstermann, U., Goppelt-Strübe, M., Frölich, J. C., Busse, R., Inhibitors of acyl-coenzyme A: lysolecithin acyltranferase activate the production of endothelium-derived vascular relaxing factor, J. Pharmacol. Exp. Ther., 238:352-359 (1986)

14. Busse, R., Pohl, U., Kellner, C., Klemm, U., Endothelial cells are involved in the vasodilatory response to hypoxia, Pflügers Arch., 397:78-80 (1983)

15. Hof, R. P., Hof, A., Vasoconstrictor and vasodilator effects in normal and atherosclerotic conscious rabbits, Br. J. Pharmacol., 95:1075-1080 (1988)

16. Verbeuren, T. J., Jordaens, F. H., VanHove, C. E., VanHoydonck, A. E., Herman, A. G., Release and vascular activity of the endothelium-derived relaxant factor in atherosclerotic rabbit aorta, Eur. J. Pharma., in press (1990)

17. Tomita, T., Ezaki, M., Miwa, M., Nakamura, K., Inoue, Y., Rapid and reversible inhibition by low density lipoprotein of the endothelium-dependent relaxation to hemostatic substances in porcine coronary arteries. Heat and acid labile factors in low density lipoprotein mediate the inhibition, Circ. Res., 66:18-27 (1990)

18. Kugiyama, K., Bucay, M., Morrisett, J. D., Roberts, R., Henry, P. D., Oxidized LDL impairs endothelium-dependent arterial relaxation, Circulation, 80 (Suppl 2):279 (1989)

19. Vedernikov, Y., Lankin, V., Tikhaze, A., Vikhert, A., Lipoproteins as factors in vessel tone and reactivity modulation, Basic Res. Cardiol., 83:590-596 (1988)

20. Kugiyama, K., Kerns, S. A., Morrisett, J. D., Roberts, R., Henry, P. D., Impairment of endothelium-dependent arterial relaxation by lysolecithin in modified low density lipoproteins, Nature, 344:160-162 (1990)

21. Esterbauer, H., Rotheneder, M., Striegel, G., Waeg, G., Ashy, A., Sattler, W., Jürgens, G., Vitamin E and other lipophilic antioxidants protect LDL against oxidation, Fat. Sci. Technol., 8:316-324 (1989)

22. Link, W. F., Solubilities of Inorganic and Metal-organic Compounds. American Chemical Society, Washington, D.C., 1965, Vol. 2, 4th Ed., p. 792,

23. Griffith, T. M., Henderson, A. H., Edwards, D. H., Lewis, M. J., Isolated perfused rabbit coronary artery and aortic strip preparations: the role of endothelium-derived relaxant factor, J. Physiol. (London), 351:13-24 (1984)

DUAL CONTROL BY NERVES AND ENDOTHELIAL CELLS OF ARTERIAL BLOOD FLOW IN

ATHEROSCLEROSIS

Geoffrey Burnstock, Anne Stewart-Lee, Antonia Brizzolara,
Annette Tomlinson and Laura Corr

Department of Anatomy and Developmental Biology and Centre
for Neuroscience, University College London, Gower Street,
London WC1E 6BT, U.K.

SUMMARY

(1)   Changes in the responses of vessels taken from Watanabe Heritable
       Hyperlipidaemic (WHHL) rabbits during the development of
       atherosclerosis at 4, 6 and 12 months were compared with those of
       vessels from control New Zealand White (NZW) rabbits at equivalent
       ages.

(2)   In vessels with severe atherosclerotic lesions (e.g. thoracic aorta)
       endothelial-mediated vasodilatation is attenuated, while direct
       responses to vascular smooth muscle are little changed.

(3)   In most other vessels (including mesenteric, hepatic, ear, coronary
       and saphenous arteries), where over 90% of endothelial cells appeared
       normal, endothelial-mediated vasodilator responses to acetylcholine
       and substance P were enhanced by 12 months in WHHL rabbits, while
       direct muscle vasoconstrictor and vasodilator responses showed
       gradual decline. Control NZW rabbits showed decline in both
       endothelial-mediated and direct muscle responses during the same
       period.

(4)   The basilar artery from WHHL rabbits showed little morphological
       evidence of serious lesions in either endothelial cells or smooth
       muscle up to 12 months, although endothelium-mediated vasodilatation
       was enhanced. This suggests that morphological criteria for
       assessing atherosclerotic damage do not necessarily correlate with
       changes in function.

(5)   Diminished sympathetic nerve-mediated vasoconstriction was
       demonstrated in 12-month-old WHHL mesenteric and hepatic arteries,
       although there was no reduction in adrenoceptor-mediated muscle
       responses.

(6)   It is suggested that the enhanced endothelial-mediated responses in
       these vessels may explain the well-known 'compensatory
       vasodilatation' characteristic of enlarged vessels in early
       atherosclerosis in which the lumen is not diminished and may even be
       enhanced. Speculations are made about the mechanism of enhanced
       endothelial-mediated vasodilatation. It is suggested that reduced

Atherosclerotic Plaques, Edited by R.W. Wissler *et al.*
Plenum Press, New York, 1991

nerve-mediated contraction may be an additional 'trophic' response contributing to 'compensatory vasodilatation' in early atherosclerosis. This study reinforces the view that different vessels respond differently in atherosclerosis and that there are marked variations with age and between the sexes in the changes occurring in the same vessel.

INTRODUCTION

There have been some dramatic changes in our understanding of the mechanisms involved in the local control of blood flow in recent years and these are reviewed briefly, before examining how atherosclerosis in the Watanabe Heritable Hyperlipidaemic (WHHL) rabbit affects these mechanisms. This study was inspired by Professor Giorgio Weber who introduced us to this atherosclerotic model in 1987 for collaborative experiments on cerebral arteries.

CONTROL OF BLOOD FLOW IN NORMAL VESSELS

There is dual control of blood flow in vessels by perivascular nerves located at the adventitial-medial border and by endothelial cells in the intima (see Lincoln and Burnstock, 1990).

Regulation of blood flow by perivascular nerves

For many years, studies of the neurohumoral control of the vasculature were dominated by the consideration of the role of noradrenaline (NA) released from sympathetic perivascular nerves (Burnstock, 1975). Attention was also drawn to the cholinergic innervation of some blood vessels (Borodulya and Pletchkova, 1976; Burnstock, 1980).

In recent years, however, non-adrenergic, non-cholinergic components of the autonomic nervous system have been discovered and, especially with the development of fluorescence immunohistochemical methods for localizing peptides and monoamines, more than 12 neurotransmitters are now considered to be involved in the neural control of the vasculature (Burnstock and Griffith, 1988). Vascular neuroeffector control mechanisms involving cotransmission and pre- and post-junctional neuromodulation have also been recognized (Burnstock, 1986, 1990a).

Combinations of transmitters have been described in different nerves supplying visceral and cardiovascular systems and some major patterns are emerging. For example, adenosine 5'-triphosphate (ATP) and neuropeptide Y (NPY) appear to coexist in various proportions with NA in sympathetic nerves supplying different target sites (Burnstock, 1986; Stjärne and Lundberg, 1986); NA and ATP appear to act as cotransmitters (Burnstock, 1988), while NPY is often utilized as a pre- and/or postjunctional modulator (Lundberg et al., 1985). Vasoactive intestinal polypeptide (VIP) often coexists with acetylcholine (ACh) in parasympathetic nerve fibres (Lundberg et al., 1979; Bloom and Edwards, 1980), while substance P (SP), calcitonin gene-related peptide (CGRP) and ATP may coexist in variable proportions in many primary afferent sensory fibres (Burnstock, 1977; Gibbins et al., 1985; Fyffe and Perl, 1984), including 'sensory-motor' perivascular nerves involved in axon-reflex activity (see Burnstock, 1990a).

Regulation of blood flow by vascular endothelial factors

Furchgott and Zawadzki (1980) introduced the concept of endothelium-mediated vasodilatation when they showed that ACh produced relaxation of the rabbit aorta when endothelium was present, but contraction via receptors on the muscle when it was removed. Later studies showed that receptors for other substances, including ATP, SP and 5-hydroxytryptamine (5-HT), were present on vascular endothelial cells; when occupied these led to vasodilatation via production of endothelium-derived relaxing factor (EDRF; see Vanhoutte and Rimele, 1983; Lincoln and Burnstock, 1990)

Identification of the source of these transmitter substances acting on endothelial cells has been problematical. It is unlikely that neurotransmitter released from the periarterial nerves, which are confined to the adventitial-medial border of most vessels, activate the smooth muscle and then diffuse all the way through the medial muscle coat without degradation, before producing vasodilatation via the endothelium. On the other hand, substances like ACh, ATP and 5-HT are rapidly degraded in the blood, so are unlikely to reach their endothelial targets from circulation. Our demonstration of immunocytochemical localization of choline acetyltransferase (ChAT), the enzyme involved in synthesis of ACh, within endothelial cells of small vessels in the rat brain led to the proposal that release of ACh from endothelial cells during ischaemia contributes to a pathophysiological mechanism of vasodilatation which protects vulnerable tissues like brain and heart from damage due to hypoxia (Parnavelas et al., 1985). We have recently extended these electron microscopic studies to other vessels and substances and shown that SP, 5-HT, ATP, angiotensin II (Ag II) and vasopressin (VP) as well as ChAT are stored and/or released during changes in flow or hypoxia from endothelial cell subpopulations (Loesch and Burnstock, 1988; Burnstock et al., 1988; Milner et al., 1989; Lincoln et al., 1990; Ralevic et al., 1990).

Neural-endothelial interactions

A hypothetical schema of the interactions of peptides and non-peptides released from perivascular nerves and from endothelial cells is presented in Fig. 1. It is proposed that transmitters, including ACh, ATP, 5-HT and SP are:

(1)   released from perivascular nerves to act on subclasses of receptors on vascular smooth muscle that lead to vasoconstriction or vasodilatation;

(2)   released from subpopulations of vascular endothelial cells to act on different subclasses of receptors on endothelial cells, leading to release of EDRF and subsequent vasodilatation.

It is suggested that these regulatory systems are involved both in normal homeostatic physiological control mechanisms when the two systems maintain a dynamic balance, and in pathophysiological situations such as ischaemia where the endothelial vasodilator mechanism is dominant as a protective device against hypoxic damage.

LOCAL VASCULAR CONTROL IN ATHEROSCLEROSIS

The WHHL rabbit, the only existing animal model for familial heritable hyperlipidaema (Kondo and Watanabe, 1975; Watanabe, 1980), was chosen as a model for atherosclerosis in this study, and New Zealand White (NZW) rabbits were used as controls. In view of the striking changes in density of innervation and expression of transmitters in different vessels at various stages in development and aging (see Cowen and Burnstock, 1986; Mione et al., 1988; Burnstock 1990b) we decided to compare responses of vessels from the WHHL and NZW rabbits between 4 and 12 months, a period

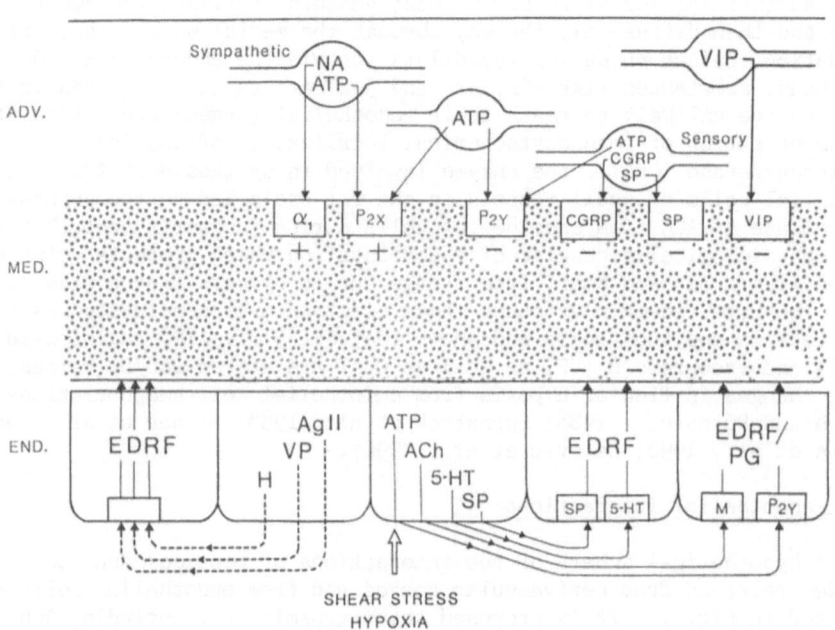

Fig. 1.   Schematic representation of potential modes of regulation of
vascular tone by endothelial-related mechanisms. NA, ATP, CGRP, SP, and
VIP can be released from nerves in the adventitia (ADV.) to act on their
respective receptors in the media (MED.) to cause vasoconstriction or
vasodilatation. ATP, ACh, 5-HT and SP released from endothelial cells
(END.) by shear stress or hypoxia act on their receptors on endothelial
cells to cause release of EDRF or prostaglandins (PG), which in turn act on
the smooth muscle to cause relaxation. In areas denuded of endothelial
cells, opposite effects may be produced by receptors on the smooth muscle.
α_1, noradrenaline receptor; P_{2X}, P_{2X}-purinoceptor; P_{2Y}, P_{2Y}-purinoceptor;
M, muscarinic receptor. Storage and possible release of Ag II, VP and
histamine (H) are also depicted (modified from Burnstock, 1989, with
permission of the publisher.)

when atherosclerotic lesions are developing. Four different types of response were measured:

(1)   responses to perivascular nerve stimulation;

(2)   responses to direct muscle vasoconstrictors, including NA, α,β-methylene ATP (a selective P_{2X}-purinoceptor agonist) and NPY (all measured as a percentage of contractions to KCl);

(3)   responses to direct muscle vasodilators including sodium nitroprusside, CGRP and VIP (measured after raising the tone with a concentration of NA giving 75% maximal contractions);

(4)   responses to endothelium-dependent vasodilators, including ACh, SP and ATP.

The vessels studied included aorta, mesenteric, coronary, hepatic, ear, saphenous and basilar arteries. Morphological and histochemical changes were monitored in these vessels by both transmission (TEM) and scanning electron microscopy (SEM) and by immunohistochemical methods at the developmental stages which were examined pharmacologically.

Aorta

In keeping with earlier reports (Ragazzi et al., 1989; Wines et al., 1989) endothelial-dependent vasodilatation to ACh was strongly diminished in the atherosclerotic aorta, while direct muscle-mediated responses were not significantly different from controls. Less than 20 to 30% of the endothelial cells appeared to be normal in these vessels at 12 months.

Mesenteric, hepatic, ear and saphenous arteries

There was a striking _increase_ in endothelial-mediated vasodilatation in this group of vessels by 12 months, although in some vessels they were diminished at 4 and 6 months. However, no significant differences in direct muscle responses to either vasoconstrictor or vasodilator agents were found.

Atheromatous lesions were present, but were largely confined to branch orifice areas, representing less than 5% of the intimal surface. Smooth muscle cells were shown in TEM to cross the elastic lamina to penetrate the intima by 6 months, before any lesions were seen in either endothelial or smooth muscle cells. By 12 months, however, damaged cells were clearly apparent. An interesting feature is that the rate of decline of endothelial-mediated vasodilator responses in control (NZW) rabbits over the period of 4 to 12 months was significantly greater in females compared with males.

Coronary arteries

These vessels tended to show intermediate features between aorta and the other vessels studied. There were diminished endothelial-mediated responses to SP at 4 and 6 months, but in keeping with the non-aortic vessels, a gradual increase in the endothelial-mediated response to SP was apparent by 12 months when it was equal to (but not greater than) the response to controls. There was a larger area of intimal lesion by 12 months than was apparent in the other non-aortic vessels.

Basilar artery

This vessel differed from the other vessels studied in that little damage, if any, to either endothelial cells or smooth muscle was detected even at 12 months in WHHL rabbits. Nevertheless there was still a marked

increase in endothelial-mediated vasodilatation to ACh by 6 months, which
was maintained at 12 months. This suggests that some substance in the
blood, perhaps originating in the heavily atherosclerotic carotid artery
might be involved in the mechanism of compensatory vasodilatation.

Summary of results and future directions

Fig. 2 summarizes the main trends in changes of responses in
atherosclerotic (WHHL) and control vessels from 4 to 12 months of age. The
striking feature is the increase in endothelial-mediated vasodilatation in
WHHL vessels compared with direct muscle responses during atherosclerosis

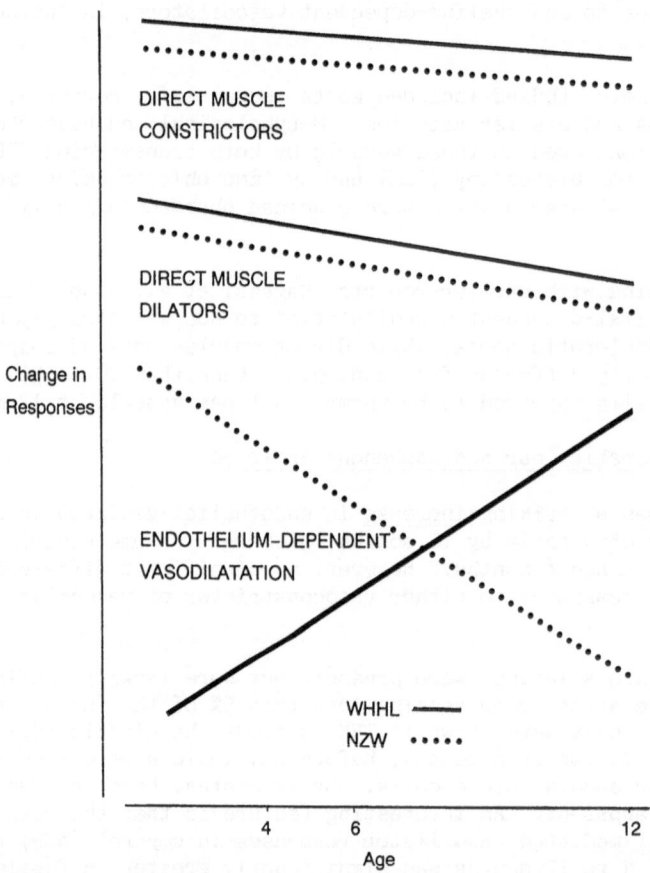

Fig. 2. Summary of the main trends in changes of responses with age in
vessels from WHHL and NZW rabbits.

in all the vessels examined except the aorta, and to some extent the
coronary arteries.

The mechanism of the enhanced vasodilatation is currently under
study. In particular, we are examining whether it might be due to: an
increase in synthesis and/or release of endothelial mediators such as ACh,
ATP, SP, VP or Ag II; an upgrading of receptors to these substances on
endothelial cells; an increase in responses of smooth muscle to EDRF; or
possibly an increased influence of superoxide dismutase. The role of
superoxide dismutase is of interest as it is present in endothelial cells
where it acts as a free radical scavenger and potentiates the activity of
EDRF (see Gryglewski et al., 1988). Free radicals are also implicated in
the suppression of prostacyclin in the vascular wall.

REFERENCES

Bloom, S.R., and Edwards, A.V., 1980, Vasoactive intestinal polypeptide in relation to atropine resistant vasodilatation in the sub-maxillary gland of the cat, J.Physiol., 300:41.

Borodulya, A.V., and Pletchkova, E.K., 1976, Cholinergic innervation of vessels of the base of the brain, Acta Anat., 96:135.

Burnstock, G., 1975, Control of smooth muscle activity in vessels by adrenergic nerves and circulating catecholamines, in: "Smooth Muscle Pharmacology and Physiology. Les Colloques de 1'INSERM, Vol. 50," INSERM, Paris, pp. 251-264.

Burnstock, G., 1977, Autonomic neuroeffector junctions-reflex vasodilatation of the skin, J.Invest.Dermatol., 69:47.

Burnstock, G., 1980, Cholinergic and purinergic regulation of blood vessels, in: "Handbook of Physiology, Section 2: The Cardiovascular System. Vol. II. Vascular Smooth Muscle," D.F. Bohr, A.D. Somlyo, H.W. Sparks, and S.R. Geiger, eds., American Physiological Society/Waverly Press, Baltimore, MD, pp. 567-612.

Burnstock, G., 1986, Purines as cotransmitters in adrenergic and cholinergic neurones, in: "Coexistence of Neuronal Messengers: A New Principle in Chemical Transmission. Progress in Brain Research, Vol. 68," T. Hökfelt, K. Fuxe, and B. Pernow, eds., Elsevier, Amsterdam, pp. 193-203.

Burnstock, G., 1988, Sympathetic purinergic transmission in small blood vessels, Trends Pharmacol.Sci., 9:116.

Burnstock, G., 1989, Vascular control by purines with emphasis on the coronary system, Eur.Heart J., 10, Suppl. F:15.

Burnstock, G., 1990a, Cotransmission. The Fifth Heymans Lecture, Gent, 1990, Arch.Int.Pharmacodyn.Ther., (In Press)

Burnstock, G., 1990b, Changes in expression of autonomic nerves in aging and disease, J.Auton.Nerv.Syst.(Suppl.), (In Press)

Burnstock, G., and Griffith, S.G., 1988, "Nonadrenergic Innervation of Blood Vessels, Vols.I (pp. 1-149) and II (pp. 1-233)", CRC Press, Boca Raton, FL.

Burnstock, G., Lincoln, J., Fehér, E., Hopwood, A.M., Kirkpatrick, K., Milner, P., and Ralevic, V., 1988, Serotonin is localized in endothelial cells of coronary arteries and released during hypoxia: a possible new mechanism for hypoxia-induced vasodilatation of the rat heart, Experientia, 44:705.

Cowen, T., and Burnstock, G., 1986, Development, aging and plasticity of perivascular autonomic nerves, in: "Developmental Neurobiology of the Autonomic Nervous System," P.M. Gootman, ed., Humana Press, Clifton, NJ, pp. 211-232.

Furchgott, R.F., and Zawadski, J.V., 1980, The obligatory role of endothelial cells in the relaxation of arterial smooth muscle by acetylcholine, Nature, 288:373.

Fyffe, R.E.W., and Perl, E.R., 1984, Is ATP a central synaptic mediator for certain primary afferent fibres from mammalian skin?, Proc.Natl.Acad.Sci.U.S.A., 81:6890.

Gibbins, I.L., Furness, J.B., Costa, M., Macintyre, I., Hillyard, C.J., and Girgis, S., 1985, Co-localization of calcitonin gene-related peptide-like immunoreactivity with substance P in cutaneous, vascular, and visceral sensory neurons of guinea-pigs, Neurosci.Lett., 57:125.

Gryglewski,R.J., Botting,R.M., and Vane,J.R., 1988, Mediators produced by the endothelial cell, Hypertension, 12:530.

Kondo, T., and Watanabe, Y., 1975, A heritable hyperlipidemic rabbit, Exp.Anim., 24:89.

Lincoln, J., and Burnstock, G., 1990, Neural-endothelial interactions in control of local blood flow, in: "The Endothelium: An Introduction to Current Research," J. Warren, ed., Alan R. Liss, New York,

Lincoln, J., Loesch, A., and Burnstock, G., 1990, Localization of vasopressin, serotonin and angiotensin II in endothelial cells of the renal and mesenteric arteries of the rat, Cell Tissue Res., 259:341.

Loesch, A., and Burnstock, G., 1988, Ultrastructural localisation of serotonin and substance P in vascular endothelial cells of rat femoral and mesenteric arteries, Anat.Embryol.(Berl.), 178:137.

Lundberg, J.M., Hökfelt, T., Schultzberg, M., Uvnäs-Wallensten, K., Köhler, C., and Said, S.I., 1979, Occurrence of vasoactive intestinal polypeptide (VIP)-like immunoreactivity in certain cholinergic neurons of the cat: evidence from combined immunohistochemistry and acetylcholinesterase staining, Neuroscience, 4:1539.

Lundberg, J.M., Pernow, J., Dahlöf, C., and Tatemoto, K., 1985, Pre- and postjunctional effects of neuropeptide Y (NPY) on sympathetic control of rat femoral artery, Acta Physiol.Scand., 125:511.

Milner, P., Ralevic, V., Hopwood, A.M., Fehér, E., Lincoln, J., Kirkpatrick, K.A., and Burnstock, G., 1989, Ultrastructural localisation of substance P and choline acetyltransferase in endothelial cells of rat coronary artery and release of substance P and acetylcholine during hypoxia, Experientia, 45:121.

Mione, M.C., Dhital, K.K., Amenta, F., and Burnstock, G., 1988, An increase in the expression of neuropeptidergic vasodilator, but not vasoconstrictor, cerebrovascular nerves in aging rats, Brain Res., 460:103.

Parnavelas, J.G., Kelly, W., and Burnstock, G., 1985, Ultrastructural localization of choline acetyltransferase in vascular endothelial cells in rat brain, Nature, 316:724.

Ragazzi, E., Chinellato, A., De Biasi, M., Pandolfo, L., Prosdocimi, M., Norido, F., Caparrotta, L., and Fassina, G., 1989, Endothelium-dependent relaxation, cholesterol content and high energy metabolite balance in Watanabe hyperlipidemic rabbit aorta, Atherosclerosis, 80:125.

Ralevic, V., Milner, P., Hudlická, O., Kristek, F., and Burnstock, G., 1990, Substance P is released from the endothelium of normal and capsaicin-treated rat hindlimb vasculature, in vivo, by increased flow, Circ.Res., 66:1178.

Stjärne, L., and Lundberg, J.M., 1986, On the possible roles of noradrenaline, adenosine 5'-triphosphate and neuropeptide Y as sympathetic cotransmitters in the mouse vas deferens, in: "Progress in Brain Research, Vol. 68," K. Fuxe, and B. Pernow, eds., Elsevier, Amsterdam, pp. 263-278.

Vanhoutte, P.M., and Rimele, T.J., 1983, Role of endothelium in the control of vascular smooth muscle function, J.Physiol.(Paris), 78:681.

Watanabe, Y., 1980, Serial inbreeding of rabbits with herditary hyperlipidemia (WHHL-rabbit). Incidence and development of atherosclerosis and xanthoma, Arteriosclerosis, 36:261.

Wines, P.A., Schmitz, J.M, Pfister, S.L., Clubb, F.J., Buja, L.M., Willerson, J.T., and Campbell, W.B., 1989, Augmented vasoconstrictor responses to serotonin precede development of atherosclerosis in aorta of WHHL rabbit, Arteriosclerosis, 9:195.

Wissler led off the discussion of Burnstock's presentation and pointed out that it was a beautiful overview. He also indicated that it might be well to take into consideration the great difference in cell populations that one sees in the diet-induced New Zealand white rabbit atheromatous lesions and the more sclerotic lesions that one sees in the homozygous WHHL rabbit when no dietary insult is present. He also pointed out that in some ways when the heterozygous WHHL rabbit is studied following a less severe atherogenic diet, it is likely to resemble (in lesion components and cellular composition) the human atherosclerotic plaque at several stages of its development. He indicated that the studies which have been done show that the heterozygous WHHL atherosclerotic lesions have a much larger complement of smooth muscle cells than the New Zealand rabbit diet-induced lesions do, according to the publications by Atkinson and coworkers at Vanderbilt University. The New Zealand diet-induced lesions are often 60-70% macrophage lesions and the WHHL heterozygous has a 70-80% smooth muscle cell population. This compares favorably with the human lesions which have an 80-90% smooth muscle cell population with an average of less than 10% monocyte derived macrophages. Burnstock indicated that he appreciated this difference in the various models of atherosclerosis in the rabbit. Heistad then discussed the findings in several studies that indicate that the microvessels are impaired as well. He pointed out that Professors Selke and Harrison have reported strikingly impaired responses in coronary microvessels, about 100-200 microns in diameter. Burnstock responded that he was quite aware of this reaction of small arteries and that the studies in his laboratory now included isolated arteries 100 microns or less in diameter. They are in the midst of analyzing their results from these studies so at the present time he indicated that he was not able to report the observations on the smaller arteries.

Heistad went on to indicate that he did not believe that superoxides were good candidates for potentiating the responses that Burnstock had reported. Burnstock responded that he thought there were papers from Moncada's group indicating that superoxide dismutase potentiates the EDRF responses. Bassenge entered the discussion and said that he believed that the effects of superoxide were indeed the opposite, that is, superoxide inhibits the response completely and superoxide dismutase preserves EDRF from being broken down. Kramsch then indicated that he was not surprised that the Watanabe rabbit showed no lesions in the basilar arteries. He noted that none of the experimental models with which he is acquainted have shown any atherosclerosis in intracranial arteries unless hypertension is also present. Weber then pointed out that in the many Watanabe rabbits that they had studied, only one quite old female had any lesions in the basilar artery.

Bond pointed out that human arteries with large plaques somehow stimulate angiogenesis and the penetration of the vasa vasorum through the media into the base of the plaque, even under conditions in which there are no penetrating vasa vasorum into that artery in a normal non-hyperlipidemic animal. He asked Burnstock whether the endothelial cells of these developing vessels might be the source of EF which caused the changes in the vascular tone of these major coronary arteries. <u>Burnstock</u> said that he did not know whether the vasa vasorum played a role and that in the lesions he had observed, the vasa vasorum had not been a major feature, but this would be worthwhile examining more closely in the future. He indicated that his group was examining regenerating endothelial cells to determine the role that vasoactive substances play during both normal development and regeneration of endothelial cells. He believes that with current techniques synthesis, storage, release, and uptake of these substances can be assessed. <u>Bond</u> also asked whether the same neurotransmitters exist in avian species as in primates. <u>Burnstock</u> said that so far there really had not been a careful comparative study of these two widely separate animals.

<u>Bassenge</u> mentioned that the serotonin seemed to cause peripheral constriction under some circumstances and peripheral dilatation in normal vessels. <u>Burnstock</u> said that this phenomenon was not troublesome to him because he knew that serotonin (or 5HT) is taken up by many sympathetic nerves and released as a false transmitter and that it does act as a very potent constrictive substance on smooth muscle cells. He indicated that if one puts 5-HT on an intact vessel, then one would expect the dilator effects through EDRF released by the endothelium, but on removal of the endothelium, 5-HT would have constrictor effects via its direct action, and <u>Burnstock</u> agreed that that was true under normal conditions in most peripheral vessels that have been studied to date.

SUMMARIZING CHAPTER

The five-day <u>Advanced Research Workshop Conference</u> has been, in Dr Wissler's words, a remarkable scientific event that has surpassed all expectations. He praised the quality of the participants' presentations concentrating on present knowledge, problems currently being addressed, and promise for the future. Wissler, as the organizing chairman, expressed his gratitude as well as that of the host, Professor Weber, for the immense contributions made by Drs Piero Tanganelli and Gene Bond. The two not only contributed greatly to organizing the program, but, together with Dr Michelle Mercuri, have served as coeditors of this published volume.

In addition, Dr Wissler thanked the audiovisual technicians, Claudio and Luciano, and acknowledged the remarkable contributions made by Dr Loretta Resi, Monica Masti, Janet Donovan, Luana Bonelli, Chris Simoes, and Vito Attino. These members of Professor Weber's staff have helped enormously to make this meeting and its monograph successful.

This chapter describes the highlights of the workshop conference as summarized by seven selected speakers from the six half-day programs. They were asked to concentrate on what, in their opinion, were the most important points emerging from each of these parts of the conference, including any new concepts or ideas they had gleaned about future developments. The chairpersons of the summarizing session were Professors Julie Campbell and Ross Gerrity.

<u>Professor Cornhill</u> summarized some of the advantages and disadvantages of the current optical methods for the study of the geometry and the composition of the arterial wall. The classical method for studying the extent of arterial atherosclerosis is based on visual estimates of the percentage of surface area involved, based in turn on inspection by several pathologists of the Sudan stained fixed arterial specimen. There is a high level of accuracy and reproducibility in the pathologist panel system for judging sudanophilia and for estimating raised lesions with varying collagen and calcium content as revealed by soft x-rays. There are also many risk factor correlations that have been demonstrated at lesion level using this kind of technology, underscoring the value of the results of the 1968 International Atherosclerosis Project involving fourteen different population groups and over 19,000 autopsies, all quantitated by these methods. According to Dr Cornhill, this technique can continue to be of value as newer approaches develop so that the results of the newer technologies can be compared with these classical findings. He emphasized the reliability of the pathologist panel system, which correlates with the computer generated data from his laboratory with the coefficients of 0.98 or 0.99. On the other hand, the pathology panel approach has problems with precision because the estimates of surface involved do not discriminate differences of less than 5% and they are cumbersome to apply to a comparison of lesions in various standard samples of artery.

Professor Cornhill expressed optimism concerning directions for measuring lesions in situ during life. He emphasized the value of the two-dimensional probability of occurrence maps, which are made possible through the use of image processing techniques. A major advantage of this approach is that it takes cross-sectional data which can be produced in a longitudinal fashion making the two-dimensional natural history of atherosclerosis clearer. He illustrated this by showing the increasing extent of raised atherosclerotic lesions in those members of the Pathobiological Determinants of Atherosclerosis in Youth (PDAY) autopsy population who show evidence of use of tobacco, revealed by postmortem blood thiocyanate determinations, and the effect this has on temporal progression. He also pointed out the advantages of being able to identify the "lesion prone" and "lesion resistant" areas. This treatment of data from several hundred cases makes it possible to state, in nonambiguous statistical terms, the probability of lesion development at any site in the arterial wall. The importance of this kind of quantitative information is obvious, especially for the increasing number of diverse studies which will be undertaken in the future. It should offer a good basis for comparing its results with those of an improved form of magnetic resonance imaging or some of the refined forms of ultrasound in living subjects, both of which appear to be imminent.

The computer assisted two-dimensional natural history studies permit the focus on specific areas such as the dorsal lateral surface of the abdominal aorta, distal to the inferior mesenteric artery, and proximal to the aortic iliac artery bifurcation. Professor Cornhill predicted that cell biologists and pathobiologists will find a rich and rewarding harvest of new information if they focus their ultrastructural, immunohistochemical, and other pathobiological studies on these specific lesion prone areas and use the lesion resistant areas for comparison.

He also made several predictions regarding magnetic resonance imaging. First of all, MRI will become more and more useful for two-dimensional studies of thickened vessel walls and should, with time, make possible the acquisition of meaningful quantitative information on the collagen, lipid, calcium, and perhaps other identifiable components in the lesions. Second, microscopic MRI will make a significant contribution to animal and pathological studies with respect to methods developed to measure temporal progression at the microscopic level. Preliminary observations indicate that artery thickness increases with age and with certain risk factors. Third, it will soon be easier to identify and measure different lesion components such as oil red O positive areas, the numbers of monocyte derived macrophages with or without foamy cytoplasm, and the regional distributions of these and other invading cells in relation to smooth muscle cell phenotypes, with and without lipid droplets.

Cornhill predicted that it will become possible to understand the differences in distributions of lesions, how these differences can be both environmentally and genetically controlled, and how hemodynamic forces can affect the location of lesions relative to the ostia of artery branches. Cornhill reiterated his hopes for a bright future for microscopic MRI, as well as the increasing value of computer-assisted image processing in a variety of applications which will have a major impact by permitting highly quantitative and previously impossible two-dimensional correlations.

Professor Dieter Kramsch summarized the part of the meeting at which he had been a major participant by evaluating progress toward reaching our goal of producing a useful, quantitative method of judging plaque severity. "Useful" means that the methodology should be beneficial to the

patient with cardiovascular disease or the subject at high risk. He
extended this to a prediction of what is likely to happen in the near
future.

Taking a page from Dr McGill's introductory lecture, Kramsch pointed
out that the plaque which brings about clinical disease and becomes life-
threatening is usually the fibrous plaque, which often contains a large
necrotic, soft grumous center and calcium. It has been shown repeatedly,
and is now being amply confirmed in the USA-PDAY study, that raised
plaques, often with a prominent fibrous component, can begin as early as
ages 15-20 in high risk populations. The World Health Organization
Surveys and the International Atherosclerosis Project indicate that when
60% of the coronary artery surface is covered with raised lesions, a
relatively high incidence of myocardial infarction can be expected.

Therefore, the optimal approach for avoiding myocardial infarction
would be to prevent the disease from ever reaching this degree of severity
and to push the disease process back to the lower portion of the sigmoid
curve where the incidence of myocardial infarctions is very low. With
this in mind, the goal should be to develop screening procedures for young
people to determine the extent of involvement of coronary arteries and
other critical arterial beds. At present, contrast media angiography is
not sensitive enough and is too invasive to be used for screening.
Therefore, it is likely to be replaced by more precise, ultrafast computer
tomography or ultrafast magnetic resonance imaging to achieve this goal.

Professor Kramsch expressed his hope that both of these methods will
receive maximum attention, and that the localization of radio-labelled LDL
to provide a measure of lesion activity might be coupled with these approaches for added advantage. He stated his belief in the future application of synchroton angiography for noninvasively following patients after
intervention, at least in the LAD and right coronary arteries. At
present, lesion tracking by conventional contrast coronary angiography is
the most practical and preferred quantitative method for measuring coronary plaques in those patients with advanced clinical ischemic disease.

Professor Kramsch was impressed by the results reported by both Dr
Landini and Dr Mercuri, indicating that B-mode ultrasound is increasingly
capable of measuring the size of carotid fibrous plaques, artery wall
thickness, the thickness of plaque intima and underlying media, the
plaque's eccentricity and/or concentricity, and its potential for forming
aneurysms. Over time it should be useful for measuring compensatory
dilatation of the artery in growing lesions and should provide information
as to what happens to the lumen size when the plaque regresses. Both of
these investigators have achieved the ability to distinguish connective
tissue signals from those produced by lipid-cholesterol ester in the necrotic wall. They are developing evidence of the possibility of differentiating diffuse lipid in a necrotic core and signals from cholesterol
crystals. Kramsch expressed the hope that this technique could be adapted
and used increasingly for patients to quantitate atherosclerotic lesion
components in the lower abdominal aorta, the iliac, and parts of the
femoral arteries.

Endovascular sonography may be approaching the stage where it can be
used for coronary artery studies as presented by Professor Liu. Although
it is invasive, it may be useful for evaluating atherosclerotic lesions in
patients at fairly long intervals, in studies of lesion regression following several forms of intervention. Reproducibility of results must be
insured so that lesions can be measured at exactly the same spot over
time. This is an important challenge and has yet to be worked out. In
contrast, esophageal echocardiography, which was presented briefly at this

meeting, appears to be totally impractical at present for assessing coronary artery stenosis, as it is not only strongly influenced by the cardiac
cycle, but also by respiratory motion. How much these can be influenced
by skillful gating is an open question.

Professor Kramsch voiced his hope that magnetic resonance spectroscopy for measuring the histopathological composition of plaques, as predicted by Drs Soma and Kuhn, might soon be useful for judging the presence
of lipids versus other components of the atherosclerotic plaque.

Dr Hay's report on the labelled LDL offers a promising method to
identify and quantitate active plaque progression. Dr Sinzinger demonstrated similar promising results with 125-iodine labelled LDL.
Sinzinger's research also shows that 111-indium labelled platelets are
demonstrably present in large quantities on the denuded subendothelial
connective tissue in bypass grafts where the endothelium sloughs off right
after grafting. The same is true in areas where angioplasty is accompanied by severe endothelial denudation. Under these conditions, platelet
adherence to the vessel may be an indication of the area where stenosis is
likely to occur in the future.

There are a number of important indicators of possible effective
therapeutic interventions in the future. One must evaluate more carefully
the question of whether preventing macrophages from entering the plaque is
beneficial or harmful in relation to the pathogenesis of progressive
atherosclerosis. Kramsch predicted that results such as those reported by
Dr Spagnoli will permit the tailoring of the patients' drug and diet
therapies to the type of lesions which they have, i.e., whether there is
predominance of connective tissue including collagen, elastin, and proteoglycans or whether there is a predominance of lipid. He predicted that
there will soon be drugs that suppress the proliferative and the collage-
nous aspects of lesion formation.

Dr Rubenstein summarized the approaches being used by the various
scientists in the field which are to some extent competitive, but most
often complementary. In other words, the risk factors considered are not
only those for coronary heart disease, but there is also a risk factor for
the scientists involved. Their approach might soon be overtaken by some-
one else's technical advance in this rapidly expanding high technology
field.

Dieter Kramsch's presentation impressed Rubenstein greatly because it
showed the accuracy of the panel of expert angiographers in reviewing
paired films side by side when the order of the films is masked and the
interventions are not known to the evaluators. In his opinion, human
panels outperform computers in the analyis of images involving cross
branching structures. Several trials have all shown lesion regression,
including a definite reduction in numbers of lesions. These include one
study with which Dr Rubenstein is closely associated under the direction
of Dr Blankenhorn at the University of Southern California, and others
conducted by Dr Dean Ornish, Dr Greg Brown, and Dr John Kane.

Three areas of Dr Paulin's presentation on MRI interested Rubenstein:
the measurement of carotid artery atherosclerosis, the usefulness of
quantitating arterial intimal-medial thickness in identifying the effects
of hypercholesterolemia, and the correlation with increasing age in individuals who were within the usual range of lipoprotein cholesterol concentrations. With greater intimal medial thickness, there is a higher tendency for the pathology to mimic the effects of elevated cholesterol.
There is also more likely to be a correlation between thickening of the
artery and the presence of plaques. Rubenstein felt that this method

could be used for longitudinal studies, but it would be necessary to know the present limits in correlating the thickening wall with the severity of atherosclerosis.

Dr Landini's presentation also impressed Rubenstein. It appears that the differences in attenuation of the ultrasound signals by collagen, fibrous tissues, and calcium are such that, at least in in vitro studies, these lesion components can be evaluated. It now seems likely that the resolution of this approach can be brought down to at least 200 microns or 0.2 mm.

As for Professor Lenzi's presentations on PET and SPECT, Rubenstein did not see any particular future for high resolution PET as applied to atherosclerotic lesions. He was, however, greatly impressed with what PET and SPECT can do to evaluate the effects on tissues of acute strokes, and the usefulness of drugs in spinal cord injuries or in ischemic brain events.

Dr Rubenstein was also impressed with Professor Liu's presentation and the resolution of the intravascular ultrasound. He praised the endo-vascular percutaneous approach, which could possibly be extended to include accurate estimations of calcium, fibrous elements, and lipids on the basis of their echoed reflectance and accoustic shadow character-istics. Rubenstein predicted that this method will become suitable for use during mechanical and pharmaceutical interventions. The challenge is to improve the size of the necessary catheters as well as the current gain setting, which may affect wall thickness measurements. It is also likely that calcium signals distort the measurements. There needs to be more study of the correlations between echogenic layering and atherosclerotic lesions, with the important caveat that the catheter must be in the right position coaxially with the axis of the artery, in order to prevent distortion.

Dr Paulin's presentation demonstrated that ultrafast cardiac MRI is rapidly developing. The current problems are imposed by the limitation of signal to noise ratio of a small Voxel element. When looking at a 1.0 mm size element there is not much time to eliminate motion blurring, thus this extraordinarily useful imaging modality cannot at present compete with x-ray based techniques for contrast angiography. It is likely that this instrument will be very useful in the study of myocardial perfusion, wall motion, and ejection parameters. It also shows promise in detecting turbulent flow in presumed regions of atherosclerosis. Dr Rubenstein noted that the program did not include presentations on MRI and peripheral arteries such as carotid or femoral. He predicted that the method will virtually eliminate competing methods for the visualization of many of the peripheral artery lesions which have been considered at this NATO confer-ence. Since it is noninvasive, involves no ionizing radiation, and provides spectacular image quality, data are needed to evaluate these approaches to the quantitation of peripheral vascular disease.

Rubenstein found Dr Mercuri's presentation valuable in validating the usefulness of the ultrasound method for plaque characterization. He noted that although Dr Kuhn's and Dr Soma's presentations indicated the ability to visualize water containing and lipid containing components of athero-sclerosis in morphologic detail down to 0.1 mm, the technical problems for clinical applications were substantial. At present they involve long examination times, vascular motion leading to blurring, poor spatial resolution under certain circumstances, and the limitation of the method to the study of small animals. He predicted that the principle of simul-taneous recording of dichromatographic images and the energies achieved when only the k-edge of iodine is visualized, will permit the development of valuable pictures of the coronary circulation in the near future. We can look forward to a very useful method coming out of their series of investigations, a method which should be valuable for long term assessment of atherosclerotic lesions and their response to interventions.

Professor Bonnet presented a rather pessimistic view as to what cardiologists can look forward to in relation to evaluating lesion severity from imaging techniques. Most cardiologists feel uncomfortable spending time and effort on measuring lesion severity in patients unless they are certain that they can obtain a reduction of coronary artery disease, mortality, and morbidity. At present, he recognized very little evidence from the various forms of therapy which suggested that they can benefit the patient. Furthermore, only those with very high levels of hypercholesterolemia should be subjected to a therapeutic approach aimed at clinical prevention.

According to Bonnet, there has not yet been a clear demonstration that antiplatelet therapy after myocardial infarction or lowering of blood pressure with beta blockers ameliorates the clinical outcome. He called for an individualized approach for each patient and an emphasis on the reduction of clinical symptoms and clinical risk for myocardial infarction. He admitted, however, that the Blankenhorn CLAS study and a few other studies using beta blockers and calcium antagonists show some promise. He noted that biologists make progress faster than do cardiologists. With our ever increasing knowledge of the atherosclerotic process, we should soon have the ability to reverse or prevent progression of the atherosclerotic plaque with new concepts of therapy.

A salient consideration for the cardiologist is whether the ends justify the treatment. A new therapy is accepted in clinical practice only if it decreases the many complications of heart disease. Bonnet doubted that it would suffice to show imaging evidence of plaque regression. Good clinical models are needed to test new drugs. He emphasized that new approaches are needed which will make it possible to obtain definitive tests with relatively few patients and little expense, approaches which do not involve repeated tests over a long period of time. In his opinion, this type of progress would overcome the biggest obstacles that cardiologists face.

Professor Sinzinger reviewed the future of measuring arterioendo-thelial integrity at specific sites in order to evaluate atherosclerotic plaque size and activity. There are a number of promising approaches, but, as of yet, they do not function at a level that will provide consistently useful information.

Circulating endothelial cells were measured as an indicator of endothelial integrity from the time of Hladovec. Ross Gerrity and others currently employ the same method, sometimes with factor 8 staining to identify the endothelial nature of the cells. In his research, aspirin has had no effect on the number of circulating endothelial cells. Two conditions with manifest vascular disease show consistent increases in the number of circulating endothelial cells: in patients who smoke or with hyperlipoproteinemia above the already elevated levels exhibited in patients with manifest atherosclerosis. Unfortunately, this method does not appear to correlate well with platelet survival insofar as that has been investigated.

Sinzinger summarized the data indicating that platelet depositions following the administration of labelled autologous platelets have been substantially reduced with prostacyclin therapy after five days of treatment. A decrease of platelet uptake at the local site is a complication

when using labelled platelets in individuals who have a peculiar hemostatic balance in relation to hypersplenism, large hematomas, and selected
types of blood dyscrasia.

Professor Sinzinger went on to describe the potential benefits of
using platelet labelling to test whether circulating prostaglandin E1 and
isosorbide dinitrate act via the cAMP to effectively prolong platelet
survival. These promising data confirm the results which have been
obtained in vitro in the aggregometer, in humans and under experimental
conditions. As yet there is no acceptable set of methods which will
provide the information needed for clinical pathopharmacological testing.
From the perspective of nuclear medicine and anticipating the future,
Sinzinger predicted that as soon as receptors or chemical structures
specific for damaged endothelium are available, these areas can be
labelled and functionally imaged to obtain the needed information on focal
progressive plaques with damaged endothelium.

Dr Gordon Campbell emphasized some of the promising cell biological
approaches which may ultimately be of value in evaluating atherosclerotic
lesions in living subjects. According to him, there are no reliable
methods for evaluating the several phenotypic changes which occur in
smooth muscle cells as the atherosclerotic plaque develops.

Future research directions in this area might become of some
practical importance. Research coming out of Bordeaux, France, and the
Soviet Union shows other cells that might be valuable indicators of early
atherogenesis. Campbell emphasized the importance of oxidized LDL,
oxidized B-VLDL, and the heparinases which may be involved in phenotypic
modulation of smooth muscle cells and in their stimulation to make many-
fold increases in the extracellular matrix.

All of these new developments may offer opportunities for immunoscintography. In the future, proteins involved in regulating the phenotype of smooth muscle cells might be very useful in indicating lesion
development and lesion progression. Cyclin or other smooth muscle cell
proliferation monitoring proteins might ultimately be used to develop an
in vivo method for signifying areas of smooth muscle cell proliferation.
Specific antibodies to fibronectin might also be valuable in recognizing
the synthetic phenotypes of smooth muscle cells.

There is no lack of new markers which may be used to identify, in any
number of new and innovative ways, areas of plaque development and
progression.

According to Professor Donald Heistad, the evidence now clearly
indicates an altered vascular tone and an increased susceptibility to
vasospasm in atherosclerosis. He pointed out the implications of this
phenomenon in relation to methods used to quantitate the extent of
atherosclerosis in living human subjects.

How is this problem dealt with? Heistad considered methods that can
be used to measure artery wall thickness and artery luminal diameter, both
of which are subject to variation during changes in vascular tone. When
making measurements of atherosclerosis in vivo, there should be proof of
maximal arterial dilatation. Research is needed to insure that reactive
hyperemia or exposure to compounds such as adenosine does not produce
further dilatation when vessels are dilated with nitroglycerin.

These considerations become particularly important when dealing with
clinical approaches in which catheters are used, because these may cause
vasospasm. Vasoconstricter responses occasionally are not abolished by

maximal vasodilitation. Heistad called for research in this area so that maximal dilatation is defined in ways that will not be subject to criticism. People doing angiography and measuring artery diameter or artery wall thickness need to provide strong evidence that vessels are maximally dilated and that vasoconstrictor responses and susceptibility to vasospasm have been effectively blocked.

A open discussion followed these summary presentations during which other information was presented.

Information was given indicating that smooth muscle cells do act as scavenger cells and have what might be regarded as scavenger receptors, which can take up large amounts of lipids once they have been processed by macrophages. Julie Campbell reported that much of the lipid carried by B-VLDL enters the smooth muscle cell by a receptor other than the Beta or Apo B receptors which are usually implicated.

Questions exist about the types of lesions most likely to lead to clinical effects. Many of the myocardial infarcts reported in rhesus monkeys with advanced coronary atherosclerosis have occurred in animals which were fed peanut oil with a high cholesterol diet, a diet which has been demonstrated to produce a more fibrous type of lesion in several species. It is clear that the pathogenesis of these infarcts, and the nature of underlying coronary artery lesions which may have produced them, are not clearly established at the present time, partly because the infarcts studied are generally several weeks to months old. This makes the underlying, acute coronary lesions responsible for the infarcts difficult to establish. Dr Heistad added to this discussion the notion that plaques which have already lost much of their necrotic core might still be dangerous, because the overlying collagen containing fibrous lesion may be very rough and ulcerated, leading to thrombosis when the endothelium is lost, even though very little lipid is present at that point.

Professor Paulin pointed out that there may be a place for the development and value of Fast CT (the Boyd technique), which uses an electron beam that is deflected magnetically rather than mechanically. This might be especially useful in measuring peripheral arterial lesions.

Professor Kramsch indicated that one of the prominent challenges of the future is to develop methods of reducing the collagen content in plaques. There are problems involved in developing the accurate and sophisticated instrumentation required for measuring plaque and arterial wall features quantitatively. This may be economically difficult in the general systems of medical care financing in various NATO countries. It is hoped that less expensive standardized methods and instruments will be available for widespread use in the not too distant future.

As the advanced research workshop conference came to a close, the organizing chairman offered an overview along the following lines.

Henry McGill, an experienced master pathologist who has described atherosclerosis as a moving target, suggested that the current multicenter cooperative study in the USA known as the Pathobiological Determinants of Atherosclerosis in Youth (PDAY) is producing important information that should ultimately help identify the various mechanisms of progression of the disease process at the cellular and molecular level in the artery wall.

Dr McGill challenged the group to fully document the importance of smooth muscle cell proliferation and the evidence that synthesis of collagen and elastin in the plaque are functions of phenotypic modulation of smooth muscle cells in the human plaque. He emphasized the recognition of the importance of extracellular lipid accumulation. Nearly everyone concurred with this concept at the most recent meeting of the American Heart Association's Committee on Lesions where intermediate lesions and their definitions were considered. The PDAY study offers an important opportunity to identify at the cellular level, and frequently at biochemical and molecular levels, the effects that each risk factor has on the progressive lesion.

Professor Bonnet, as an active cardiologist, maintained that there are a myriad of important clinical aspects the cardiologist needs to consider when he evaluates a patient for future examination and potential therapy. He urged caution and careful consideration before subjecting patients to repeated invasive examinations and therapeutic interventions by pharmaceutical agents and limited diets.

Dr Gene Bond offered a thought-provoking clarification on the present status of ultrasound and its clear-cut advantages for evaluating not only changes in arterial wall lesions, but also the degree of disease and the effects of therapy. He emphasized the dilatability of the artery as atherosclerosis develops and the necessity for learning more about which kinds of lesions are most likely to lead to narrowing of the lumen as opposed to increasing the diameter of the lumen.

Both Professors Spagnoli from Rome and Tanganelli from Siena indicated the benefits of studying the pathological specimens from endarterectomies. Dr Spagnoli pointed out that the lesions are very heterogeneous. He called attention to the importance of the quantitative relationships of the grumous core of the advanced atherosclerotic plaque to the fibrous cap, as well as its potential importance in relation to the patient's clinical effects. As methodological improvements develop, it will be important to measure lesions much smaller than the ones usually examined by angiography at present. There is increasing evidence that the danger of some of these small lesions is not fully recognized.

Dr Cornhill illustrated the present PDAY study results, using highly sophisticated and reproducible computer assisted morphometry, including micromorphometry and the quantitation of the various components of the developing plaque. When these methodologies can be applied to the developing plaque in vivo, we will be able to satisfy many of the needs addressed by Professor Bonnet in his second presentation, in which cases with identified risk factors were studied.

Professor Dieter Kramsch identified the advantages of contrast media angiography as it is now being applied in quantitative studies of interven-tion into the atherosclerotic process. Drs Poli and Landini reported in their presentations that the developing field of measuring the constitu-ents of arterial wall plaque may add an additional dimension to the ones which are at present demonstrated with noninvasive ultrasound techniques.

Dr Barbieri discussed what is to be expected of the laser as it develops as a diagnostic instrument and is used to measure the therapeutic results by placing a receiver inside the artery.

Professor Liu's presentation of the "sound at the end of the tunnel" introduced new ways in which ultrasound may help in the evaluation of coronary artery disease from new vantage points, and with less interference from surrounding structures. With time, the array system inside the coronary artery may give us very useful quantitative information which is difficult to obtain from other vantage points.

Dr Paulin put to rest for all time the notion that MRI won't work on small arteries by showing us a mouse coronary artery. He believes MRI will replace the thallium scan in the near future.

Drs Dix and Rubenstein described their highly sophisticated methods to develop resource centers where arteries can be measured in very short periods of time, using a subtraction technique and focusing on the circulating iodine in the coronary arteries.

Dr Mercuri brought his results with ultrasound back to the very middle of this highly sophisticated new frontier as he reported in detail what one can see and quantitate inside the artery wall. As he pointed out, this is where the action is. More knowledge in this area is needed in order to understand what happens to plaques during the regression period or following therapies of many types.

Dr Assmann shared his knowledge of the genetic problems now being explored and the molecular biology being woven into the whole field of atherogenesis at the cellular and molecular level. This opens the door to learning more about lesion progression and lesion components based on very subtle changes in lipoproteins and in apolipoproteins as they occur in many newly discovered defects.

Dr Rick Hay and Dr Sinzinger are exploring what can be learned by following the localization of platelets and lipoproteins in the artery wall and in the lesions, and what this may help us learn about plaque stability and the functional morphology of the atherosclerotic process.

Dr Alessandra Bini carried the discussion to other circulating factors that may be important in atherogenesis. She emphasized the importance of knowing more about fibrin and fibrin split products and their importance in relation to the progressive plaque. This led to a discussion of the role of endothelial damage in the microarchitecture of plaques and the need for better tools to identify concentric plaques which have much greater medial involvement than the usual advanced atherosclerotic lesion.

These presentations emphasized the need for a better way to measure extracellular lipid in the artery wall of the living patient, to follow the course of early plaques, and to understand and measure the numbers and proportions of macrophages in these plaques. The Campbells' presentations pointed out the future promise of learning more about the phenotypic changes in the function of the smooth muscle cell in the plaque and the factors that influence the development of these changes.

We finally came to a detailed consideration of how arterial tone and dilatation influence the interpretation of lesions in the artery wall. The master investigators in the field are interested in the paracrine and autocrine factors that may control the tone of the artery. They put forth the challenge of developing better methods of controlling arterial tone so that we will not be misled in sequential studies of lesions.

It is clear that sequential quantitative arterial angiography is developing rapidly. We can look forward to increasingly informative data which can be used to evaluate accurately what is happening in the artery lumen, on the artery surface, and in the artery wall as atherosclerosis develops and during intervention.

Sequential observations
  non-invasive, 210
Sestamibi, 99
Sex, 286
Shrinkage effect, 40
Sidak's multiplicative inequality,
      28
Smoking, 34
Smooth muscle, 240, 285
Spasm, 47
Spectroscopy
  fluorescence, 84, 85
  NMR, 118, 147
Spin-echo technique, 113
Stenosis
  diameter, 49
  percent, 57
Studies
  reproducibility, 24,
  validation, 23
Substance P, 285
Superoxide dismutase, 290
Synchrotron radiation, 125
Synthetic state, 238

Tagging, 119
Tc-99m, 173
Teboroxime, 99
Techniques
  histochemical, 213
  immunohistochemical, 213
Thallium-201, 99
Therapeutic window, 78
Therapy
  diet, 59
Thermal system, 86
3-D display, 116
Thrombosis, 1, 30, 192
Thrombotic process, 47
Tissue
  characterization, 96, 141
  connective, 4, 31,
  elastic, 4
  fibrous, 96
  microscopy, 147
Tomography
  positron emission, 77
  single photon emission
        computerized, 77
  ultrafast computed, 59
Tracers, 99
Transmitters, 286
Tropomyosin, 218
Turbo-flash technique, 117
Tyramine cellobiose, 173

Ulceration, 1
Ultrasound, 63, 92, 141
  animal, 18
  attenuation, 69
  backscattering, 69

Ultrasound (continued)
  B-mode scanning, 21, 39, 141
  endovascular, 93
    advantages, 96
    indications, 98
    principles, 93

Vascular smooth muscle, 285
Vascularization, 1, 5,
  and aging, 31
Vasoactive intestinal polypeptide,
      286
Vasoconstriction
  sympathetic nerve, 285
Vasoconstrictor, 285
Vasodilatation, 285
  compensatory, 285
Vasodilator
  endothelial-mediated, 285
  reserve, 93
  response, 285
Vasopressin, 287
Vessel wall dilatation, 55
Video Densitometric Station, 142
Videodensitometry, 143
Vinculin
  meta-, 219

Watanabe Heritable Hyperlipidaemic
        (WHHL) rabbit, 285
Wave
  continuous, 82
  pulsed, 82
Wigglers, 126, 133

Young patients, 31
Young people, 210